Assembling the Tropics

From popular fiction to modern biomedicine, the tropics are defined by two essential features: prodigious nature and debilitating illness. That was not always so. In this engaging and imaginative study, Hugh Cagle shows how such a vision was created. Along the way, he challenges conventional accounts of the Scientific Revolution. The history of "the tropics" is the story of science in Europe's first global empire. Beginning in the late fifteenth century, Portugal established colonies from sub-Saharan Africa to Southeast Asia and South America, enabling the earliest comparisons of nature and disease across the intertropical world. *Assembling the Tropics* shows how the proliferation of colonial approaches to medicine and natural history led to the assemblage of the tropics as a single, coherent, and internally consistent global region. This is a story about how places acquire medical meaning, about how nature and disease become objects of scientific inquiry, and about what is at stake when that happens.

HUGH CAGLE is Assistant Professor of the History of Science at the University of Utah, where he is also Director of the International Studies program.

Studies in Comparative World History

Editors

Michael Adas, *Rutgers University*
Heather Streets Salter, *Northeastern University*
Douglas Northrop, *The University of Michigan*

Other Books in the Series

Assembling the Tropics

Science and Medicine in Portugal's Empire,
1450–1700

HUGH CAGLE
University of Utah

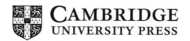

CAMBRIDGE
UNIVERSITY PRESS

CAMBRIDGE
UNIVERSITY PRESS

University Printing House, Cambridge CB2 8BS, United Kingdom

One Liberty Plaza, 20th Floor, New York, NY 10006, USA

477 Williamstown Road, Port Melbourne, VIC 3207, Australia

314–321, 3rd Floor, Plot 3, Splendor Forum, Jasola District Centre,
New Delhi – 110025, India

79 Anson Road, #06–04/06, Singapore 079906

Cambridge University Press is part of the University of Cambridge.

It furthers the University's mission by disseminating knowledge in the pursuit of
education, learning, and research at the highest international levels of excellence.

www.cambridge.org
Information on this title: www.cambridge.org/9781107196636
DOI: 10.1017/9781108164856

First published 2018

Printed in the United Kingdom by TJ International Ltd. Padstow Cornwall

A catalogue record for this publication is available from the British Library.

Library of Congress Cataloging-in-Publication Data
Names: Cagle, Hugh, author.
TITLE: Assembling the tropics : science and medicine in
Portugal's empire, 1450-1700 / Hugh Cagle.
OTHER TITLES: Studies in comparative world history.
DESCRIPTION: Cambridge, United Kingdom ; New York, NY :
Cambridge University Press, 2018. | Series: Studies in comparative world history |
Includes bibliographical references and index.
IDENTIFIERS: LCCN 2018021310 | ISBN 9781107196636
(hardback : alk. paper)
SUBJECTS: | MESH: Tropical Medicine–history | Colonialism–history |
Public Health Practice–history | Science–history | History, 15th Century |
History, 16th Century | History, 17th Century | Portugal
CLASSIFICATION: LCC RC961 | NLM WC 11 GP7 | DDC 616.9/883–DC23
LC record available at https://lccn.loc.gov/2018021310

ISBN 978-1-107-19663-6 Hardback

For Leslie.
Anumang bagay ay maisasakatuparan niya.

The double, the shadow, the negative image of the great adventure of the New World.

Caetano Veloso, *Verdade tropical*

Contents

Illustrations

Figures

Maps

Acknowledgments

This book has taken a long time to write. It began at Rutgers in 2008 as an entirely different project. In the intervening years, I have carried it with me – writing and then revising it – virtually everywhere I've been. I remember where fragments of chapters finally came together. On a plane to Goa. On another to Barcelona. A bus in Lima. Trains between New York and New Brunswick, London, and Cambridge, and Lisbon, Guimarães, and Porto. There were late nights at coffee shops scattered across Manhattan, long days at another in Sunnyside (Queens), and early mornings at several others in Rio and Salt Lake. I imagine the book still bears the traces of its disjointed authorship. But I really have no idea. It has been with me for too long, and I am now much too close to it, to know for sure. For its errors and failings, I alone am responsible. But much that is good about it has come from the wisdom, kindness, and generosity of very many people.

Michael Adas is first among them. Perhaps more than anyone else, Michael understands what a circuitous path mine has been. I never would have begun the project were it not for his encouragement, unwavering support, and his subtle, brilliant mentorship. James Delbourgo's candor, imagination, and good will have made this book, and the intellectual life around it, immeasurably better. The late Philip Pauly first introduced me to the history of science. Gail Triner and Chris Brown generously signed onto the project as it was just getting underway and were patient enough to see me through it even as I struggled to match feasible questions with archival evidence.

I never would have found my way to Rutgers had it not been for two people. Steve Marks encouraged me long ago to travel adventurously and to take my writing more seriously. I can finally thank him in print. Betsy Kuznesof took a chance on me as a Latin American Studies student and has remained a dear friend ever since. Her professionalism, grace, and unfailing intellectual rigor continue to inspire.

Historical research, not to mention writing, is a long and lonely business. But I've had the good fortune to share time in Lisbon and elsewhere with Palmira Fontes da Costa, Mariana Cândido, Yacine Daddi Addoun, Drew Thompson, Jelmer Vos, Kalle Kananoja, Claudia Souza, Alfredo César Melo, and Tim Walker. Years ago, on my first trip to Lisbon, Liam Brockey was kind enough to advise me on archival research there and to help me think through some preliminary questions about Jesuit networks. One memorable morning in July 2015, António de Almeida Mendes helped me reconstruct the footprint of medieval Lisbon and then showed me how to navigate its streets. Across the Atlantic in Rio, I thank Vera Santos and João Duarte for a delightful evening just as this project was winding down.

In London and beyond, I have benefited from the friendship and expertise of Bridie Andrews, Winston Black, Ann Carmichael, Fabian Crespo, Luke Demaitre, Theresa Earenfight, Nahyan Fancy, Carol Pal, Stephen Pemberton, George Sussman, Carlos da Silva Junior, Dora Vargha, and the incomparable Monica Green. I first met Monica through the 2012 NEH seminar that she ran with Rachel Scott at the Wellcome Collection. Monica's work is a model of genuine interdisciplinarity. I thank her in particular for helping me get a handle on medieval medicine, the biomedical literature pertaining to the diseases mentioned in the text, and the interpretive dilemmas of retrospective diagnosis.

In Goa, the inimitable Blossom Madeira made my time at the Historical Archives of Goa (HAG) far more productive than I could possibly have hoped. Agnelo Fernandes offered good cheer and indispensable guidance to the content and organization of the archive. Special thanks to Rameshwar and to Bapa, who made sure I knew where to go and got me there safely. To pin down details on Goa's topography, a very kind gentleman helped me find my way to Carambolim Lake. I never knew his name but the collection of certain details in Chapter 3 would have been impossible without his help. My time in Goa and elsewhere would have been much less fruitful were it not for Tim Walker, whose guidance and knowledge of so many aspects of early modern Portuguese medicine I have been the grateful beneficiary of on numerous occasions.

Iona McCleery has been an insightful colleague and stalwart collaborator ever since I began working in the history of medicine. I thank her here for the conversations and good company in London, Lisbon, St. Albans, and Kalamazoo. Conversations with Allison Bigelow, Surekha Davies, Pablo Gómez, Felipe Valencia, Matt Crawford, and Molly Warsh kept me reading, reflecting, and writing even when the will was wanting and the way was uncertain. Tom Robertson and Carmen Gitre, too, offered advice and encouragement when it was sorely needed. With a single, well-placed question, Jorge Cañizares helped me reconceptualize cross-cultural interaction in Brazil. My interpretation of missionaries and disease is significantly better thanks to Linda Newson. Luce Giard showed me how to disagree with grace and compassion. A very special thanks to Ramón Oteo, whom I met long ago at the Universitat Rovira i Virgili: Dondequiera que estés, sé que todavía sigues leyendo. Espero que te llegue esto.

Many other friends and colleagues have commented on the manuscript in whole or in part, responded patiently to hasty emails, shared material, made recommendations, and otherwise offered much-needed guidance. Sincerest thanks go to Crislayne Alfagali, Arturo Arias, Santa Arias, Antonio Barrera, Luís Filipe Barreto, Herman Bennett, Joe Blackmore, Ann Blair, Pedro Cardim, Judith Carney, Tito Carvalho, Fiona Clark, Tim Coates, Diogo Curto, Greg Cushman, Júnia Ferreira Furtado, Luis Fernando Restrepo, Anita Guerrini, Annemarie Jordan Gschwend, Stefan Halikowski-Smith, Florence Hsia, Henrique Leitão, Kate Lowe, Dániel Margócsy, Stuart McManus, Joe Miller, Eric Myrup, Marcy Norton, Katrina Olds, Ricardo Padrón, Juan Pimentel, Cynthia Radding, Gabriela Ramos, Maria Leônia Chaves de Resende, Isabel dos Guimarães Sá, Neil Safier, Fernando Salmón, Kevin Sheehan, Jim Sweet, John Thornton, José Pardo Tomás, Camilla Townsend, Paula de Vos, Chi-ming Yang, and Ines Županov.

Special thanks as well to Gary and the crew at Aubergine, where so many of the ideas here were first written up – how I miss the coffee and good cheer, the morning foot traffic and the crowds of a spring afternoon. Tremendous thanks to Pedro Pinto in Lisbon for helping me secure permission to reproduce images from the Arquivo Nacional da Torre do Tombo and the Biblioteca Nacional de Portugal. I am grateful as well to Maria Inês Cordeiro at the BNP, Silvestre Lacerda and Aura Carrilho at the ANTT, Maria Ana Paiva at the Krishnada Shama Goa State Central Library, Elizabeth Bray at the British Museum, Domniki Papadimitriou at the Cambridge University Library, Ian Graham at the John Carter Brown Library, and Brigitte Brot at the Bibliothèque et archives de l'Assemblée Nationale in Paris.

Audiences in Atlanta, Baltimore, Belfast, Lima, London, Seattle, New York, Philadelphia, Lisbon, Heidelberg, Charleston, New Brunswick, Chicago, Park City, Salt Lake City, Toronto, Lawrence, Madison, New Orleans, San Diego, Sussex, Charlottesville, Rio de Janeiro, Guimarães, and Porto offered insightful and challenging questions that variously improved this book.

Travel and research are costly affairs. Generous support for this project came from the Fundacão Luso-Americano, the Gulbenkian Foundation, Harvard University, the Mellon Foundation, Rutgers University, and the University of Texas – Austin. I also benefited from faculty fellowships from the University Research Council and the Tanner Humanities Center, both of the University of Utah. Directors and staffs at libraries and archives on four continents were incredibly generous with their time and – what is often forgotten in a world of digital databases – their incomparable archival expertise. Tremendous thanks to the library and archival staff at the following institutions: the University of Cambridge, the University of Kansas, NYU, Princeton, Rutgers, Queens College, UT-Austin, the New York Academy of Medicine, the Historical Archives of Goa, the Goa Public Library, the Biblioteca Nacional de Portugal, the Arquivo Nacional da Torre do Tombo, the British Library, the British Museum, the John Carter Brown Library, the Beinecke Rare Book and Manuscript Library at Yale University, the French Bibliothèque et archives de l'Assemblée Nationale, and the Wellcome Collection. The interlibrary loan staff at the University of Utah deserve special recognition for their patience and persistence over these last years.

Tremendous thanks, too, to my colleagues in the departments of History, Languages and Literature, and Art History at the University of Utah. I am especially grateful to Jim Lehning, Ben Cohen, Nadja Durbach, Gema Guevara, Eric Hinderaker, Becky Horn, Jessen Kelly, Chris Lewis, Colleen McDannell, Isabel Moreira, Bradley Parker, Susie Porter, Jerry Root, and Elena Shtromberg, and to graduate students Mariana Alliatti and Travis Ross.

At Cambridge University Press, Debbie Gershenowitz and Kristina Deusch were unfailingly patient and supportive as the final manuscript came together, and as I flooded them with sundry last-minute questions. Special thanks to Andreia Carvalho, whose close reading and subject expertise made the book materially better. Julie Hrischeva, Niranjana Harikrishnan, and Laura Lawrie moved the book through the final phases of production with skill and efficiency.

My deepest gratitude must go to Leslie; to Hugh and Nan; to Alex and Pelin, Aubrie, and Casey and Megan; to Eva, Antón, and Carmen; to Chris, Maite, and Pere; and to Valerie, Gary, and Rose. This project is finally finished. Thank you.

A Note on Spelling and Translation

Portuguese orthography is notoriously irregular. In the pages that follow –
and with occasional exceptions – I have changed the spelling and accentu-
ation of various Portuguese words to correspond to the guidelines set
forth in the orthographic accord of 1990. For personal names, I have
generally followed the spelling currently used to catalog materials at the
Biblioteca Nacional de Portugal in Lisbon. Where Spanish is concerned,
I have – again, with some exceptions – followed the *Diccionario Real de
la Lengua Española*. All translations are my own unless otherwise noted.
Where the Spanish Hapsburgs are mentioned, I have followed convention
and used the Anglicized version of their names, with roman numerals
indicating their succession in the Portuguese line (so I use "Philip I" not
"Filipe I" or "Philip II of Spain").

Abbreviations

APO	Cunha Rivara, ed., *Archivo Portuguez-Oriental*, 6 vols.
BL	Machado, *Bibliotheca Lusitana*, 4 vols.
DHAM-AC	Diretoria do Arquivo, *Documentos históricos do Arquivo Municipal. Atas da Câmara*, 10 vols.
DI	Wicki, ed., *Documenta Indica*, 18 vols.
HCJB	Leite, *História da companhia de Jesus no Brazil*, 10 vols.
MB	Leite, ed., *Monumenta brasiliae*, 5 vols.
MH	Comissão Executiva das Comemorações do V Centenário da Morte do Infante D. Henrique, ed., *Monumenta Henricina*, 14 vols.
MMA ser. 1	Brásio, ed., *Monumenta Missionaria Africana*, 1st series, 15 vols.
MMA ser. 2	Brásio, ed., *Monumenta Missionaria Africana*, 2nd series, 5 vols.
MRP	Andrade and Duarte, ed., *Morão, Rosa e Pimenta*.
PVCB	Abreu, ed., *Primeira visitação do Santo Ofício às partes do Brasil. Confissões da Bahia, 1591–1592*.
PVCP	Mello, ed., *Primeira visitação do Santo Ofício às partes do Brasil. Confissões de Pernambuco, 1594–1595*.
PVDB	Abreu, ed., *Primeira visitação do Santo Ofício às partes do Brasil. Denunciações da Bahia, 1591–1593*.
PVDP	Garcia, ed., *Primeira visitação do Santo Ofício às partes do Brasil. Denunciações de Pernambuco, 1593–1595*.
SVB	França and Siqueira, eds., *Segunda visitação do Santo Ofício às partes do Brasil*.

I

Reading between the Lines

The name of the game will be to leave the boundaries open and to close them only when the people we follow close them.

Bruno Latour[1]

THE DEATH OF DR. VOGEL

When the combined interests of commerce, abolition, and exploration catalyzed British support for the massive Niger Expedition of 1841, the ambitious Theodor Vogel managed to get himself appointed to the distinguished post of chief botanist.[2] It was a minor coup. The young Prussian had never actually been to the tropics. In fact, he had never been any closer to West Africa than western Germany, where the nearest thing to the tropical Niger was the distinctly temperate Rhine.[3] Nor had he much exposure to West African flora. His expertise was based on the study of a Brazilian collection conveniently ensconced in a herbarium in Berlin. But

---

[1] Bruno Latour, *Science in Action: How to Follow Scientists and Engineers through Society* (Cambridge, MA: Harvard University Press, 1987), 175.

[2] The following account is taken from a combination of Vogel's botanical and private journals, large sections of which are reproduced in *Niger Flora; or, An Enumeration of the Plants of Western Tropical Africa, Collected by the Late Dr. Theodore Vogel, Botanist to the Voyage of the Expedition Sent by Her Britannic Majesty to the River Niger in 1841, under the Command of Capt. H. D. Trotter, R. N., &c.*, ed. W. J. Hooker (London: Hippolyte Bailliere, 1849).

[3] Parts of which were as likely as not to freeze in the winter, as observed by the seventeenth-century Jesuit Athanasius Kircher and described in John Glassie, *A Man of Misconceptions: The Life of an Eccentric in an Age of Change* (New York: Riverhead Books, 2012), 27–30.

that was enough – and it was a measure of just how coherent the tropics now were in the minds of European naturalists: where expertise was concerned, plants collected from the expansive Brazilian interior could stand in for those that lined a discrete corner of the sub-Saharan world.

By the time he reached the yawning delta of the Niger, after layovers spread from Funchal to Accra, Vogel had assembled a collection of plants so numerous that they crowded him out of his cramped stateroom. The sweltering climate, he griped, made his specimens "fall to pieces and mold continuously."[4] He preserved as many of them as possible in his journal, its pages a thicket of binomial nomenclature: *Tamarix senegalensis, Cassia obovata, Elais guineensis, Sarcocephalus esculentus, Anona murciata*.[5] Had he lived, the ambitious young doctor would have consolidated his reputation as an authority on the distinctive botany of the immense tropical world.

But of course, he did not live. "Tropical fevers," Vogel wrote, worried everyone on the expedition.[6] His colleagues in medicine thought these fevers were the result of the combined heat, humidity, and dense vegetation of the tropics. Widespread putrefaction, they believed, caused miasma – the pernicious, earthy exhalations of mist and haze that seemed to pervade the tropics. How, exactly, miasma caused fevers, what the differences were between them, and how each should be treated were among the questions then driving medical transformations within metropolitan Europe.[7] In Europe's expanding tropical colonies, fevers were so ubiquitous, so baffling, and so virulent that, in clinical terms, subtle distinctions could often seem meaningless.[8] By all accounts, tropical fevers were deadlier than most.

Vogel's fever began on September 6, far up the Niger, only days from his destination at the confluence of the Benue. Over the following weeks, his condition grew worse. By September 18, he could muster little more than clipped sentences and tortured grammar. "I continue unwell" he

[4] Hooker, ed., *Niger Flora*, 11.

[5] Hooker, ed., *Niger Flora*, 24–37. These are, respectively, salt cedar, senna, African oil palm, Guinea peach, and soursop.

[6] Hooker, ed., *Niger Flora*, 17.

[7] A classic statement is Michel Foucault, *The Birth of the Clinic: An Archaeology of Medical Perception*, trans. A. M. Sheridan (New York: Pantheon Books, 1973 [1963]). Perhaps the best recent survey is Christopher Hamlin, *More Than Hot: A Short History of Fever* (Baltimore, MD: Johns Hopkins University Press, 2014).

[8] Philip D. Curtin, *Death by Migration: Europe's Encounter with the Tropical World in the Nineteenth Century* (New York: Cambridge University Press, 1989).

wrote, "head-ache and fever."[9] His ship turned downstream, headed for the sea, and a safe harbor on the island of Fernando Po.

At just over three degrees and three minutes north latitude, and tucked deep into the Gulf of Guinea, Fernando Po (now Bioko, Equatorial Guinea) sits almost exactly on the equator, in the very heart of the tropics. There, in Clarence Cove, Vogel spent the last ten weeks of his life – bedridden, febrile, and delirious. His botanical collection was brought ashore where it was variously invaded, occupied, and purloined by an assortment of unspecified bugs. Vogel mused that he had turned from gathering plants to collecting insects.[10] On December 17, 1841, amid his dwindling collection and an insurgent nature, Theodore Vogel, chief botanist of the British Niger expedition of 1841, "succumbed," as one of his colleagues put it, "to the destructive influence of the climate."[11] His death helped mark the disastrous conclusion to one of Victorian Britain's most ambitious West African ventures.[12]

It did not take a tropical botanist to understand something of the world that Vogel confronted. For many in nineteenth-century Europe and the United States, the tropics could be found almost anywhere. Empires actual and aspirational (the United States had no formal tropical holdings until 1898[13]) had already begun to bring the tropics home. Plants, animals, objects, and people from across the tropical world had become the subjects not only of specialized inquiry but also of general public fascination. Crowds at Kew marveled at enormous Amazonian lilies; rhododendrons from India lined a park near the Thames.[14] The Berlin

---

[9] Hooker, ed., *Niger Flora*, 61, 69. The emphasis in the latter appears in the original.

[10] Hooker, ed., *Niger Flora*, 72.   [11] Hooker, ed., *Niger Flora*, 1.

[12] Hooker, ed., *Niger Flora*, vii–ix; Philip D. Curtin, *The Image of Africa: British Ideas and Action, 1780–1850*, 2 vols. (Madison, WI: University of Wisconsin Press, 1964); Daniel R. Headrick, *The Tools of Empire: Technology and European Imperialism in the Nineteenth Century* (New York: Oxford, 1981); David Lambert, *Mastering the Niger: James MacQueen's African Geography and the Struggle over Atlantic Slavery* (Chicago, IL: University of Chicago Press, 2013).

[13] American geopolitical ambitions during and after the early Republic are surveyed in Michael Adas, *Dominance by Design: Technological Imperatives and America's Civilizing Mission* (Cambridge, MA: Belknap Press, 2006), the notes to which reference an array of more specialized studies in both the Pacific and the Caribbean. According to Hooker, ed., *Niger Flora*, 33, Vogel noted an already-ambiguous political relationship between the United States and Liberia during his short stay in Monrovia.

[14] Richard Drayton, *Nature's Government: Science, Imperial Britain, and the Improvement of the World* (New Haven, CT: Yale University Press, 2000), chapter 6; and, more broadly, Beth Fowkes Tobin, *Colonizing Nature: The Tropics in British Arts and Letters, 1760–1820* (Philadelphia, PA: University of Pennsylvania Press, 2005).

zoo filled with monkeys and giraffes, while pythons and parrots were hawked in the back alleys of Hamburg.[15] Parisians paid to ride pachyderms. In the woods of Maine, Americans hunted them. Crowds in Washington eyed the cranium of a Fijian "chief"; live "Nubians" captured the Parisian public's attention.[16] Meanwhile, traveling menageries sporting tropical creatures – zebras, hippos, and rhinos – toured between New York, Boston, and Philadelphia.[17] The spoils of empire were, by turns, signs of affluence, measures of metropolitan reach, symbols of imperial power, and emblems of colonial mastery.[18]

Such public displays juxtaposed tropical objects and dramatized tropical difference – and the tropics were not just different, they were pathologically so. Tropical heat and humidity seemed to pervert human nature, excite the passions, and damage the intellect. Unchanging climates and vegetable abundance obviated daily labor and left time for intercourse verbal and otherwise. Tropical inhabitants were viewed as lazy, lascivi-

---

[15] Nigel Rothfels, *Savages and Beasts: The Birth of the Modern Zoo* (Baltimore, MD: Johns Hopkins University Press, 2002), chapter 2; and Herman Reichenbach, "A Tale of Two Zoos: The Hamburg Zoological Garden and Carl Hagenbeck's Tierpark," in *New Worlds, New Animals: From Menagerie to Zoological Park in the Nineteenth Century*, eds. R. J. Hoage and William A. Deiss (Baltimore, MD: Johns Hopkins University Press, 1996), although the author makes the wildly inaccurate claim that recently arrived rhinoceroses were the first to come to Europe "since ancient times" (55). On the rhinoceros in Europe see, for example, Juan Pimentel, *El Rinoceronte y el Megaterio: Un ensayo de morfología histórica* (Madrid: Abada Editores, 2010); and Donald F. Lach, *Asia in the Making of Europe*, 3 vols. (Chicago, IL: University of Chicago Press, 1967), vol. 1, 169, 488, and 569, n. 398.

[16] Ann Fabian, *The Skull Collectors: Race, Science, and America's Unburied Dead* (Chicago, IL: University of Chicago Press, 2010), chapter 4; Michael A. Osborne, *Nature, the Exotic, and the Science of French Colonialism* (Bloomington, IN: Indiana University Press, 1994), 7, 115–116, 126.

[17] Michael A. Osborne, "Zoos in the Family: The Geoffroy Saint-Hilaire Clan and the Three Zoos of Paris," in *New Worlds*, eds. Hoage and Deiss, 39–41; Richard W. Flint, "American Showmen and European Dealers: Commerce in Wild Animals in Nineteenth Century America"; in *New Worlds*, eds. Hoage and Deiss, 98; and Vernon N. Kisling Jr., "The Origin and Development of American Zoological Parks to 1899," in *New Worlds*, eds. Hoage and Deiss, 112–113.

[18] Here I draw on a good deal of postcolonial scholarship. But the act of collecting as part of both personal and imperial self-fashioning was not a strictly European phenomenon and those who engaged in it, including British and French connoisseurs, did not necessarily draw such hard and fast distinctions as the scholarly dichotomy between "colonized" and "colonizer" might suggest. See Maya Jasanoff, *Edge of Empire: Lives, Culture, and Conquest in the East, 1750–1850* (New York: Vintage, 2005).

ous, unclean, and immoral.[19] Visions of unruly nature and debilitating illness fostered research programs and propelled global bioprospecting campaigns.[20] They helped legitimate imperial dominance and inspired techniques of colonial rule.[21] Metropolitan physicians identified diseases of the tropics. Medical geographers plotted them on their maps.[22] Colonial authorities outfitted themselves with pith helmets and quinine. They built hill stations and hydrotherapy spas, installed personal hygiene regulations and sanitation regimes. They separated the sick from the healthy and – after germ theory made it possible to map disease agents onto native bodies – they increasingly separated European settlers from indigenous inhabitants.[23] In the tropics, where the line between nature and humanity

[19] David N. Livingstone, "Tropical Climate and Moral Hygiene: The Anatomy of a Victorian Debate," *The British Journal for the History of Science* 32 (1999): 93–110; Alan Bewell, *Romanticism and Colonial Disease* (Baltimore, MD: Johns Hopkins University Press, 2003); Gavin Bowd and Daniel Clayton, "Tropicality, Orientalism, and French Colonialism in Indochina: The Work of Pierre Gourou, 1927–1982," *French Historical Studies* 28 (2005): 297–327; David Brody, *Visualizing American Empire: Orientalism and Imperialism in the Philippines* (Chicago, IL: University of Chicago Press, 2010).

[20] Lucile H. Brockway, *Science and Colonial Expansion: The Role of the British Royal Botanic Gardens* (New Haven, CT: Yale University Press, 1979); Helen Tilley, *Africa as a Living Laboratory: Empire, Development, and the Problem of Scientific Knowledge, 1870–1950* (Chicago, IL: University of Chicago Press, 2011); Philip D. Curtin, *Disease and Empire: The Health of European Troops in the Conquest of Africa* (New York: Cambridge University Press, 1998); Michael A. Osborne, *The Emergence of Tropical Medicine in France* (Chicago, IL: University of Chicago Press, 2014); and Abena Dove Osseo-Asare, *Bitter Roots: The Search for Healing Plants in Africa* (Chicago, IL: University of Chicago Press, 2014).

[21] Osborne, *Nature, the Exotic, and the Science of French Colonialism*; Richard H. Grove, *Green Imperialism Colonial Expansion, Tropical Island Edens and the Origins of Environmentalism* (New York: Cambridge University Press, 1995); Mark Harrison, *Climates and Constitutions: Health, Race, Environment and British Imperialism in India, 1600–1850* (New York: Oxford University Press, 1999); David Arnold, *The Tropics and the Travelling Gaze: India, Landscape, and Science, 1800–1856* (Seattle, WA: University of Washington Press, 2006); Alice L. Conklin, *In the Museum of Man: Race, Anthropology, and Empire in France, 1850–1950* (Ithaca, NY: Cornell University Press, 2013).

[22] David Arnold, ed., *Warm Climates and Western Medicine: The Emergence of Tropical Medicine, 1500–1900* (Atlanta, GA: Rodopi, 1996); Nancy Leys Stepan, *Picturing Tropical Nature* (Ithaca, NY: Cornell University Press, 2001).

[23] Dane Kennedy, *The Magic Mountains: Hill Stations and the British Raj* (Berkeley, CA: University of California Press, 1996); Eric T. Jennings, *Curing the Colonizers: Hydrotherapy, Climatology, and French Colonial Spas* (Durham, NC: Duke University Press, 2006); David Arnold, *Colonizing the Body: State Medicine and Epidemic Disease in Nineteenth-Century India* (Berkeley, CA: University of California Press, 1993); Warwick Anderson, *Colonial Pathologies: American Tropical Medicine, Race, and Hygiene in the Philippines* (Durham, NC: Duke University Press, 2006); Mariola Espinosa, *Epidemic*

seemed to collapse, installing that and other boundaries became keys to survival. The whole region was to be tamed by European and American science, medicine, technology, and discipline.

EMPIRES AND THEIR TROPICS

The tropics have been central to Western political, cultural, and intellectual life for centuries. From the pre-Romantic fiction of Daniel Defoe's *Robinson Crusoe* to the structural anthropology of Claude Lévi-Strauss, and from bygone debates over miasma to vector-based models for the transmission of disease, the tropics have remained constant – a single coherent region defined by two essential features: profuse and unruly nature, and debilitating febrile illness.[24]

That was not always so. This book, in its broadest terms, is about the birth of that perspective – about how a single, coherent, global region now called "the tropics" was first conjured into being. Much like Fernand Braudel's "Mediterranean," Edmundo O'Gorman's "America," or Edward Said's "Orient," "the tropics" is a historical artifact[25] – a totalizing spatial framework cobbled together and made to seem natural as a consequence of centuries of European empire.[26] Hollywood movies (such as *Outbreak*) and science fiction novels (most famously, *The Hot Zone*) no less than academic specializations (from tropical medicine to

Invasions: Yellow Fever and the Limits of Cuban Independence, 1878–1930 (Chicago, IL: University of Chicago Press, 2009); John W. Cell, "Anglo-Indian Medical Theory and the Origins of Segregation in West Africa," *American Historical Review* 91 (1986): 307–335.

[24] That was true even as nineteenth-century observers quarreled over how best to gauge coherence and readily conceded the fact of internal variation. See Warwick Anderson, "Climates of Opinion: Acclimatization in Nineteenth-Century France and England," *Victorian Studies* 35 (1992): 135–157; and David Arnold, "'Illusory Riches': Representations of the Tropical World, 1840–1950," *Singapore Journal of Tropical Geography* 21 (2000): 6–18.

[25] Fernand Braudel, *The Mediterranean and the Mediterranean World in the Age of Philip II*, 2 vols., trans. Siân Reynolds (Berkeley, CA: University of California Press, 1995 [1949]); Edmundo O'Gorman, *La invención de América* (Mexico City: Fondo de Cultura Económica, 1986); Edward Said, *Orientalism*, (New York: Pantheon, 1978).

[26] As is the case with globalizing perspectives generally, according to Martin W. Lewis and Kären E. Wigen, *The Myth of Continents: A Critique of Metageography* (Berkeley, CA: University of California Press, 1997).

evolutionary biology) continue to normalize the concept.[27] Yet it has never been merely a reflection of the natural order of things and there was nothing inevitable about its creation.

The origins of the tropics lay in the ancient Aristotelian concept of the "torrid zone." By the mid-nineteenth century, these two terms had become virtually interchangeable. But whereas the tropics and the torrid zone refer to an identical area of the globe – one demarcated by the Tropic of Cancer north of the equator and the Tropic of Capricorn to its south[28] – they are not the same thing. The fundamental difference is environmental. The tropics brim with life; the torrid zone, at least in the narrowest Aristotelian sense (beset with the searing intensity of the sun directly overhead), was bereft of it.[29]

How, when, and why these views were reconciled, and what was at stake when that happened, are principal concerns of this book. A dominant narrative shared by the histories of science, medicine, and geography alike date the invention of "the tropics" to European imperial pursuits at the end of the eighteenth century. The central figure in this account is Vogel's elder countryman, the Prussian Alexander von Humboldt, who, together with the botanist Aimé Bonpland, trekked through the Andes between 1799 and 1804. Humboldt had a predilection for instrumentation and measurement, and a penchant for lyrical descriptions of equinoctial vegetation. His travels, lyricism, and faith

---

[27] Priscilla Wald, *Contagious: Cultures, Carriers, and the Outbreak Narrative* (Durham, NC: Duke University Press, 2008), chapters 1 and 4; and Gary Y. Okihiro, "Unsettling the Imperial Sciences," *Environment and Planning D: Society and Space* 28 (2010): 745–758. See also, for example, the widely-cited essay by the influential geneticist Theodosius Dobzhansky, "Evolution in the Tropics," *American Scientist* 38 (1950): 209–221. I thank Tito Carvalho for this reference.

[28] These lines mark, respectively, the northern- and southern-most positions at which it is still possible to observe the sun directly overhead. They presently correspond to 23 degrees and 51 minutes north and south latitude. Because the Earth's rotational axis itself rotates (the motion of precession: much like a spinning top, the Earth wobbles), the sun's apparent motion shifts over long spans of time and therefore the precise latitudes of the northern and southern tropics also shift.

[29] The classic statement appears in Aristotle, *Meteorologica*, trans. H. D. P. Lee (Cambridge, MA: Harvard University Press, 1952), bk. 2, pt. 5. For a discussion, see Denis Cosgrove, "Tropic and Tropicality," in *Tropical Visions in an Age of Empire*, eds. Felix Driver and Luciana Martins (Chicago, IL: University of Chicago Press, 2005), 199–202.

in precision measurement inspired similar intertropical itineraries.[30] Vogel's was among them.[31]

Humboldt gave short shrift to disease, although fever ("yellow fever" in particular) made its way into volume three of his widely read *Personal Narrative*.[32] He need not have said more. Imperial rivalries, renewed settler colonialism in Africa and Asia, the intensification of global trade, and the compilation of colonial health statistics had all begun to focus European attention on the problem of disease in many parts of the intertropical world.[33] The climate and vegetation that Humboldt helped make emblematic of that world always implied the presence of miasma

---

[30] Mary Louise Pratt, *Imperial Eyes: Travel Writing and Transculturation*, 2nd edn. (New York: Routledge, 2008), chapter 6; Hugh Raffles, *In Amazonia: A Natural History* (Princeton, NJ: Princeton University Press, 2001); Michael Dettelbach, "Global Physics and Aesthetic Empire: Humboldt's Physical Portrait of the Tropics," in *Visions of Empire: Voyages, Botany, and Representations of Nature*, eds. David Philip Miller and Peter Hanns Reill (New York: Cambridge University Press, 1996), 258–292; Malcolm Nicholson, "Alexander von Humboldt and the Geography of Vegetation," in *Romanticism and the Sciences*, eds. Andrew Cunningham and Nicholas Jardine (Cambridge: Cambridge University Press, 1990); John Hemming, *Naturalists in Paradise: Wallace, Bates, and Spruce in the Amazon* (London: Thames and Hudson, 2015); Stepan, *Picturing Tropical Nature*; Arnold, "Illusory Riches"; Driver and Martins, eds., *Tropical Visions*.

   In addition, Aaron Sachs, *The Humboldt Current: Nineteenth-Century Exploration and the Roots of American Environmentalism* (New York: Penguin, 2006), credits Humboldt with shaping domestic American attitudes toward nature. The life and travels of the Prussian engineer-turned-explorer continue to inspire literature aimed at general audiences. See, for example, Andrea Wulf, *The Invention of Nature: Alexander von Humboldt's New World* (New York: Alfred A. Knopf, 2015); and Daniel Kehlmann, *Measuring the World: A Novel*, trans. Carol Brown Janeway (New York: Vintage Books, 2006).

[31] According to D. Graham Burnett, *Masters of All They Surveyed: Exploration, Geography, and a British El Dorado* (Chicago, IL: University of Chicago Press, 2001), 123, n. 21, Vogel would have been part of a community of expatriate Prussian naturalists who had gathered in London by the late 1830s.

[32] These are scattered throughout Alexander von Humboldt, *Personal Narrative of Travels to the Equinoctial Regions of the New Continent, during the Years 1799–1804*, trans. Helen Maria Williams, 3 vols. (London: Longman, Hurst, Rees, Orme, and Brown, 1814–1822), vol. 3, 32, 301, 310, 380–381, 387, 390–406, 466, 468. According to Nicolaas A. Rupke, "Humboldtian Medicine," *Medical History* 40 (1996): 293–310, his work also inspired a short-lived area of medicine.

[33] David Arnold, "Introduction: Tropical Medicine before Manson," in *Warm Climates*, Arnold, ed., 1–19; Mark Harrison, "A Global Perspective: Reframing the History of Health, Medicine, and Disease," *Bulletin of the History of Medicine* 89 (2015): 639–689; Daniel R. Headrick, *Power over Peoples: Technology, Environments, and Western Imperialism, 1400 to the Present* (Princeton, NJ: Princeton University Press, 2012); Curtin, *Death by Migration*; Curtin, *Disease and Empire*; Harrison, *Climates and Constitutions*; Stepan, *Picturing Tropical Nature*.

and therefore pervasive illness. As Humboldt's work found readers across Europe, and as the figure of the afflicted explorer became an icon of scientific heroism,[34] fever became the signal disease of the intertropical world. It was foremost among the ills that contemporary physicians began to identify as "diseases of warm climates." And in the 1880s, even as the emerging field of tropical medicine dispensed with environmental explanations in favor of germ theory and parasitology, fever remained the focus.[35]

Yet long before metropolitan readers began to immerse themselves in the ink of Humboldt's prodigious pen – before the extension of colonial empires in the nineteenth century, before the beginnings of English and French settlement in Asia and the Americas, decades even before the Columbian voyages of the 1490s – a tentative link had been drawn between intertropical latitudes, prodigious nature, and debilitating fevers. The connection came not as British, French, or Spanish ships sailed across the Atlantic to the Americas but as ships sailing under Portuguese auspices ventured southward, into the Atlantic, along the West African coast.

Beyond the Senegal River, the unexpected virulence of fevers amid verdant landscapes and abundant wildlife called into question a set of ancient and authoritative accounts of both nature and disease. Instead of the scorched and desolate landscape imagined by Aristotle, fifteenth-century travelers found one that was lush and verdant. Bountiful nature was supposed to be a sign of health and vitality. Yet travelers found themselves besieged by debilitating, often deadly, fevers. Seemingly irresolvable questions had been opened. What could explain the coincidence of fecund landscapes and virulent fevers? How could an entire region that

---

[34] Nigel Leask, *Curiosity and the Aesthetics of Travel Writing, 1770–1840* (New York: Oxford University Press, 2002); Christopher Lawrence and Michael Brown, "Quintessentially Modern Heroes: Surgeons, Explorers, and Empire, c. 1840–1914," *Journal of Social History* 50 (2016): 148–178; Johannes Fabian, *Out of Our Minds: Reason and Madness in the Exploration of Central Africa* (Berkeley, CA: University of California Press, 2000).

[35] Deborah J. Neill, *Networks in Tropical Medicine: Internationalism, Colonialism, and the Rise of a Medical Specialty, 1890–1930* (Stanford, CA: Stanford University Press, 2012); Michael A. Osborne, *The Emergence of Tropical Medicine in France* (Chicago, IL: University of Chicago Press, 2014); Michael Worboys, "Germs, Malaria, and the Invention of Mansonian Tropical Medicine: From 'Diseases in the Tropics' to 'Tropical Diseases,'" in *Warm Climates*, ed. Arnold, 181–207; Michael Worboys, "The Emergence of Tropical Medicine: A Study in the Establishment of a Scientific Specialty," in *Perspectives on the Emergence of Scientific Disciplines*, eds. Gerard Lemaine, Roy Macleod, Michael Mulkay, and Peter Weingart (The Hague: Mouton, 1976), 75–98.

was otherwise teeming with life be so inhospitable? And how could travelers survive in such bedevilling circumstances? Prevailing notions of miasma seemed unable to explain the problem. Familiar medicines seemed inadequate to resolve it. In environmental and epidemiological terms, fifteenth-century voyages into the Atlantic were as disorienting as later voyages across it.[36]

The proposition that intertropical lands might everywhere be endowed with profuse and exploitable nature would soon raise the stakes of exploration. Southerly sailing came to be seen as an asset by European statesmen and seafarers alike.[37] But in the closing decades of the fifteenth century, it was not at all clear that the situation in West Africa should be taken as characteristic of the entire intertropical world. The true extent of intertropical abundance remained unknown. The causes and distribution of fevers were uncertain. What in the postcolonial, biomedical present has come to seem self-evident was, for some two centuries, anything but so. The many disorientations provoked by fifteenth-century voyages, and the strategies devised by travelers to cope with them, are the subject of Chapter 2.

The history of the tropics is the story of what happened next. The Portuguese established colonies from sub-Saharan Africa to Southeast Asia and South America, enabling the earliest global comparisons of nature and disease across the vast intertropical world. From Malacca in Southeast Asia to Olinda and Salvador da Bahia in Northeastern Brazil, a loosely connected network of Portuguese physicians and apothecaries emerged. For the first time ever, persons with a common intellectual inheritance and similar training spanned the intertropical world. Everywhere, unfamiliar nature and debilitating fevers became a focus of colonial inquiry and vigorous debate. Yet in Portugal's colonies, encounters with nature and disease inspired a range of geographical imaginings. For physicians such as Garcia de Orta in India or Aleixo de Abreu in Brazil,

---

[36] With an emphasis on geography and cross-cultural encounter, a similar point has been made, for example, by Luís Filipe Barreto, *Descobrimento e renascimento: Formas de ser e pensar nos séculos XV e XVI* (Lisbon: Imprensa Nacional-Casa da Moeda, 1983); Fernández-Armesto, *Before Columbus: Exploration and Colonization from the Mediterranean to the Atlantic, 1229–1492* (Philadelphia, PA: University of Pennsylvania Press, 1987); and Alida C. Metcalf, *Go-Betweens and the Colonization of Brazil, 1500–1600* (Austin, TX: University of Texas Press, 2005), chapter 2.

[37] Nicolás Wey Gómez, *The Tropics of Empire: Why Columbus Sailed South to the Indies* (Cambridge, MA: MIT Press, 2008); Maria da Graça Mateus Ventura, ed., *Viagens e viajantes no Atlântico quinhentista* (Lisbon: Edições Colibri, 1996).

the intertropical world was vast and internally differentiated – nature and disease were widely variable, the tropics a patchwork of distinctive places.[38] In neither theater of empire did Portuguese authors imagine themselves as inhabiting an environmentally or epidemiologically coherent intertropical zone.

Meanwhile, plants, animals, objects, and people from across the Portuguese colonial world flooded into Lisbon.[39] Finely carved African ivory, silken Indian headdresses, brightly glazed martabans from Pegu, Chinese porcelain, Japanese armor, and silver-ornamented coconuts from the Maldives filled shops along the bustling Rua dos Mercadores.[40] A skilled goldsmith from India, Rauluchantim, arrived to make finery for the Portuguese Crown. Some dozen elephants and three rhinoceroses ambled ashore into the heart of Lisbon during the sixteenth century. Civet cats scampered across the grounds of the royal menagerie. Baboons scaled its trees. Gray parrots from Guinea, parakeets from South Asia, and macaws from the far side of the Atlantic all spread their wings in the aviary of the Alcaçova palace – their plumage spanning the rainbow from luminous yellows to regal blues and reds.[41] Gardens greened with the leaves of exotic flora. Bananas and plantains from Guinea, taro from South Asia, and tobacco from the Americas grew on the estates of imperial ministers, royal factors, and returned colonial governors.[42] Abbeys

[38] Such a multiplicity of visions of imperial geography also characterized the Spanish case, as described by Ricardo Padrón, *The Spacious Word: Cartography, Literature, and Empire in Early Modern Spain* (Chicago, IL: University of Chicago Press, 2004).

[39] Annemarie Jordan Gschwend and K. J. P. Lowe, eds., *The Global City: On the Streets of Renaissance Lisbon* (London: Paul Holberton, 2015).

[40] Donald F. Lach, *Asia in the Making of Europe*, vol. 2, bk. 1, 10–16; Annemarie Jordan Gschwend, "Catarina de Áustria: Colecção e *Kunstkammer* de uma Princesa Renascentista," *Oceanos* 16 (1993): 62–70; Annemarie Jordan Gschwend, "As Maravilhas do Oriente: Colecções de Curiosidades Renascentista em Portugal/The Marvels of the East: Renaissance Curiosity Collections in Portugal," in *A Herança de Rauluchantim/The Heritage of Rauluchantim*, ed. N. V. Silva (Lisbon: Museu de São Roque, 1996), 82–127.

[41] Gschwend, "A Procura Portuguesa"; and Palmira Fontes da Costa, "Secrecy, Ostentation, and the Illustration of Exotic Animals in Sixteenth-Century Portugal," *Annals of Science* 66 (2009): 59–82.

[42] Garcia de Orta, *Colloquies on the Simples and Drugs of India*, trans. Clements Markham (London: Henry Southern and Company, 1913), 200 and n. 1; Carolus Clusius, *Rariorum aliquot stirpium per Hispanias* (Antwerp: Christopher Plantin, 1576), 131, 254, 280, 289, 299, 444; Rose Standish Nichols, *Spanish and Portuguese Gardens* (London: Constable and Company, 1922), 225–226; Damião de Góis, *Chronica do felicissimo rei Dom Emanuel* (Lisbon: Francisco Correa, 1566–1567), part 1, chapter 56, 52–52v; *MB* vol. 1, 423, n. 10 and 424, n. 14.

and apothecaries alike stocked tamarind and senna from West Africa, along with Asian drugs, spices, and aromatics ranging from amber to zedoary. Dispensaries sold them to the sick. Infirmaries served them to the poor. The spoils of empire delighted the senses, filled the bellies, and fortified the souls of even the kingdom's unlikeliest subjects.[43]

Global seafaring, cross-cultural encounter, and colonization had shown not only that tremendous human diversity[44] but also climatic, geographic, environmental, and epidemiological diversity characterized the very part of the world that Aristotle had insisted was a single, coherent, and uniformly lifeless region. Yet none of the exotic plants, animals, and people pouring into Lisbon were taken as an index of essential intertropical similarity and used to articulate a vision of environmental and epidemiological coherence.[45]

The tropics – its nature and its characteristic qualities – was not a discovery but a political project. Intertropical objects and their varied provenances had to be imbued with new meaning. How and why disparate places spread across the midriff of the terraqueous globe finally became aggregated and assimilated to one another is the subject of Chapter 8. Across the latter half of the seventeenth century, I argue, a coterie of politically connected, university-trained physicians turned the empire into an epistemic, curative, and professional resource. Manuel de Azevedo, Simão Pinheiro Mourão, and João Curvo Semedo are not well known even among specialists of early modern medicine. But they were among a number of physicians in Lisbon who tried to resolve the intractable medical questions surrounding the causes of fever and the relationship between nature and disease – the questions first posed by those early

---

[43] Lach, *Asia in the Making of Europe*, vol. 2, bk. 1, 11–12; Isabel M. R. Mendes Drummond Braga, *Assistência, saúde pública e prática médica em Portugal: Séculos XV–XIX* (Lisbon: Universitária Editora, 2001); Lisbeth de Oliveira Rodrigues and Isabel dos Guimarães Sá, "Sugar and Spices in Portuguese Renaissance Medicine," *Journal of Medieval Iberian Studies* 7 (2015): 176–196.

[44] Surekha Davies, *Renaissance Ethnography and the Invention of the Human: New Worlds, Maps, and Monsters* (New York: Cambridge University Press, 2016); João-Pau Rubiés, *Travel and Ethnology in the Renaissance: South India through European Eyes, 1250–1625* (New York: Cambridge University Press, 2000); Anthony Pagden, *The Fall of Natural Man: The American Indian and the Origins of Comparative Ethnology* (New York: Cambridge University Press, 1982).

[45] Some may object that such a framework was indeed present earlier as evidenced in works such as Shakespeare's *The Tempest*. But there as elsewhere in the early seventeenth century, disease was mentioned with reference to putrid airs in localized swamps rather than as a generalized condition of the intertropical world. Mine is, in essence, an account of how that view became generalized.

Atlantic encounters. For them, naming and defining the tropics was part of a strategy of personal and professional advancement. They embraced what they saw as the exceptional therapeutic value of intertropical nature but argued that intertropical diseases demanded metropolitan curative acumen. Drawing attention to epidemics of fever in both Portugal and its colonies, they stressed the combination of university learning and inter-tropical itineraries as grounds for both authoritative medical knowledge and superior clinical practice. They attempted to showcase their learning through increasingly elaborate treatises on fever, its causes, categoriza-tion, and treatment. In metropolitan Portugal, claims of intertropical coherence became foundational for claims about the authority and neces-sity of learned medicine throughout the empire.[46]

By itself, a story that links fifteenth-century epidemiological encounters in the Atlantic to seventeenth-century intertropical imaginings in Lisbon is important for several reasons. Most narrowly, this story challenges a prominent depiction of learned medicine in early modern Portugal. Rather than an era in which single-minded Portuguese physicians remained mired in an implacable, backward-looking Galenism,[47] I show that metropolitan physicians of the seventeenth century vigorously and creatively disputed the cause and treatment of fevers then plaguing the Portuguese colonial world. As part of a bid to shore up the ever-tenuous authority of learned medicine in Portugal and its empire, I argue, these debates were a prelude to the better-known pursuits of the eighteenth century, when metropolitan physicians partnered with powerful church-men to prosecute lay healers in Inquisitorial courtrooms.[48]

More broadly, because these earlier contests for clinical primacy unfolded in the pages of published books and pamphlets, their story draws attention to the largely uncharted place of medicine in the history

---

[46] That ideological changes underpin the formulation of new visions of the globe is a pattern of metageographical thinking more generally according to Lewis and Wigen, *Myth of Continents*, xi.

[47] Augusto da Silva Carvalho, *A Medicina Portuguesa no século XVII* (Lisbon: Academia das Ciências de Lisboa, 1940); Ian Maclean, *Learning and the Market Place: Essays in the History of the Early Modern Book* (Boston: Brill, 2009), chapter 13.

[48] Timothy D. Walker, *Doctors, Folk Medicine, and the Inquisition: The Repression of Magical Healing in Portugal during the Enlightenment Era* (Boston: Brill, 2005); and Braga, *Assistência*.

of Portuguese print culture, and to the as-yet unexamined role of physicians in a transformational era of Portuguese imperial politics.[49] This story also highlights the ways in which the earliest decades of Atlantic exploration shaped not just early modern therapeutics (itself now the subject of a rich literature[50]) but also metropolitan medical and philosophical frameworks. Medical theory was not impervious to the epidemiological feedback generated by some of the earliest Atlantic voyages. Rather, West African encounters helped propel shifts in medical thinking that implied more sweeping claims about the inner workings of the natural world.[51] In the seventeenth century, Portuguese physicians promoted the view that fever was a form of contagion. As a disease, fever became the consequence of noxious particles rather than a

[49] A lucid exploration of political and intellectual life can be found in Diogo Curto, *O Discurso político em Portugal (1600–1650)* (Lisbon: Universidade Aberta, 1988). For the history of the book in Portugal, see, for example, the bibliography compiled by Manuela D. Domingos, ed., *Estudos sobre História do Livro e da Leitura em Portugal, 1995–2000* (Lisbon: Biblioteca Nacional, 2002); and the essays surveying printed work on medicine in Palmira Fontes da Costa and Adelino Cardoso, eds., *Percursos na História do Livro Médico* (Lisbon: Edições Colibri, 2011). On physicians and politics generally see Laurinda Abreu, "A organização e regulação das *profissões médicas* no Portugal Moderno: entre as orientações da Coroa e os interesses privados," in *Arte Médica e Imagem do Corpo: de Hipócrates ao final do século XVIII*, eds. Adelino Cardoso, et al. (Lisbon: Biblioteca Nacional de Portugal, 2010), 97–122; and Francis A. Dutra, "The Practice of Medicine in Early Modern Portugal: The Role and Social Status of the *Físico-mor* and the *Surgião-mor*," in *Libraries, History, Diplomacy, and the Performing Arts: Essays in Honor of Carleton Sprague Smith*, ed. Israel J. Katz (Stuyvesant, NY: Pendragon Press, 2001), 135–169.

[50] See, for example, Mauricio Nieto Olarte, *Remedios para el imperio: historia natural y la apropiación del Nuevo Mundo* (Bogota: Universidad de los Andes, 2006); Crisina Gurgel, *Doenças e curas: o Brasil nos primeiros séculos* (São Paulo: Editora Contexto, 2010); Pratik Chakrabarti, *Materials and Medicine: Trade, Conquest and Therapeutics in the Eighteenth Century* (Manchester: University of Manchester Press, 2010); Timothy D. Walker, "The Medicines Trade in the Portuguese Atlantic World: Acquisition and Dissemination of Healing Knowledge from Brazil (c. 1580–1800)," *Social History of Medicine* (2013): 403–431; Matthew James Crawford, *The Andean Wonder Drug: Cinchona Bark and Imperial Science in the Spanish Atlantic, 1630–1800* (Pittsburgh, PA: University of Pittsburgh Press, 2016); and Londa Schiebinger, *Plants and Empire: Colonial Bioprospecting in the Atlantic World* (Cambridge, MA: Harvard University Press, 2004).

[51] The point is usually made with reference not to fever along the African coast but to the plague pandemic of the fourteenth century and the outbreak of venereal syphilis in Mediterranean Europe in the wake of the first Columbian voyages. See Roger French, *Medicine before Science: The Business of Medicine from the Middle Ages to the Enlightenment* (New York: Cambridge University Press, 2003); and Jon Arrizabalaga, John Henderson, and Roger French, *The Great Pox: The French Disease in Renaissance Europe* (New Haven, CT: Yale University Press, 1997).

humoral imbalance. The episode not only dramatizes the little-known ways that Lisbon's physicians participated in wider contemporary debates over the causes and classification of fever.[52] But claims that endowed disease with a discrete ontological existence were also consonant with the emergent mechanical philosophy of the New Science, which raises questions about the relationship of Portuguese physicians to their counterparts in London and elsewhere.[53]

Most important, here, is the link between medical ontology and global geography. The seventeenth century was an era in which a raft of novel spatial frameworks came into being within metropolitan Europe.[54] The tropics, I contend, was one of them, and debates surrounding fever were central to its creation.[55] The point is not merely that colonial diseases shaped metropolitan medical debates and permitted new geographical distinctions – or even that lines of geographical distinction supported lines of professional exclusion. The intertwined processes of imperial expansion and colonial settlement did not simply enable encounters with disparate febrile environments. In ways both material and discursive, those processes helped to create such environments.[56] The Portuguese empire mobilized peoples, pathogens, and therapeutics, and compelled them to cluster in locations spread across the intertropical world.[57] In so

---

[52] On the contemporaneous emergence of fever as a focus of English medical debate, see Mark Harrison, *Medicine in an Age of Commerce and Empire: Britain and Its Tropical Colonies, 1660–1830* (New York: Oxford University Press, 2010).

[53] On the larger question of the participation of physicians in the New Science, see Harold J. Cook, "The New Philosophy and Medicine in Seventeenth-Century England," in *Reappraisals of the Scientific Revolution*, eds. David C. Lindberg and Robert S. Westman (New York: Cambridge University Press, 1990), 397–365. On the relationship between the often separate histories of science and medicine that this approach is meant to address, see Nancy Siraisi, "Medicine, 1450–1620, and the History of Science," *Isis* 103 (2012): 491–514.

[54] Lewis and Wigen, *Myth of Continents*; Benjamin Schmidt, *Inventing Exoticism: Geography, Globalism, and Europe's Early Modern World* (Philadelphia, PA: University of Pennsylvania Press, 2015).

[55] Though marginal to the account of Grove, *Green Imperialism*.

[56] Classic studies include Alfred W. Crosby, *The Columbian Exchange: Biological and Cultural Consequences of 1492* (Westport, CT: Greenwood, 1972); and Alfred W. Crosby, *Ecological Imperialism: The Biological Expansion of Europe, 900–1900* (New York: Cambridge University Press, 1986); but for an approach that moves beyond what many have seen as Crosby's biological determinism, see Mark Harrison, *Contagion: How Commerce Has Spread Disease* (New Haven, CT: Yale University Press, 2012).

[57] A standard of account of which is A. J R. Russell-Wood, *The Portuguese Empire, 1415–1808: A World on the Move* (Baltimore, MD: Johns Hopkins University Press, 1992).

doing, the empire also permitted physicians to assemble those elements together on the pages of books and manuscripts, to collectively name and define them, and to seek personal advantage and build professional alliances based on that vision[58] – all while helping to alter the techniques of colonial rule.[59] In Portugal's empire, global geography, febrile disease, and professional medicine proved mutually constitutive.

CULTURES OF INQUIRY AND THE LOCATION OF EXPERTISE

Read another way, this book is about the investigative practices of disparate colonial communities spread across the intertropical world. Although a vision of intertropical coherence constituted an intellectual and political project among physicians in metropolitan Lisbon, its history cannot simply be found among the European books, curiosities, and medical debates of the sixteenth and seventeenth centuries any more than it can among the research laboratories, public parks, and traveling menageries of the nineteenth and twentieth centuries. In Lisbon, if perplexing fevers and exotic plants and animals all became emblems of tropicality in the late seventeenth century, it was because physicians there mobilized and reconfigured knowledge to serve their own ends – knowledge that originated in places throughout the intertropical world.

A history of the tropics is necessarily one of proliferating centers and cosmopolitan colonies.[60] Just as successive cycles of encounter, reportage, and tabulation linked Europe to the wider world and led to the production of new knowledge in imperial Lisbon, so too did empire have similar effects inPortugal's colonies.

In the commercial city of Goa in India and on the plantations of Pernambuco in Brazil, distinctive cultures of inquiry took shape. They were composed of an idiosyncratic amalgam of participants. They allocated authority and expertise – and they focused investigative and curative efforts – in unpredictable ways. And they endowed nature and disease

---

[58] I have in mind the dynamic elaborated in Bruno Latour, *Pandora's Hope: Essays on the Reality of Science Studies* (Cambridge, MA: Harvard University Press, 1999), chapter 3.

[59] Physicians' efforts helped "territorialize" the intertropical world in the sense developed by Robert D. Sack, *Human Territoriality: Its Theory and History* (New York: Cambridge University Press, 1986).

[60] The concept of cosmopolitanism for the early modern world has been worked out by a number of historians, but for the history of science in particular, see Kapil Raj, "The Historical Anatomy of a Contact Zone: Calcutta in the Eighteenth Century," *The Indian Economic and Social History Review* 48 (2011): 55–82.

with meanings of their own. Imperial networks may have mobilized objects like ivory sculptures, plants like coconut palms, and creatures like elephants and macaws but their meanings were unstable and plastic rather than "immutable."[61]

What, then, were the varied meanings given to nature and disease in Portugal's colonies? How were they constituted? How and why were they packed into the pages of books and letters in the first place? By whom? How were expertise and authority configured? What kinds of intellectual projects motivated colonial natural inquiry and what spatial frameworks were they part of? To answer these questions, this story sweeps out across Portugal's empire. It retraces the passages of books and letters, animals and plants from imperial Lisbon back to the colonial port cities that set them in motion.

In following the successive processes of recontextualization by which things and creatures were repeatedly given new meanings, *Assembling the Tropics* establishes important material and ideological relationships between the Atlantic and Indian Ocean worlds. In so doing, this story challenges a range of more conventional historical-spatial frameworks (center-periphery models, oceanic worlds, and area studies perspectives).[62] The story also refuses the centripetal pull of imperial histories of science, especially Iberian science, that focus primarily on metropolitan outlooks and transformations.[63]

Here the dominant narrative is about a scientific revolution. During the sixteenth and seventeenth centuries, contentious debates over the content and inner workings of the natural world within Europe are supposed to have led to paradigmatic transformation in Western definitions of nature and in the procedures judged appropriate for natural inquiry. What had once been an animate, even mischievous cosmos is supposed to have been endowed instead with an inert, regular, and mechanical existence.[64] Thick, leather-bound tomes by ancient authors no longer vouchsafed claims to

[61] Contrary to the model of "immutable mobiles" in Latour, *Science in Action*, especially 223-228. See also David Turnbull, "Travelling Knowledge: Narratives, Assemblage, and Encounters," in *Instruments, Travel and Science: Itineraries of Precision from the Seventeenth to the Twentieth Century*, eds. Marie-Noëlle Bourguet, Christian Licoppe, and H. Otto Sibum (London: Routledge, 2002), 273–294.

[62] Building on discussions by Lewis and Wigen, *Myth of Continents*; and Harrison, "A Global Perspective."

[63] The key concept here of course is that of "centers of calculation" from Latour, *Science in Action*.

[64] But see Lorraine Daston, "The Nature of Nature in Early Modern Europe," *Configurations* 6 (1998): 149–172.

truth. Sensory experience and instruments did. In Galileo's telescope or Boyle's air pump, nature could be made to testify on its own behalf. Reasoning from universal axioms gave way to reasoning from particular instances. Knowledge was to be built from mechanically produced, experimentally verified, collectively attested, and discreet matters of fact.[65]

The contemporaneous creation of overseas empires have more recently been implicated in these transformations. Unanticipated encounters overseas, no less than telescopic observations of the heavens at home, expanded Europeans' sense of what was possible in nature. The intensification of global trade, which placed a premium on discerning eyes, noses, mouths, and hands, further eroded the bookish predilections of naturalists and enhanced the value of evidence drawn from the senses.[66]

Faced with the long-standing exclusion of Spanish and Portuguese endeavours from this standard account,[67] scholars from a range of disciplinary backgrounds have begun to highlight Iberian contributions to fields ranging from metallurgy and medicine to natural history, navigation, and cosmography. They have traced the varied routes by which exotica, iconography, instruments, and print media circulated back and forth across the Pyrenees, and in the process have stressed the importance of the Spanish and Portuguese empires to the wide range of cultural and intellectual transformations unfolding within early modern Europe.[68]

---

[65] Foundational are Steven Shapin and Simon Schaffer, *Leviathan and the Air Pump: Hobbes, Boyle, and the Experimental Life* (Princeton, NJ: Princeton University Press, 1985); and Lorraine Daston and Katherine Park, *Wonders and the Order of Nature, 1150–1750* (New York: Zone Books, 2001).

[66] A bellwether of the shift was Anthony Grafton with April Shelford and Nancy Siraisi, *New Worlds, Ancient Texts: The Power of Tradition and the Shock of Discovery* (Cambridge, MA: Belknap Press, 1992). See more recently Harold J. Cook, *Matters of Exchange: Commerce, Medicine, and Science in the Dutch Golden Age* (New Haven, CT: Yale University Press, 2007); and Dániel Margócsy, *Commercial Visions: Science, Trade, and Visual Culture in the Dutch Golden Age* (Chicago, IL: University of Chicago Press, 2014).

[67] An omission, moreover, that helps sustain lasting assertions about the impoverished character of Iberian and Latin American society, culture, and politics: Jeremy Adelman, ed., *Colonial Legacies: The Problem of Persistence in Latin American History* (New York: Routledge, 1999). A central issue is the so-called "black legend" of Iberian colonial violence and political tyranny, the invention of which is covered in Benjamin Schmidt, *Innocence Abroad: The Dutch Imagination and the New World, 1570–1670* (New York: Cambridge University Press, 2001).

[68] Broadly representative of the range of approaches are Ana Cristina Araújo, *A Cultura das Luzes em Portugal: Temas e problemas* (Lisbon: Livros Horizonte, 2003); Miguel de Asúa and Roger French, *A New World of Animals: Early Modern Europeans on the Creatures of Iberian America* (Burlington, VT: Ashgate, 2005); Miruna Achim, *Lagartijas medicinales: Remedios americanos y debates científicos en la ilustración* (Mexico City: Consejo Nacional para la Cultura y las Artes, 2008); Neil Safier, *Measuring the New World: Enlightenment Science and South America* (Chicago, IL: University of Chicago

Under the unifying rubric of Iberian science, some have argued that it was in Spain, Portugal, and their empires that empirical, experimental, and utilitarian approaches to the study of nature first emerged. Iberian empires, rather than metropolitan virtuosi, birthed modern science and its ontologies.[69]

These are large claims that deserve, and have garnered, a great deal of attention.[70] Most studies in this vein have focused on Spain and its empire. But the perspective has patterned interpretations of the Portuguese world too. If they are studied at all, most of the authors and institutions that appear in the pages that follow – Garcia de Orta in India, Jesuit missionaries in both South Asia and South America, Aleixo de Abreu in the South Atlantic – have been pitched as prefigurations of an epistemic or clinical modernity to come.[71] Yet tethering these histories to

Press, 2008); María M. Portuondo, *Secret Science: Spanish Cosmography and the New World* (Chicago, IL: University of Chicago Press, 2009); Daniela Bleichmar, Paula de Vos, Kristin Huffine, and Kevin Sheehan, eds., *Science in the Spanish and Portuguese Empires, 1500–1800* (Stanford, CA: Stanford University Press, 2009); Daniela Bleichmar, *Visible Empire: Botanical Expeditions and Visual Culture in the Hispanic Enlightenment* (Chicago, IL: University of Chicago Press, 2012); Mauricio Nieto Olarte, *Las máquinas del imperio y el reino de Dios: reflexiones sobre la ciencia, tecnología y religión en el mundo Atlántico del siglo XVI* (Bogotá: Universidad de los Andes, 2013); and Eliane Cristina Deckman Fleck, *Entre a caridade e a ciência: a prática missionária e a científica da Companhia de Jesus (América platina, séculos XVII e XVIII)* (São Leopoldo: Oikos and Editora Unisinos, 2014).

[69] Jorge Cañizares-Esguerra, *How to Write the History of the New World: Histories, Epistemologies, and Identities in the Eighteenth-Century Atlantic World* (Stanford, CA: Stanford University Press, 2001); Jorge Cañizares-Esguerra, "Iberian Science in the Renaissance: Ignored How Much Longer?," *Perspectives on Science* 12 (2004): 86–124; Antonio Barrera-Osorio, *Experiencing Nature: The Spanish American Empire and the Early Scientific Revolution* (Austin, TX: University of Texas Press, 2006); Victor Navarro Brotóns and William Eamon, eds., *Más allá de la Leyenda Negra: España y la Revolución Científica* (Valencia: Instituto de Historia de la Ciencia y Documentación López Piñero of the University of Valencia and CSIC, 2007). For a broader discussion, see Stephen Toulmin, *Cosmopolis: The Hidden Agenda of Modernity* (Chicago, IL: University of Chicago Press, 1992).

[70] These debates have had an influence well beyond the history of science. See, for example, David J. Weber, *Bárbaros: Spaniards and Their Savages in the Age of Enlightenment* (New Haven, CT: Yale University Press, 2005).

[71] Onésimo Teotónio de Almeida, "Portugal and the Dawn of Modern Science," in *Portugal, the Pathfinder: Journeys from the Medieval toward the Modern World, 1300–ca. 1600*, ed. George Winius (Madison, WI: University of Wisconsin Press, 1995), 341–361; Lopes Rodrigues, *Anchieta e a Medicina* (Bello Horizonte: Edições Apollo, 1934); Steven J. Harris, "Long-Distance Corporations, Big Sciences, and the Geography of Knowledge," *Configurations* 6 (1998): 269–304; Steven J. Harris, "Jesuit Scientific Activity in the Overseas Missions, 1540–1773," *Isis* 96 (2005): 71–79; Miguel de Asúa, "Los jesuítas y el conocimiento de la naturaleza Americana," *Stromata* (2003): 1–20; and F

an (ultimately dubious[72]) origins story of modernity comes at considerable cost. Colonial cultures of inquiry were never merely extensions of metropolitan concerns, priorities, questions, investigative techniques, and representational conventions.[73] The fullness of their stories is valuable not because those stories reflect seemingly modern clinical and investigative dispositions but because they are emblematic of the profusion of practices born in the crucible of early modern empires. The era in question did not witness a single scientific revolution nor was Europe the only site of dramatic investigative and curative transformation. Early modern empires produced a proliferation of ways of knowing, suffering, diagnosing, and healing.[74]

In the middle chapters of this book, I attempt to rediscover colonial cultures of natural inquiry on their own terms – to identify their various preoccupations, sort out their priorities, and watch as some of their protagonists fashioned epistemic tools and representational conventions of their own. Colonial encounters unsettled older epistemologies, yes, but they rarely produced a stable consensus around new ones. When it came to the investigation of nature generally and to the explanation and treatment of disease in particular, authority was up for grabs. While it was certainly true that the climatic, environmental, and epidemiological particularities of the colonial world propelled the consolidation of cultural and racial typologies used to legitimize Iberian imperial expansion and colonial rule,[75] it was also true that rhetorics of strict cultural conformity

---

[rancisco]. Guerra, "Aleixo de Abreu (1568–1630), Author of the earliest book on Tropical Medicine describing Amoebiasis, Malaria, Typhoid Fever, Scurvy, Yellow Fever, Dracontiasis, Trichuriasis and Tungiasis in 1623," *The Journal of Tropical Medicine and Hygiene* 71 (1968): 55–69.

72 Bruno Latour, *We Have Never Been Modern* (Cambridge, MA: Harvard University Press, 1993); Daston, "The Nature of Nature in Early Modern Europe"; Ralph Bauer, "A New World of Secrets: Occult Philosophy and Local Knowledge in the Sixteenth-Century Atlantic," in *Science and Empire in the Atlantic World*, eds. James Delbourgo and Nicholas Dew (New York: Routledge, 2008), 99–126.

73 A point variously illustrated by Barbara E. Mundy, *The Mapping of New Spain: Indigenous Cartography and the Maps of the Relaciones Geográficas* (Chicago, IL: University of Chicago Press, 1996); and Crawford, *Andean Wonder Drug*.

74 A point illustrated most recently for the Caribbean by Pablo F. Gómez, *The Experiential Caribbean: Creating Knowledge and Healing in the Early Modern Atlantic* (Chapel Hill, NC: University of North Carolina Press, 2017).

75 Jorge Cañizares-Esguerra, *Nature, Empire, and Nation: Explorations of the History of Science in the Iberian World* (Stanford, CA: Stanford University Press, 2006), chapter 4; Marcy Norton, *Sacred Gifts, Profane Pleasures: A History of Tobacco and Chocolate in the Atlantic World* (Ithaca, NY: Cornell University Press, 2008); Rebecca Earle, *The*

masked quotidian colonial realities that fostered invention and collaboration.[76] Familiar, text-centered approaches to the investigation of nature and Hippocratic-Galenic perspectives on the cause treatment of disease jostled for adherents alongside a raft of unfamiliar but appealing alternatives. Portuguese governors in Goa patronized Hindu temples; Jesuit missionaries in Brazil enacted the shamanic rituals of their native Tupi opponents.[77] Everywhere, claims about nature and disease that were committed to paper were often partial and probabilistic rather than total and certain.[78] Knowledge about nature and disease was never self-evident or of obvious value to metropolitan officials. Only deliberate strategies of self-fashioning and presentation could render knowledge produced in Goa or along the coast of Brazil intelligible, credible, and valuable to readers an ocean away.[79] And that act of translation was laborious, uncertain, even dangerous.

Chapters 3 to 5 use the work of Garcia de Orta to examine the networks and preoccupations that shaped medicine and natural history in the cosmopolitan colony of Portuguese Goa. In Goa, the heart of Portugal's trading empire in Asia, commerce propelled epistemic innovation, but it also produced intractable problems of knowledge that perpetuated the bookish learning of old. Orta's *Colóquios dos simples e drogas e coisas medicinais da Índia* exemplifies the kind of inquiry enabled by Portuguese empire in Asia. Rather than a masterful triumph

Body of the Conquistador: Food, Race and the Colonial Experience in Spanish America, 1492–1700 (New York: Cambridge University Press, 2012).

[76] A similar point has been made by Stuart Schwartz, *All Can Be Saved: Religious Tolerance and Salvation in the Iberian Atlantic World* (New Haven, CT: Yale University Press, 2008).

[77] Similar episodes from the Portuguese Atlantic appear in James H. Sweet, *Domingos Álvares: African Healing and the Intellectual History of the Atlantic World* (Chapel Hill, NC: University of North Carolina Press, 2011); Cécile Fromont, *The Art of Conversion: Christian Visual Culture in the Kingdom of Kongo* (Chapel Hill, NC: University of North Carolina Press, 2014).

[78] John V. Pickstone, "Working Knowledges before and after circa 1800: Practices and Disciplines in the History of Science, Technology, and Medicine," *Isis* 98 (2007): 489–516; Serge Gruzinski, *The Mestizo Mind: The Intellectual Dynamics of Colonization and Globalization*, trans. Deke Dusinberre (New York: Routledge, 2002).

[79] James A. Secord, "Knowledge in Transit," *Isis* 95 (2004): 654–672; Kapil Raj, *Relocating Modern Science: Circulation and the Construction of Knowledge in South Asia and Europe, 1650–1900* (New York: Palgrave Macmillan, 2007); Lissa Roberts, "Situating Science in Global History: Local Exchanges and Networks of Circulation," *Itinerario* 33 (2009): 9–30.

of Renaissance empiricism or a vessel in which unmediated South Asian therapeutic knowledge was passed off as Orta's own,[80] I contend that the dynamic intra-Asian exchanges that predated Portuguese arrival also shaped colonial natural inquiry. The *Colóquios* embodied the connected histories[81] of Renaissance naturalists in Italy, Portuguese apothecaries in Cochin and Malacca, and Hindus and Muslims, women and men, ayurveda and unani specialists, Javanese midwives, and the Konkani-speaking servants who inhabited Goa, passed through the Orta household, and populated Orta's book. To assemble the *Colóquios*, I argue, Orta collected people.[82] The credibility of the former hinged on the diversity of the latter. And that made getting those claims into print especially tricky in the only city outside of metropolitan Portugal to be home to a standing tribunal of the Inquisition.

Chapters 6–8 focus on Brazil and the Atlantic world. They explore the overlapping practices of medicine and natural history as they took shape in the midst of missionary incursions, epidemic disease, plantation agriculture, and chattel slavery. Here the time span is longer and the cast of characters is larger. Beginning in 1549, I argue, contests between Jesuit missionaries and native Tupi shamans (*pajés*) over the explanation and treatment of disease helped pattern subsequent colonial approaches to both medicine and the study of nature. Contrary to most other work on the subject, the upshot was not, I contend, a committed empiricism among seamlessly interconnected Jesuit missions but a learned ignorance of colonial nature, sustained by an epistolary network of factious Company men.[83] At the turn of the

---

[80] Prominent interpretations to this effect include, respectively, Teresa Nobre de Carvalho, *Os desafios de Garcia de Orta. Colóqios dos Simples e Drogas da Índia* (Lisbon: Esfera do Caos, 2015); and Grove, *Green Imperialism*. For alternative formulations see the essays in Palmira Fontes da Costa, ed., *Medicine, Trade and Empire: Garcia de Orta's Colloquios on the Simples and Drugs of India (1563) in Context* (Burlington, VT: Ashgate, 2015); and in António Manuel Lopes Andrade, Carlos de Miguel Mora, and João Manuel Nunes Torrão, eds., *Humanismo e Ciência: Antiguidade e Renascimento* (Coimbra: The University of Aveiro and the University of Coimbra Press, 2015).

[81] The formulation has been worked out by Sanjay Subrahmanyam, *Explorations in Connected History: From the Tagus to the Ganges* (New York: Oxford University Press, 2005).

[82] James Delbourgo, "Listing People," *Isis* 103 (2012): 735–742.

[83] Among the interlocutors here are Rodrigues, *Anchieta e a Medicina*; Harris, "Long-distance Corporations"; Harris, "Jesuit Scientific Activity"; Asúa, "Los jesuítas"; and Andrés I. Prieto, *Missionary Scientists: Jesuit Science in Spanish South America, 1570–1810* (Nashville, TN: Vanderbilt University Press, 2011).

seventeenth century, the physician Aleixo de Abreu and the sugar planter Ambrósio Brandão penned competing visions of the cause and treatment of fevers in the Portuguese Atlantic. They debated the prospect of an epidemiologically coherent Atlantic world, not an intertropical one. Brandão's work in particular dramatically expanded the catalog of colonial nature and suggests that the longstanding portrait of Brazilian planters as willfully disengaged from contemporary intellectual life is in need of revision. The example of Brandão shows how and why sugar planters might become planter-naturalists.

The expertise that enabled and sustained Portugal's global empire was not purveyed by benighted physicians and naturalists from metropolitan Portugal. That expertise was instead created by – and remained located within – colonial cultures of inquiry in both Asia and the Atlantic.

ON METHOD AND TERMINOLOGY

In the chapters that follow, I identify and try to make sense of important differences between the Asian and Atlantic theatres of Portuguese colonization. But this is not an attempt at systematic comparison. I have not assembled what I would consider commensurate bodies of archival evidence. Rather, I have emphasized local and regional particularities as part of an effort to historicize and reinterpret some of the best-known books and manuscripts on nature and disease from the sixteenth and seventeenth century Lusophone world, and to bring to light some of the least-known but potentially most illuminating ones.

To investigate these diverse histories of early modern natural inquiry, I draw on scholarly literatures ranging from the history of the book to colonialism and historical epidemiology. I have drawn on print media, maps, and manuscripts. Early modern printed books have proven useful not only for their content but also as objects whose physical attributes (size, organization, illustration) provide clues to the meanings they were meant to carry.

When referring to the Jesuits, I use the archaic "Company of Jesus" rather than the current "Society of Jesus." This is not only how early modern Jesuits themselves referred to the Catholic missionary order of which they were a part, but it also connotes the centralized organization, bureaucratic character, clear stratification, and direct lines of communication taken to characterize the order and which are central to modern studies of its epistemic practices. These are characteristics that I variously call into question.

My concern for the perspectives of the people of the past has led me to eschew retrospective diagnosis.[84] Where appropriate, the notes reference important findings in ongoing debates over the possible identity of the diseases in question. But early modern diagnostic categories were often more capacious than familiar post-germ-theory terminology would suggest. For the period in question, the same language could be applied to diseases now understood as entirely different. My interest is in the contests for the definition of those categories. So, with few exceptions, as overlapping stories of disease and natural history unfold, I have preferred terms such as 'fever,' 'dysentery,' and 'pox' to the anachronistic use of modern diagnostic categories like 'malaria,' 'cholera,' 'smallpox,' and 'measles' – even as I acknowledge that these, too, have histories that predate modern nosology, and even though it may be argued that in some cases symptoms described in contemporary sources were pathognomonic. Finally, wherever possible, I have used the term 'naturalist' to refer to anyone engaged in a process that I refer to as 'natural inquiry.' Though they, too, are somewhat anachronistic, I have preferred these to the distinctly unsuitable 'scientist' and 'science.'[85]

---

[84] On handling this contentious issue, I have relied on Andrew Cunningham, "Identifying Disease in the Past: Cutting the Gordian Knot," *Asclepio* 54 (2002): 13–34; Jon Arrizabalaga, "Problematizing Retrospective Diagnosis in the History of Disease," *Asclepio* 54 (2002): 51–70; Piers Mitchell, "Retrospective Diagnosis and the Use of Historical Texts for Investigating Disease in the Past," *Journal of International Palaeopathology* 1 (2011): 81–88; and Bruno Latour, "On the Partial Existence of Existing *and* Nonexisting Objects" in *Biographies of Scientific Objects*, ed. Lorraine Daston (Chicago, IL: University of Chicago Press, 2000), 247–269. Characteristic of an alternative approach would be J. R. McNeill, *Mosquito Empires: Ecology and War in the Greater Caribbean, 1620–1914* (New York: Cambridge University Press, 2010).

[85] Brian W. Ogilvie, *The Science of Describing: Natural History in Renaissance Europe* (Chicago, IL: University of Chicago Press, 2006), takes a more a nuanced approach to the term. I follow Daston and Park, *Wonders*, in this more general usage. For a consideration of similar linguistic tangles, see Andrew Cunningham, "Getting the Game Right: Some Plain Words on the Identity and Invention of Science," *Studies in History and Philosophy of Science Part A* 19 (1988): 365–389.

PART I

THE COAST OF AFRICA, 1450–1550

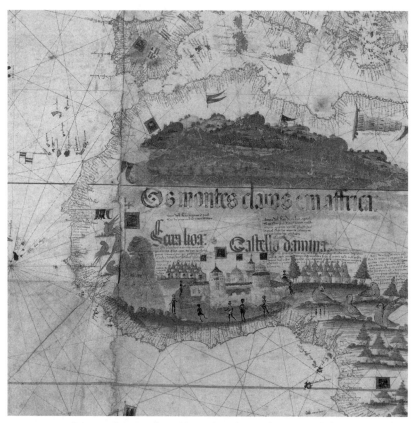

FIGURE 2.1 Image of a New World. Rather than a barren and desiccated land, the world beyond the Senegal was home to brightly colored creatures, like these green (left) and grey (right) parrots. It was also home to thriving trade routes. And it was in an attempt to strengthen their involvement in regional commerce that the Portuguese built the São Jorge da Mina Castle in 1482. Detail of West Africa from the Cantino Atlas.

© Getty Images.

2

Dead Reckonings

When, therefore, a physician comes to a district previously unknown to him, he should consider its situation and its aspect to the winds ... The nature of the water supply must be considered ... Then think of the soil ... Lastly consider the life of the inhabitants themselves.

Unknown author of *Airs, Waters, Places*[1]

BEYOND THE SENEGAL

On the island of Principe, deep in the Gulf of Guinea, Duarte Pacheco Pereira lay prostrate and ill beneath the equatorial sun. It was 1488. This was not the first time that Pereira had sailed to the Gulf of Guinea, though he might have wondered whether it would be his last.[2] A knight of the royal household and servant to D. João II of Portugal, he had come on this occasion as the commander of a supply vessel bound for the São Jorge da Mina castle. That Gold Coast redoubt was Portugal's first permanent mainland trading post south of the Senegal River. The castle – later known to sailors of all nations as "El Mina" – would become a notorious slave port from which African captives were forced across the Atlantic. For men like Pereira, the trade in slaves was but one element in an emergent commercial nexus that linked North African manufactories, and European metal foundries to sub-Saharan weavers, dyers, and smiths.

---

[1] G. E. R. Lloyd, ed., *Hippocratic Writings* (New York: Penguin 1983), 148.

[2] João de Barros, *Da Ásia de João de Barros e de Diogo de Couto*, New ed. (Lisbon: Regia Officina Typografica, 1777–1778), "Decada Primeira," pt. 1, bk. 3, ch. 4: 191.

The so-called Guinea route (carreira da Guiné) that linked Lisbon to the São Jorge da Mina castle was a lucrative but risky affair. Pereira and his crew hoped to return to Lisbon with not only slaves but a cargo of gold and ivory, and perhaps malagueta pepper, tamarind, senna,

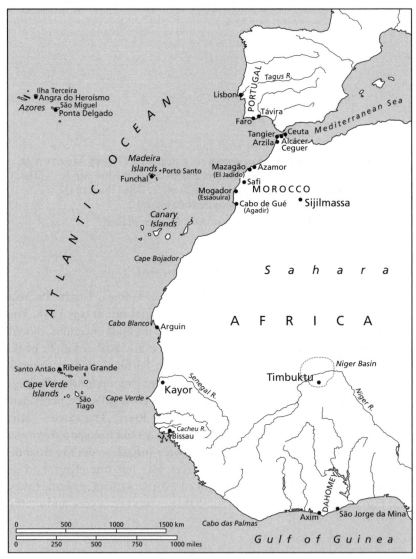

MAP 2.1 Portuguese Settlements and Principal Ports of Trade in West Africa and the Atlantic Islands. Adapted by David Cox from Bethencourt and Curto, eds., *Portuguese Oceanic Expansion*, xvii.

spikenard, and kola nuts as well.[3] But now, too weak to command his ship and too ill to move, Pereira had been left on the diminutive island of Principe to convalesce or die. All along the Guinea Coast, death from fever and other afflictions had become a common experience for seafarers from western Christendom.

It is a familiar image. Citing a raft of febrile diseases, one historian of the slave trade has described West Africa as "one of the most formidable disease environments in the world."[4] Yet for Pereira, and for many other seafarers in the early decades of Atlantic sailing, the Gulf of Guinea was not a place of perilous fevers. It was one of unparalleled health and Edenic verdure. Between about 1450 and 1500, a shift in perception would unfold in which a natural world once associated with human health and physical vitality came increasingly to be associated instead with debilitating illness and death. The transformation was neither immediate nor total. But by the closing decades of the fifteenth century both views had become clearly discernible. Each coexisted in tension with the other.

Alvise da Cadamosto, the famed Venetian merchant-traveler, began the first of two well-known voyages to that world – and inaugurated the era of sub-Saharan maritime trade that nearly killed Pereira – when on March 22, 1455, he set sail from Lagos in southern Portugal, ultimately arriving at the Wolof state of Kayor on the bank of the Senegal River.[5] In less than a fortnight, he had drawn within sight of the African coast just north of Cabo Blanco, where the vast Sahara juts timidly into the Atlantic, forming a long, narrow peninsula.[6] The scene made a strong impression on the young merchant, who described the "very great desert"

---

[3] Toby Green, *The Rise of the Trans-Atlantic Slave Trade in Western Africa, 1300–1589* (New York: Cambridge University Press, 2011); John Vogt, *Portuguese Rule on the Gold Coast, 1469–1682* (Athens, GA: University of Georgia Press, 1979); and George E. Brooks, "Kola Trade and State-Building: Upper Guinea Coast and Senegambia, 15th–17th Centuries" (Working Paper 38, African Studies Center, Boston University, 1980).

[4] Kenneth F. Kiple, *The Caribbean Slave: A Biological History* (New York: Cambridge University Press, 1984), 13, 20–22.

[5] Alvise Cadamosto [Alvise da Cà da Mosto], "The Voyages of Alvise Cadamosto and Pero de Sintra," in *The Voyages of Cadamosto and Other Documents on Western Africa in the Second Half of the Fifteenth Century*, trans. G. E. R. Crone (London: Hakluyt Society, 1937 [1507]). Note that in the text, I use the popularized spelling of his name ("Cadamosto") following Crone, the editor of the edition in which the translated version of the account appears.

[6] Cadamosto, "Voyages," 14–15.

in the frankest of terms: it was "everywhere sandy, white, arid, and all equally low-lying."[7] The peninsula itself was "without signs of grass or trees whatsoever" – part of a denuded, featureless landscape that stretched southward for what Cadamosto reckoned to be some three hundred and eighty miles.

It was that very monotony – an arid, empty, and lifeless coast – that made the sight of the Senegal River so spectacular. The Senegal marked the southern limit of the Sahara, where the expansive desert met the grasslands of the Sahel and where well-watered riverbanks produced dense, verdant foliage. The natural abundance of those banks appeared so suddenly – and stood in such marked contrast with the desert to the north – that Cadamosto could not but be struck by it. His description of the peoples on either side of the Senegal is at once stunning and revealing:

This river separates the Blacks from the brown people called the Azanaghi, and also the dry and arid land, that is, the above mentioned desert, from the fertile country of the Blacks. ... It appears to me a very marvelous thing that beyond the river all men are very black, tall and big, their bodies well formed; and the whole country green, full of trees, and fertile; while on [the north] side the men are brownish, ... lean, ill-nourished, and small in stature; the country ... [is] arid.[8]

There is a strongly diagnostic quality to this passage: beyond the Senegal, nature is abundant and the people there are healthy.

Cadamosto was not alone in this opinion. Before 1455 and for decades to come, authors of the best-known accounts of the early West African voyages were unanimous in their view that a land of health and vitality lay beyond the gentle currents of the Senegal River. One of the most lurid accounts of the region came from the pen of a man who, unlike Cadamosto, had never actually been there. Gomes Eanes de Zurara, the Crown-appointed historian of Portugal and keeper of the royal archive, wrote the closing chapter of his *Chronica do descobrimento e conquista de Guiné* in about 1453. Most of his text was given over to stories he had collected of Portuguese comings and goings in the Atlantic. But even Zurara, more often concerned with detailing Portuguese exploits than puzzling through the novelty of either human societies or the natural world, could not stop himself from dwelling on the reported abundance of the Senegal. He praised the "delicious" fruit, the tall green trees and, above all, "the pleasant scent of the air" which, like the freshwater flooding into the ocean from the Senegal itself, lingered along the

---

[7] Cadamosto, "Voyages," 16.   [8] Cadamosto, "Voyages," 27–28.

shoreline, where Portuguese mariners smelled and drank of the area's strange and exquisite nature.[9]

Pereira would offer similar praise. In 1506, years after his ill-fated voyage to the Mina castle and in response to inquiries from Manuel I about the geography of the terraqeous globe, Pereira produced the *Esmeraldo de situ orbis*. For Pereira – as for Zurara and Cadamosto before him – the Senegal River stood out. It was a distinguishing feature of the overseas world and Pereira was rather specific about its location and meaning: for Pereira, the Senegal marked the northern edge of "western Lower Ethiopia," an ill-defined but immense region that stretched southward all the way to the Cape of Good Hope. "In Ethiopia," Pereira wrote confidently, "no one dies of pestilence." It was hardly a revelation. The health of "Ethiopia" was an established fact or, as Pereira put it, "certain and known."[10]

Yet in 1506 Pereira's confidence was already the relic of an earlier age. A half-century of travel, trade, and slaving along the West African coast had given rise to competing and even contradictory interpretations of the region. The *Esmeraldo* registered that transformation. No matter how confidently Pereira asserted the health of the world beyond the Senegal, he was forced to double back on his own opinion. When he averred in no uncertain terms that "in Ethiopia no one dies of pestilence," there was already so much evidence to the contrary that in the course of the same passage he was compelled to concede that, in fact, the opposite also seemed to be true: at least some parts of the coast past the Senegal, he wrote, were "unhealthy," for they provoked "fevers."[11] Around Cabo das Palmas and near the fabled mines that

[9] Gomes Eanes de Zurara, *Chronica do descobrimento e conquista de Guiné* (Paris: J. P. Aillaud, 1841), 277–278. He got much of his information from João Fernandes, who traveled overland throughout the Sahara for seven months in 1445 and visited many of the main markets there. See Zurara, *Chronica*, ch. 77: 364–370. On difficulties with the precise dating of this manuscript, see P. E. H. Hair, "The Early Sources on Guinea," *History in Africa* 21 (1994): 87–126.

[10] Duarte Pacheco Pereira, *Esmeraldo de situ orbis*, ed. Augusto Epiphanio da Silva Dias (Lisbon: Typographia Universal, 1905 [ca. 1506]), 79–80. Unfortunately, the *Esmeraldo* only survives in the form of two copies from the eighteenth century, both of which are incomplete; see Francisco Contente Domingues, "Science and Technology in Portuguese Navigation: The Idea of Experience in the Sixteenth Century," in *Portuguese Oceanic Expansion, 1400–1800*, eds. Francisco Bethencourt and Diogo Ramada Curto (New York: Cambridge University Press, 2007), 464.

[11] Pereira, *Esmeraldo*, bk. 1, ch. 27: 82, and bk. 2, ch. 1: 102.

lent the Gold Coast its alluring sobriquet, Pereira dryly noted that "white men die here."[12]

The ambiguity marked earlier accounts too. Amid passages of West African verdure and good health, Zurara summarily noted an encounter with a would-be African captive found sick and near death on the same stretch of coast.[13] On Cadamosto's second West African voyage in 1456, illnesses suffered on shore became standards of shipboard conversation and inspired ad hoc strategies for staying well. As often as not, they failed to do the trick. On route to negotiate terms of trade with the Mande traders of the Gambia River, Cadamosto and his party refused to eat the local dates for "fear of dysentery." Some of the men became sick anyway, suffering "from a high fever [that was] sharp and continuous." Cadamosto and his crew "left suddenly" in order "to proceed to the mouth of the river," whence they made a fast retreat back out to sea.[14] It was a striking move in an age when the illnesses that accompanied shipboard life itself had become increasingly apparent.[15] The region was plainly becoming difficult to assess.

As reports of disease from crewmen, shipmasters, and merchants accumulated, fever and dysentery became known perils of putting ashore. In 1481, those concerns made even the building of the São Jorge da Mina castle a contentious proposition. When the newly crowned king, João II, called together a meeting of his councilors to advise on the project, he got what one observer described as a collection of "very contrary opinions."[16] Some thought the project should go ahead; others plainly did not. Opinions divided over what the chronicler Rui de Pina described as the "ill effects of the land."[17] Commercial ambitions trumped epidemiological concerns and the fort was built anyway.

---

[12] Pereira, *Esmeraldo*, bk. 2, ch. 5: 114–115. On the constitution of ethnic identities based on culture and color, see Herman Bennet, "'Sons of Adam': Tet, Context, and the Early Modern African Subject," *Representations* 92 (2005): 16–41. I suggest that this is an example of the kind of schizophrenia that is in other ways characteristic of the *Esmeraldo* according to Luís Filipe Barreto, *Descobrimentos e renascimento: Formas de ser e pensar nos séculos XV e XVI* (Lisbon: Imprensa Nacional-Casa da Moeda, 1983).

[13] Zurara, *Chronica*, 194.   [14] Cadamosto, "Voyages," 69.

[15] Francisco Contente Domingues and Inácio Guerreiro, *A vida a bordo na carreira da Índia (século XVI)*, separata of the *Revista da Universidade de Coimbra* (Lisbon: Instituto de Investigação Científica Tropical), 1988.

[16] *MMA*, ser. 1, vol. 1, doc. 3: 8.

[17] Rui de Pina, "Chronica d'Elrey D. João II," in *Crónicas de Rui de Pina*, ed. M. Lopes de Almeida (Porto: Lello and Irmão Editores, 1977), 894, which must have been the source used by Barros when he repeated the story in *Da Ásia*, "Decada Primeira," pt. 1, bk. 3, ch. 8: 223. See P. E. H. Hair, *The Founding of the Castelo de São Jorge da Mina: An Analysis of the Sources* (Madison, WI: African Studies Program and the University of Wisconsin Press, 1994), 114–115.

Accounts of ill-health from Portuguese outposts on the African coast soon became a regular part of the epistolary traffic of the Portuguese Atlantic – an ebb and flow of administrative correspondence so dense that Portuguese scattered among the trading posts of coastal West Africa occasionally complained of the need for more paper and ink.[18] Among these was a lengthy 1513 missive from Francisco de Góis, governor of the Mina castle. A short note scrawled overleaf by a Crown official neatly summed up the letter's contents: whoever was to serve the king at the Mina castle would need to be "old in wisdom but young in body" (*velho na sabedoria e moço*) (Figure 2.2).[19]

In 1539, partly in response to letters like that, João de Barros finally penned a definitive rejection of the Edenic vision.[20] Like Zurara earlier, Barros was the Crown-appointed keeper of the royal archive. Unlike Zurara, Barros had spent time at the São Jorge da Mina castle – and he was a good deal more poetic with the pen.[21] Experience in a region that Barros, like Pereira, termed "Ethiopia," led him to suggest that "God . . . has placed [here] a striking angel with a flaming sword of deadly fevers" that prevented his countrymen "from penetrating into the interior [and on] to the springs of this garden."[22] A natural world once associated with human health and physical vitality had come instead to be associated with debilitating fever and death.

---

[18] As can be traced through several exchanges: ANTT, CC, pt. 1, mç. 38, n. 3; ANTT, CC, pt. 1, mç. 50, n. 14; ANTT, CC, pt. 2, mç. 16, n. 97; ANTT, CC, pt. 2, mç. 17, n. 81; ANTT, CC, pt. 2, mç. 18, n. 85; ANTT, CC, pt. 2, mç. 18, n. 101; ANTT, CC, pt. 2, mç. 60, n. 89.

[19] ANTT, CC, pt. 1, mç. 13, n. 48.

[20] I have borrowed the notion of the "Edenic" as central to Portuguese endeavors from Sérgio Buarque de Holanda, *Visão do paraiso: Os motivos edenicos no descobrimento e colonização do Brasil*, 2nd ed. (São Paulo: Companhia Editora Nacional, 1969).

[21] Despite many claims, a careful reading does not make clear in what capacity Barros spent his time at São Jorge. For a careful discussion of Barros's activities as they relate to the castle see Hair, *Founding*, 114–15.

[22] Barros, *Da Ásia*, "Decada Primeira," pt. 1, bk. 3, ch. 12: 266. See also Barros, *Da Ásia*, "Decada Primeira," pt. 1, bk. 3, ch. 8: 223. Barros's comments were not published until 1552 but the words had been penned no later than 1539. Barros's *Da Ásia* was published along with subsequent volumes by Diogo do Couto and António Bocarro under the better-known title of *Decadas da Ásia*. The publication of these was intermittent and irregular. Although the first volume of *Da Ásia* was printed in 1552 and the second in 1553, the third volume was not printed until 1563 and the fourth only posthumously in 1613 or 1615. Still useful as a survey of Portuguese reportage is C. R. Boxer, *Three Historians of Portuguese Asia: Barros, Couto and Bocarro* (Macau: Imprensa Nacional, 1948), and especially 7–8.

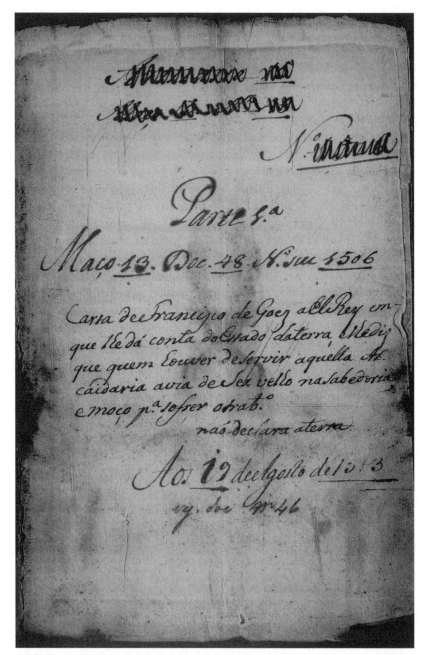

FIGURE 2.2 Symptoms of the Problem. Francisco de Góis wrote of ill-health in this letter, dated August 19, 1513, from the São Jorge da Mina Castle. "Carta de Francisco de Góis [Goes] dando conhecimento ao rei do estado da terra." ANTT-CC, Parte I, mç.13, n. 48, f. 4v.
Courtesy of the Arquivo Nacional da Torre do Tombo.

POINTS OF ORIENTATION

After the opening decades of the sixteenth century, European perceptions of the disease environment of West Africa would never again be the same. For the practice of medicine in Portugal's colonies, the repercussions would be profound and far-reaching. Encounters with the disease environment beyond the Senegal inspired an abiding preoccupation with the causes and treatment of fever. Febrifuges became central to cross-cultural medical interaction. But these shifts were not immediate and they took shape in response to particular interpretive challenges posed by both the peculiarities of the coastal disease environment,[23] and by a tangle of European myth and miscomprehension surrounding the lands immediately below the Sahara. Even though the combination of verdure and fever encountered beyond the Senegal would become emblematic of the entire intertropical world, much of the interpretive and explanatory confusion inaugurated by those encounters was not generalizable at all.

Africa beyond the Senegal was laden with medical meaning long before Iberian shiphands ever hoisted sail in the Atlantic. Much like the sailors who would arrive to the Caribbean believing they had reached the islands of Asia, those Portuguese who sailed beyond the Senegal did so with a distinct set of expectations about the world they had entered. Their vision of the Africa that lay beyond the Senegal was one that combined Ptolemaic geography with a natural world drawn from the pages of Pliny's *Natural History* – and one that merged the Christian legend of Prester John with the Biblical account of an earthly paradise.

The world beyond the Senegal was one possessed of natural wonders and fanciful creatures – where lifesaving waters poured from a hidden spring and where the gentle currents of a mighty river gave life to a profusion of exotic plants and animals. Although the precise inventory of texts that inspired Iberian imaginings of the region is more or less well known, its medical implications are not. Claims about the geography and

---

[23] The most pervasive febrile killers were (and remain) malaria and yellow fever. On the characteristics of the disease environment and the nature of acquired resistance, see James L. A. Webb Jr., *Humanity's Burden: A Global History of Malaria* (New York: Cambridge University Press, 2009), 18–41; and Kenneth F. Kiple, *The Caribbean Slave: A Biological History* (New York: Cambridge University Press, 1984), chapters 1–3. Zurara, *Chronica*, details the trade-and-raid pattern of early Portuguese engagement in the region, which would have complicated any distinction between diseases of the ship and the shore. On Portuguese shipboard illness during the sixteenth and seventeenth centuries see Domingues and Guerreiro, *A vida a bordo*.

environment of the region implied epidemiological claims as well. The lands and waters believed to characterize the West African littoral also endowed it with particular curative significance. By the middle of the fourteenth century, that significance had come to suffuse not only the literary, devotional, and material culture of the Aviz court,[24] but it was understood equally well by Atlantic-bound mariners too. Aboard ship in the Atlantic, no less than at court in Lisbon, West Africa was commonly understood to be a land of verdure, abundance, and health, and it was precisely that vision that would make it a source of both epidemiological confusion and therapeutic tinkering.

Ptolemy, following Aristotle, had described the globe as a giant sphere whose habitable northern and southern hemispheres (the antipodes) were divided by an immense, sun-scorched, and generally lifeless torrid zone. The details of this geography – the precise number of terrestrial zones and whether or not the driest desert reaches were as impassible as they were rumoured to be, for example – were long a matter of debate among Scholastic philosophers.[25] But according to Ptolemy, somewhere below the known trading networks of North Africa – and beyond the burnt, desiccated, and lifeless torrid zone – lay a vast, ill-defined region he referred to as "Ethiopia," a land traversed by the extensive, meandering sinews of the Nile. For fifteenth-century seafarers, this geography loomed large. Cadamosto had initially feared sailing southward precisely because it would bring him to the torrid zone – concerns that were echoed among the nobility in Lisbon who, for that very reason, opposed the Atlantic voyages altogether.[26] When Cadamosto spoke of the "Blacks of Lower Ethiopia," and when Pereira referred to the Senegal as a landmark on the fringes of "western Lower Ethiopia," they were using the toponymy of Ptolemaic geography.[27]

[24] I have explored these aspects in more depth in Hugh Cagle, "Beyond the Senegal: Inventing the Tropics in the Late Middle Ages," *Journal of Medieval Iberian Studies* 7 (2015): 197-217.

[25] Alessandro Scafi, *Mapping Paradise: A History of Heaven on Earth* (Chicago, IL: University of Chicago Press, 2006); Seymour Phillips, "The Outer World of the European Middle Ages," in *Implicit Understandings: Observing Reporting and Reflecting on the Encounters between Europeans and Other Peoples in the Early Modern Era*, ed. Stuart B. Schwartz (New York: Cambridge University Press, 1994), 23-63. See Also J. H. Parry, *The Discovery of the Sea* (Berkeley, CA: University of California Press, 1981), 53-57, 60. For Iberian debates, see Wey Gómez, *Tropics of Empire*.

[26] Cadamosto, "Voyages," 5-6; Wey Gómez, *Tropics of Empire*, 304.

[27] Cadamosto, "Voyages," 1; Pereira, *Esmeraldo*, bk. 1, ch. 27: 79-80. See also Barros, *Da Ásia*, "Decada Primeira," pt. 1, bk. 3, ch. 12: 265-266.

While Ptolemy had described in broad outlines the lay of the southerly lands for fifteenth-century Iberian travelers, Pliny's *Natural History* told in encyclopaedic fashion the kinds of creatures they should expect to find there.[28] And for Pliny no less than for Ptolemy, the Nile was a principal fluvial landmark. The *Natural History* described the strange and even terrifying animals nurtured by its waters, and of the exotic trees and other plants that grew along its banks – flora and fauna that were not to be found anywhere else in the world.[29]

As on the page, so too at sea: these texts turned the Nile into an indispensable point of orientation. Suspicion ran high that one of the many branches rumoured to extend from that mythical, mysterious river debouched into the Atlantic. The Senegal River seemed the obvious candidate. And indeed, Zurara and Pereira alike, citing Pliny, readily elaborated on the fantastical flora and fauna they fully expected the Portuguese to find further up the Senegal as a result of its upriver confluence with the rich and transformative waters of the Nile.[30] Such associations played themselves out in cartographic fits: streams flowed and pooled ambiguously across contemporary maps, as master cartographers, journeymen, and apprentices variously grappled with competing and contradictory reports from texts and travelers (Figure 2.3).[31]

The immense but uncertain African landscape charted by Ptolemy, together with Pliny's account of the natural world of the Nile, accommodated in turn the most fanciful details of the famous Prester John legend and its association with the biblical earthly paradise. If by the seventh century, as Paul Freedman has noted, biblical and classical traditions were often joined to portray the kingdom of Prester John and the earthly

[28] Trevor Murphy, *Pliny the Elder's Natural History: The Empire in the Encyclopedia* (New York: Oxford University Press, 2004).

[29] Although it stretches to thirty-seven books and references to the Nile are spread throughout, see especially Pliny the Elder, *The Natural History of Pliny*, 6 vols., trans. John Bostock and H. T. Riley (London: George Bell and Sons, 1855–1857), vol. 1, bk. 5, ch. 10; vol. 2, bk. 6 ch. 35, bk. 8, chs. 32 and 37–39, and bk. 9, ch. 84; and vol. 3, bk. 13, ch. 28.

[30] Zurara, *Chronica*, ch. 60: 277–287, ch. 61: 289, and ch. 62: 296–301; Pereira, *Esmeraldo*, bk. 1, ch. 37: 79–80.

[31] Men like Diogo Gomes, for example, who accompanied Cadamosto up the Gambia river and who (very late in life) was interviewed by the Bohemian cosmographer Martin Behaim, then in the employ of Afonso V. Russell, *Prince Henry*, 374, n. 23; Armando Cortesão, *Cartografia e cartógrafos Portugueses dos séculos XVI e XVII* (Lisbon: Imprensa Nacional, 1935), 344–349.

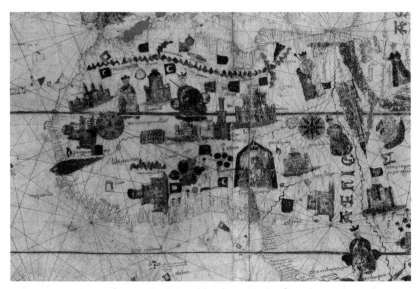

FIGURE 2.3   River of Deceit. In maps like this one, the fluvial connection between the Senegal and the Nile is made plain. Mistaken for a mythical West African branch of the Nile, the verdure and natural abundance of the Senegal seemed to promise health. Yet mariners confronted fevers and death. Detail from the *Carta de Juan de la Cosa*. MNM 00257.
Courtesy of the Museu Naval, Madrid.

paradise in the East, the same was true, according to Alessandro Scafi, of intertropical Africa beginning in the early fifteenth century.[32]

This placement, too, was understood equally well by members of the Aviz court and ocean-bound sailors – a consequence of the efforts of the preeminent propagandist of the early Atlantic. Once referred to as "Henry, the Navigator," the Portuguese Infante D. Henrique, Duke of Viseu, never actually sailed into the Atlantic himself. But his vigorous and calculating promotion of the West African voyages helped spread the notion of a verdant, salubrious, and populous sub-Saharan world among the merchants, pilots, and shiphands who put to sea.

The Venetian Cadamosto was among them. Were it not for a chance encounter with the prince in August of 1454, Cadamosto would not have dared to board a ship for the Guinea Coast. Such a voyage would have

---

[32] Both were part of the process by which Greco-Roman learning was assimilated to Christian theology as discussed in Paul Freedman, *Out of the East: Spices and the Medieval Imagination* (New Haven, CT: Yale University Press, 2008), especially 93. Scafi, *Mapping Paradise*, 218–230.

meant skirting the notorious Cape Bojador, the treacherous stretch of land that lay opposite the Canary Island of Fuerteventura and which, as far as Cadamosto knew, "had never before been sailed." The prince feted merchants like Cadamosto with tales of geographical conquest (Bojador had been safely rounded years earlier, in 1434, by one of D. Henrique's squires, Gil Eanes), of bustling ports, and of lucrative trade.[33]

The prince's vision of the world that lay beyond the Senegal was based on his reading of the late-fourteenth-century *Libro del conosçimiento de todos los reinos*,[34] a book that chronicled the fictional journey of its author, an anonymous Spanish Franciscan, across the Maghreb and the Sahara. The further its author traveled from western Christendom, the longer and more nuanced his descriptions became. Cursory accounts of Tripoli, Tunis, and Fez gave way to extensive and detailed passages about Sijilmasa and Timbuktu, and the wealth of the Saharan markets.[35]

The *Libro* itself was but an elaboration of a much older and much more widely known account of the same region – one apparently penned by a Jewish traveler in Central Asia in the middle of the twelfth century. It told of a realm possessed of temperate winds, revivifying waters, thick forests, and such wondrous creatures as elephants, gryphons, and red and white lions. Signally, the letter also told of the four rivers that were believed to flow from the earthly paradise itself: the Geon, Phison Tigris, and Euphrates. The gentle currents of not one but two of these crossed the kingdom of a devout Christian ruler who would soon be known as Prester John. In the Prester's kingdom, the Phison fed a spring that conferred eternal youth. The Geon, as the Nile, watered the Prester's dense, verdant forests and endowed his realm with aromatic stands of pepper and spices.[36]

The kingdom of Prester John was a land of health and abundance second only to the earthly paradise itself – a relationship made explicit by

---

[33] Cadamosto, "Voyages," 5; Patricia Seed, "Navigating the Mid-Atlantic; or, What Gil Eanes Achieved," in *The Atlantic in Global History, 1500–2000*, eds. Jorge Cañizares Esguerra and Erik R. Seeman (Upper Saddle River, NJ: Prentice Hall, 2007), 77–89; Peter Russell, *Prince Henry*, 109–134.

[34] This is the interpretation of Russell, *Prince Henry*, 123–126. See also Wey Gómez, *Tropics of Empire*, 71–78.

[35] *Libro del conosçimiento de todos los reinos y tierras y señoríos que son por el mundo y de las señales y armas que han cada tierra y señorío por si y de los reyes y señores que los poseen* (Madrid: Alejandro Pueyo, 1920), especially 63–79.

[36] Jean Delumeau, *History of Paradise: The Garden of Eden in Myth and Tradition*, trans. Matthew O'Connell (Urbana, IL: University of Illinois Press, 2000 [1992]), 72–77.

their very proximity and common hydrography. As the legend of the Prester's kingdom circulated, a raft of particular details – the precise number of rivers and their names, the stock of exotic creatures, or the extent of the Prester's material wealth and military power – were dropped, countered, or embellished. But the crucial features of this legendary kingdom – its proximity to the earthly paradise, the rejuvenating quality of its rivers, the vegetable abundance of its forests, the wondrous quality of its creatures, the fragrant character of its plants, and the sweet water of its springs – all remained intact. In circulation, the Prester John legend gained reach and purchase on imaginations throughout western Christendom. By the middle of the fifteenth century, versions of the letter, now widely rumored to have been composed by the Prester himself, were available in several European vernaculars. Fragments of it found their way into other travelers' tales. All made reference to the natural world; each in its own way suggested something of the abundance and good health of the Prester's realm.[37]

The *Libro del conosçimiento* was one of these.[38] And as the letter and the *Libro* circulated on paper, intermittent diplomacy made the once-rumored kingdom of Prester John a very real part of Iberian political life.[39] The rulers of Coptic Ethiopia, widely presumed to be the heirs of the fabled patriarch, found their emissaries welcomed across the Mediterranean, from Florence to the Aragonese court.[40] Yet relations with an actual Christian kingdom of North Africa did little to diminish the orientation provided by the longstanding legend. As growing numbers of Portuguese visited the Coptic dominions, they continued to pen their impressions of the therapeutic quality of its nature.[41]

---

[37] Delumeau, *History of Paradise*, 79–96.

[38] So too was the *Libro del Infante don Pedro de Portugal*. Rumors that the Infante of Coimbra, Prince Pedro, had journeyed to the Prester's realm during his travels in the late 1420s found their way into print in 1515. No fewer than 123 separate editions of the book greeted early modern Iberian readers. See Carmen Mejía, "*El libro del Infante don Pedro de Portugal*: estudio crítico y problemas de transmisión," *Revista de Filología Románica* 15 (1998): 215–232.

[39] Russell, *Prince Henry*, 126; and John K. Thornton, "The Portuguese in Africa," in *Portuguese Oceanic Expansion*, eds. Bethencourt and Curto, 138–139.

[40] John K. Thornton, *A Cultural History of the Atlantic World, 1250–1820* (New York: Cambridge University Press, 2012), 15–19, surveys these connections.

[41] This was true even among those more concerned with Portuguese Asia, as for example Gaspar Correia, *Lendas da Índia*, 4 vols., ed. M. Lopes de Almeida (Porto: Lello and Irmão, 1975 [ca. 1556]), vol. 3, 73–74.

The mythical kingdom oriented Portuguese imperial ventures in ways not entirely metaphorical. By the early sixteenth century, the coming and going of Portuguese ships had threaded together an incipient seaborne trading empire that spanned the South Atlantic and Indian Oceans. In an institution that would become the *Casa da Índia*, an imperial map took shape – born of the careful accumulation of corrected sea charts distributed and collected expressly for that purpose. In the exact middle of what has become well known as the Cantino planisphere stood the atlas's principal compass rose. From it, in light emerald and crimson hues, stretched the dense web of rhumb lines by which pilots plotted their courses. And there – in the very centre of it all, just beneath the central massive orienting compass – the approximate location of the once-mythical kingdom was duly recorded: *terra de Preste Juam*, the "land of Prester John" (Figure 2.4).

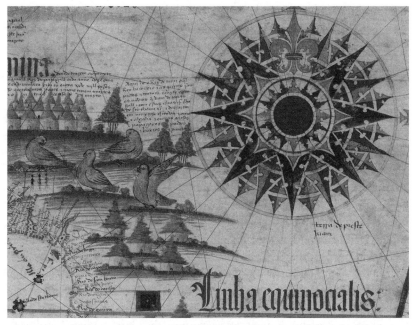

FIGURE 2.4 Visions of Paradise. The "terra de preste juam" (Land of Prester John), helped orient the earliest Iberian assessments of West African epidemiology. The mythical realm remained a point of imperial orientation long after the Edenic vision of West Africa had proven untenable. Detail from the Cantino Atlas.
© Getty Images.

The *Libro* 's description of West Africa did more than offer a vision of the sub-Saharan world as both populous and abundant, it helped consolidate the relationship between a set of iconic places – the Nile and its multiple, undulating branches, the kingdom of Prester John, and the earthly paradise – and it articulated their defining qualities of natural abundance, curative nature, and bodily health. Shipboard along the Guinea Coast, even the senses seemed to supply confirmation of both the proximity of the kingdom and the curative capacity of its nature. Although curiosity and corporeal pleasure had been stigmatized as manifestations of vanity or hedonism and deemed worthy of condemnation, their meanings and moral charge had begun to shift. Late antique writings of Church patriarchs and the late medieval devotional literature of the Portuguese court embraced the senses as pathways to spiritual growth and the expression of piety.[42] So when Zurara, Cadamosto, Pereira, and Barros described not only the sight but the scent and even the flavor of the world beyond the Senegal, they were offering sensory confirmation of existing knowledge through a heavily validated epistemology of experience – one that permitted the somatically rich world of West Africa to confirm an established Christian cosmography.

HIPPOCRATIC PATHOLOGIES

Taken together, the widespread legend of Prester John, the mythical kingdom's proximity to the earthly paradise, the exotic and curative nature of both, their imagined common hydrography, and even the pleasant scent of coastal forests all collectively constituted a body of knowledge about the sub-Saharan world – a body of knowledge, moreover, whose medical implications were comprehended by sailors southbound in the Atlantic no less than by courtiers in Lisbon. The undeniable, widely-shared experience of debilitating fevers challenged this vision of the world beyond the Senegal.

Yet the assimilation of the fact of fevers into a shared vision of that world had implications that were broader still. The proposition that illness could derive from exposure to verdant, fecund environments tugged at a set of fundamental associations that late medieval and early modern travelers relied upon to help make sense of the observable natural

---

[42] Freedman, *Out of the East*, chapter 3; Lorraine Daston, "Curiosity in Early Modern Science," *Word and Image* 11 (1995): 391–404; Mário Martins, "Experiência religiosa e analogia sensorial," *Brotéria: Cultura e informação* 78 (1964): 552–561.

world more generally. West African epidemiological encounters threw into question canonical ideas about the material causes of human sickness. That is what gave regional encounters more global implications.

The theoretical apparatus of learned medicine had crystalized as part of the broader body of ancient medical writing that constituted the Hippocratic-Galenic corpus. In the late fifteenth century, that corpus had become the subject of humanist reinvention and dissemination – first in Italy and then elsewhere. Over the course of the early sixteenth century, the influence of Galen and his humoral view of the body became especially pronounced. A number of historians have discussed the ways in which both Hippocratic environmentalism and especially Galenic humoral theory disciplined the interpretive practices of both the Spanish and English in the Americas.[43] As a single corpus of learned opinion, Hippocratic-Galenic medicine framed earlier impressions of, and experiences in, West Africa as well. But in the fifteenth century, at least among observers and participants of the West African voyages, Hippocratic environmentalism, rather than Galenic huomralism, predominated.

The Hippocratic view that both the human and natural worlds were subject to the same forces, both life-giving and debilitating was one with deep and prestigious roots in the intellectual history of the Latin West.[44] It was given what was perhaps its clearest expression in the Hippocratic treatise, *Airs, Waters, Places*.[45] The text received a great deal of attention among Scholastics because it provided a single, comprehensive method for making sense of a discreet range of observable natural phenomena – from the presence and apparent health of people, plants, and animals, to differences in their physical form, to the causes of disease and death, and even the diversity of human social, cultural, and political life across Eurasia. The brief but influential Hippocratic text, in other words, explained observable human and environmental differences in terms of observable, natural causes.

[43] Karen Ordahl Kupperman, "The Puzzle of the American Climate in the Early Colonial Period," *American Historical Review* 87 (1982): 1262–1289; Andrew Wear, *Knowledge and Practice in English Medicine, 1550–1680* (New York: Cambridge University Press, 2000), 199–202; Andrew Wear, "Place, Health, and Disease: The *Airs, Waters, Places* Tradition in Early Modern England and North America," *Journal of Medieval and Early Modern Studies* 38 (2008): 443–465; and Earle, *Body of the Conquistador*.

[44] On environmental influences broadly speaking, see Clarence J. Glacken, *Traces on the Rhodian Shore: Nature and Culture in Western Thought from Ancient Times to the End of the Eighteenth Century* (Berkeley, CA: University of California Press, 1967), especially 429–460.

[45] Lloyd, ed., *Hippocratic Writings*, 148–165.

From the Hippocratic perspective articulated in *Airs, Waters, Places*, the way to gage whether a place was healthy or not was to examine the airs that circulated there and the quality of its soil and water. Where these were good, the flora and fauna would be abundant and the people healthy.[46] Although the unknown author of *Airs, Waters, Places* insisted on an order of interpretation – air, then soil and water, and then the vitality of local plant, animal, and human inhabitants – fifteenth- and sixteenth-century chroniclers such as Cadamosto, Zurara, Pereira, and Barros did not. Seafarers understood it in terms of another equation: unhealthy places were barren but healthy ones were lush and life there was abundant.

In effect, the natural world became a set of mutually reinforcing signs. Cadamosto's comparison of the lands and peoples on either side of the Senegal River was an instantiation of precisely this framework.[47] And so too were Pereira's numerous reflections on the region.[48] More than any other observer, Barros used this basic interpretive framework to make sense of the unfamiliar, dense, and thickly layered ecology of the sub-Saharan world. In one sweeping passage, he moved easily from a description of the millet fields, mangroves, and elephants of the region between the Senegal and the Gambia rivers to construct a comprehensive classification of all of the lands that lay along the vast southern fringes of the Sahara – a typology based on water and soil, and the plant and animal life they yielded.[49] The Hippocratic framework articulated in *Airs, Waters, Places* permitted considerable interpretive flexibility. That only made it more useful.[50] When travelers explained why things were so, they anchored their accounts to the pervasive influence that environmental factors had on the constitutions of plants, animals, and people alike.

[46] Lloyd, ed., *Hippocratic Writings*, 148–65.　　[47] Cadamosto, "Voyages," 27.

[48] Pereira, *Esmeraldo*, bk. 2, ch. 5: 114–15.

[49] Barros, *Da Ásia*, "Decada Primeira," pt. 1, bk. 3, ch. 8: 220.

[50] The link between immoderate climates and immoderate qualities in plant, animal, and human populations can be extended in more subtle (and not necessarily positive) ways as well. Pereira reported on the strange and threatening creatures found beyond the Senegal. He was especially impressed by the snakes that were "very big" and "very wide," among which were some that measured "a quarter of a league" in length; they had large eyes and a mouth and fangs "corresponding to their size." They inhabited the lakes and coastal waters but were known to "leave great destruction in their wake" (*por honde leuam seu caminho muito dano fazem*) when they slithered out of water, which was "in their nature" to do – though he admitted that they rarely appeared and that such things would be difficult to believe among those who lacked the "experience of such things" (*a pratica d'estas cousas*). See Pereira, *Esmeraldo*, bk. 1, ch. 27: 82.

Both above and below the Senegal, the all-encompassing tautology of the Hippocratic framework seemed at first to hold true. The divergent qualities of the environments above and below the Senegal appeared entirely comprehensible. In the overheated Sahara north of the Senegal – characterized by an arid and debilitating climate, an appropriately barren landscape, and enfeebled inhabitants – sickness and death were unsurprisingly common. Hence Zurara's portrait of the region: "there are neither people nor settlements whatsoever and the land is no less arid than the deserts of Libya, where there is neither water, nor trees, nor anything green."[51] When it came to human health, Cadamosto was more pointed. The Arab and Azanaghi inhabitants of the Saharan coast "sicken in this place and die ... on account of the great heat." He went on to give the summary (if also notably precise) explanation that "at certain seasons of the year," the extreme heat "causes the blood to putrefy."[52] Above the Senegal, the cause of death was not mystery.

As with the Sahara, so too beyond the Senegal: the quality of the environment – a warm climate and fertile landscape continually replenished by good water – nurtured a region that was as beautiful as it was bountiful, and fostered what at first seemed to be a pervasive vitality in the resident plant, animal, and human populations. Hence, again, Cadamosto's remark that, "all men are ... tall and big, their bodies well formed; and the whole country [is] green, full of trees, and fertile."[53] In similar fashion, Barros drew attention to the fresh water borne to the coast by the Senegal and Gambia Rivers, to which he attributed the evident abundance of life: "the animals which drink the waters of these rivers are so numerous and of so many varieties that even elephants go in herds."[54]

Here was a place whose location fit easily within the geography of Ptolemy, a land that appeared to possess all of the qualities suggested by Pliny, accommodated by biblical tales, and popularly enshrined in the legend of Prester John – one, moreover, whose qualities were cogently explained by the Hippocratic environmentalist epistemology. Pervasive illness beyond the Senegal not only flew in the face of ancient and authoritative accounts that linked the kingdom of Prester John to the Biblical

---

[51] Zurara, *Chronica*, ch. 8: 51.   [52] Cadamosto, "Voyages," 21.

[53] Cadamosto, "Voyages," 27. Likewise, in a simile that was aptly bellicose for the chronicler of conquests, Zurara reported that the shells of the sea tortoises that swam along the coast were "as big as a battle shield." Pereira was captivated by the countless, brightly-colored birds. See Zurara, *Chronica*, ch. 44: 209–210, ch. 59: 274–275; and Pereira, bk. 2, ch. 5: 114–115.

[54] Barros, "Decada Primeira," pt. 1, bk. 3, ch. 8: 217–219.

earthly paradise, it challenged the very framework that seemed to explain the internal operations of the natural world itself. From the perspective of the former, pervasive fevers made the problem a highly local one. From the perspective of the latter, the problem was far greater, as it threw into question the relationship between nature and disease globally.

And that was the real problem. No matter where the Portuguese might go ashore, even the healthiest looking places might turn out to be otherwise. Encounters in the early Atlantic upset the framework that made unfamiliar places epidemiologically intelligible.

FEVERS AND FEBRIFUGES IN THE EARLY ATLANTIC

Judith Carney and Richard Rosomoff have shown how the fertility and vegetable abundance of the Senegambia, together with the agricultural and curative expertise of West African men and especially women, were recruited to the service of the transatlantic slave trade.[55] But well before that trade was underway, I have argued, it was that very abundance that had proven so epidemiologically disorienting. The once authoritative association between particular environments and health or disease had been fundamentally challenged by the coincidence of verdure and fevers along the Guinea Coast.

In the face of widespread sickness and death, as experience below the Senegal so plainly and consistently failed to meet expectations, two things happened. First, albeit slowly and unevenly, an imperial medical infrastructure came into being. On paper if not in practice, and sometimes more grudgingly than others, the Crown and its ministers provisioned outposts with some combination of a makeshift hospital, a physician, an apothecary, and a surgeon.[56] At times, as at Sofala on the East African Coast, funding from the royal account came decades after conditions on the ground required it. Royal approval in these cases was little more than

---

[55] Judith Carney and Richard Nicholas Rosomoff, *In the Shadow of Slavery: Africa's Botanical Legacy in the Atlantic World* (Berkeley, CA: University of California Press, 2009).

[56] See the varied arrangements made for Mozambique, Sofala, Aden, Hormuz, Diu, Bassein, Cannanore, and Malaca in Pandoronga S.S. Pissurlencar, *Regimentos das fortalezas da Índia: Estudo e Notas* (Bastorá: Tipografia Rangel, 1951). According to Jaime Walter, "O Infante D. Henrique e a medicina," *Studia* 13/14 (1964): 33–34, the whole system, if it can be called that, traced its roots to Faro and Tavira, two small towns on the southernmost shore of Portugal itself, and to a time when North Africa and the Canary Islands marked the extent of Portugal's Atlantic reach.

formalized acquiescence – the accommodation of arrangements already in place.[57] Sometimes a colonial hospital deemed vital would fall into disrepair despite the protestations of sea captains, sailors, and officials assigned there. This happened at Mozambique Island, which was often the first safe port for India-bound ships once they rounded the treacherous Cape of Good Hope.[58] And, on occasion, local circumstances made a port city a popular place to convalesce even when no unusual need seemed to require it. This happened in Cannanore on the Malabar Coast, where diplomatic relations and easy access to abundant local produce made it a favored spot among among ailing Portuguese sailors.[59]

Yet to see these varied arrangements for the provision of medical care as part of a coherent imperial approach to colonial health is to overstate the case. Across Portugal's intertropical empire, a particular clinical institution – the hospital – may have multiplied, but explanatory and therapeutic diversity prevailed. That was the second consequence of early Atlantic epidemiological encounters: they spurred natural inquiry and therapeutic improvisation, in which the explanation and treatment of fever were central. [60] Sickness according to Cadamosto may have derived in some way from the diminutive fruits of the region, hence his refusal to eat the dates of the Gambia. Cadamosto's fellow traveler, Diogo Gomes, looked for a more conventional, environmental explanation. He related what the merchants of the Gambia River entrepot of Cantor had explained to him: that inhabitants of the Guinea Coast "did not live long on account of the impure air," which was due in turn to the gold mines there.[61]

---

[57] Pissurlencar, *Regimentos*, 196–197; and follow the correspondence in *Documentos sobre os Portugueses em Moçambique e na África Central, 1497–1840* (Lisbon: National Archives of Rhodesia and Nyasaland, and the Centro de Estudos Históricos Ultramarinos, 1962–1969), vol. 3: 526–533, vol. 5: 538–573, and vol. 7: 196–211.

[58] The hospital at Mozambique Island was the subject of much wrangling between the Crown and appointees on the island. See Francisco de Sousa, *Oriente Conquistado a Jesus Cristo pelos Padres da Companhia de Jesus da Província de Goa*, ed., M. Lopes de Almeida (Porto: Lello and Irmão, 1978), 34, 55, 317, 319.

[59] Correia, *Lendas*, vol. 1: 729 and 961, vol. 2: 26, 118, 537, 969–970, and vol. 3: 17.

[60] I return to this in chapters 7 and 8 but, particularly for Portuguese Africa, see Kalle Kananoja, "Bioprospecting and European Uses of African Natural Medicine in Early Modern Angola," *Portuguese Studies Review* 23 (2015): 1–25.

[61] Gomes was a nobleman, pilot, and member of the royal household who was dispatched to the Senegambia region in the early 1480s to secure trading agreements for the Portuguese. His testimony was taken first in German but was subsequently translated into the Latin and, only in the nineteenth century, was copied into both Portuguese and English. I have relied on Crone's description and publication of the English version in Crone, ed., *Voyages of Cadamosto and Other Documents*, xlv and 95.

Barros articulated a much more elaborate explanation – one similarly fashioned to fit, however awkwardly, the environmental framework of the Hippocratic corpus. He wondered if perhaps the Senegal's life-giving water might in fact be the cause. In reference to the Senegal and one of its upriver tributaries, the Gufitembó, he explained that "when anyone drinks water from one [river] and then the other, he begins to vomit." Such illness, he supposed, was due to the fact that the two rivers were different in their very nature – "competitors and contrary" – as indicated by their contrasting colors (the Senegal appeared white, the Gufitembó red). But, as though puzzled and evidently unconvinced by his own explanation, Barros added that "neither of [the rivers], separately, cause this . . . [nor do they do so] even after they have run together."[62] Observers may not have agreed on the probable causes of fever but could indeed agree that the conventional signs of health could no longer be trusted.

Atlantic travelers wasted little time in inquiring how the people they met managed to survive. Cadamosto took care to note that the inhabitants of the "empire of Mali" drank one large ampule of saline solution daily in order to avoid the ill effects of the scorching temperatures.[63] If his seafaring contemporaries took such claims about salt seriously, they would have had little trouble acquiring it. Salt was already a major item of coastal trade and European travelers and their descendants would soon take it up. Diasporic Portuguese and Luso-African traders (*lançados* and, by the end of the fifteenth century, *tangomãos*) connected the Cape Verdes and other Atlantic islands to the mainland markets of the coast and the interior. They insinuated themselves into a trade in salt, kola nuts, and other *materia medica* that they did not create and could not control but upon which coastal commercial fortunes, and perhaps even lives, depended.

Therapeutic and commercial exchange begot artistic patronage that may have contributed to an emergent material culture of healing in the early Atlantic world. Craftsmen from the Upper Guinea Coast and the Kingdom of Benin produced countless finely-carved ivory sculptures.

---

[62] Barros, "Decada Primeira," pt. 1, bk. 3, ch. 8: 215. In his translation of this section of Barros's text, Crone, ed., *Voyages of Cadamosto and Other Documents*, 137 n. 1, explains that the river is probably the modern Feleme and that the red color was due to the laterite from which the gold was mined.

[63] Cadamosto, "Voyages," 21–22. Salt for the concoction came from Mali's extensive salt mines, which supplied the trans-Sahara commerce including the famous (if also apocryphal) silent trade. See Philip D. Curtin, *Cross-Cultural Trade in World History* (New York: Cambridge, 1984), 12–13.

These were prized among European traders, who hauled them back home as gifts for their patrons and financiers. Salt cellars were a favourite and are perhaps the single most numerous type of these Afro-Portuguese ivories to have survived. Given Cadamosto's comment and the prominence of the salt trade not only among the traveling merchants of Mali but among diasporic Portuguese and Luso-Africans too, those diminutive monuments to Atlantic exchange probably offered not only pleasure to the tongue but protection to the body.[64]

Duarte Pacheco Pereira engaged in a bit of medicinal prospecting too. It might have been as he lay dying beneath the equatorial sun, or maybe as he commanded supply ships running between Lisbon and the Mina castle, but sometime before he penned the *Esmeraldo*, he learned of two medicaments he thought worthy of note. Both were in use among the Jolof and Mandinka near the mouth of the Senegal River. And both found their way into his manuscript. One, a stone he called "alaquequas" (agate), was already a familiar element of Mediterranean *materia medica*. Pereira believed it was used to stanch the flow of blood. The other was entirely unfamiliar to him. Pereira described it as a wood; it was "dark as a buffalo's horn within ... and hard as a bone." He called it "balamban" and recorded in the *Esmeraldo* that it was "made into a powder, mixed with water ... [and given] as a drink to those with cough."[65]

Pereira's description of balamban may have been the earliest recorded exchange of novel *materia medica* in the long history of European seaborne empires. In the eighteenth century, balamban resurfaced in the reports of Swedish, British, and Portuguese naturalists who continued to reconnoiter their own corners of the Guinea Coast. A lucrative and thriving trade in balamban grew up on São Tomé, where for centuries slaves harvested it in the highlands and sold it on coastal markets. But balamban was not used for cough as Pereira had described. It had become vital to Portuguese colonial medicine on São Tomé and throughout the Gulf of Guinea as a treatment for fever.[66]

---

[64] On the development of the Guinea trade see Brooks, "Kola Trade"; on the various ways in which salt figured into see Green, *Rise of the Atlantic Slave Trade*, 102, 159, 235, and 249; and on the ivories, see William Fagg, *The Afro-Portuguese Ivories* (London: Batchworth Press), 1959.

[65] Pereira, *Esmeraldo*, bk. 1, ch. 27: 82.

[66] Conde de Ficalho, *Plantas Úteis da África Portuguesa*, 2nd ed. (Lisbon: Imprensa Nacional, 1947 [1884]), 191. Adam Afzel observed its use during his travels to the region in the late eighteenth century and recorded his observations in *Plantarum Guineensium* (Uppsala: Typis Edmannianis, 1804).

COSMOGRAPHIC INSCRIPTIONS AND
INTERTROPICAL POSSIBILITIES

In 1563, Duarte Pacheco Pereira's brother-in-law António Galvão lay dying in a bed in Lisbon's Hospital de Todos-os-Santos. In his last years, Galvão had written a long and reflective history of "discoveries ancient and modern." The *Tratado dos descobrimentos* celebrated not only the development of Portugal's empire but the colonizing exploits of the English, French, and Spanish as well. What is clear from Galvão's *Tratado* is that Portugal stood out in one peculiar way. Metropolitan officials in each of these empires had devised techniques for measuring the extent of their dominions. But their methods differed. English and Spanish contemporaries often preferred the Roman example. They measured the extent of their dominions in terms of distance from an imperial capital – London or Madrid.[67] Theirs were empires that radiated outward from a center. By contrast, for Galvão in the *Tratado dos descobrimentos*, the chosen point of reference was not a point at all. It was a line. The positions of Portuguese colonines were recorded not in terms of their distance from Lisbon but as degrees of arc above or below the equator. The equinoctial line rather than Lisbon served as the essential spatial referent.[68] Portuguese such as Galvão had long conceived of their empire in precisely these terms – not merely as political or commercial projections outward but as a horizontal extension across the midriff of the terracqueous globe. Decades earlier, for his *Esmeraldo*, Pereira had tabulated with maximum precision the locations of Portuguese colonies using not linear distances from Lisbon but the latitudes they occupied.[69]

This was a perspective that drew attention to the empire's expansion across the vast intertropical world, and it was a world that officials in the Casa da Índia in those years could see for themselves. Carefully plotted

---

[67] Karen Ordahl Kupperman, *The Jamestown Project* (Cambridge, MA: Belknap Press, 2007), 109–112; Padrón, *The Spacious Word*, 63–84. My point is not that these were mutually exclusive ways of conceiving of imperial space but rather, as Padrón explores, that individuals and their circles preferred to think and represent empire in particular ways. Itinerary maps that emphasized point-to-point vectors remained important to the creation, maintenance, and self-conception of both Iberian empires and to cartographic imaginations throughout Europe in the sixteenth century.

[68] I work from the second edition of 1731: António Galvão, *Tratado dos descobrimentos antigos, e modernos*, 2nd ed. (Lisbon: Officina Ferreiriana, 1731 [1563]). For more on Galvão, see Sanjay Subrahmanyam, "On World Historians in the Sixteenth Century," *Representations* 91 (2005): 26–57.

[69] He devoted much discussion to this perspective. See Pereira, *Esmeraldo*, bk. 1, chs. 6–9.

and drawn across the Cantino atlas, a pair of thin red lines (the northern and southern tropics) encompassed that world – one that was now dotted with the banners of the Crown, which marked the positions of Portuguese enclaves overseas.

The empire's geographical situation had purchase on Portuguese imaginations well beyond the guarded chambers of the Casa or the personal libraries and private chambers of men like Pereira and Galvão. By the time Galvão lay in hospital in Lisbon, the peculiar image of the armillary sphere had multiplied across Lisbon's publicly visible spaces. This esoteric instrument modeled the circles of the celestial globe: the equator, the ecliptic, and the northern and southern tropics. Used variously by natural philosophers, cosmographers, and pilots, the armillary sphere was also the royal emblem of Manuel I and it was a distinguishing feature of Manueline architecture.[70] It adorned the courtyards of the imperial capital's newest monasteries, the façades that lined Lisbon's main thoroughfares, and the defensive fortifications that guarded the city's waterfront.[71] The instrument was familiar among Manuel's maritime subjects too. Not only was it a tool for training new pilots in the art of blue water navigation, but Atlantic bound travelers carried drawings of it with them into the Atlantic. The image traveled aboard ships bound for the Guinea Coast, and found its way among the objects that changed hands beneath the curtain walls of the São Jorge da Mina castle. It was also given to the ivory craftsmen of Benin, who reproduced it on the sculptures that circulated along the coast and which made the journey back to Europe (Figure 2.5).

Whatever the artisans who made them saw in such a symbol (and that has become a prominent question in the study of these objects[72]), Portuguese patrons at sea and at court would have been reminded not simply of the mythical West African region from which the ivory objects came – embodied, metonymically, in the exotic material itself – but of the wider

[70] Jim Bennett, "Early Modern Mathematical Instruments," *Isis* 102 (2011): 697–705; Jay A. Levinson, ed., *Circa 1492: Art in the Age of Exploration* (New Haven, CT: Yale University Press, 1991), 145–146.

[71] Ana Maria Alves, *Iconologia do Poder Real no Período Manuelino* (Lisbon: Imprensa Nacional, 1985); Susannah Humble Ferreira, "Inventing the Courtier in Early Sixteenth-Century Portugal," in *Contested Spaces of Nobility in Early Modern Europe*, eds. Matthew P. Romaniello and Charles Lipp (Burlington, VT: Ashgate, 2011), 85–102.

[72] Question of identity and cultural hybridity are the focus of most recent studies of the Luso-African ivories. An early probing example is Suzanne Preston Blier, "Imaging Otherness in Ivory: African Portrayals of the Portuguese ca. 1492," 75 (1993): 375–396. Thorny questions of attribution are addressed in Fagg, *Afro-Portuguese Ivories*.

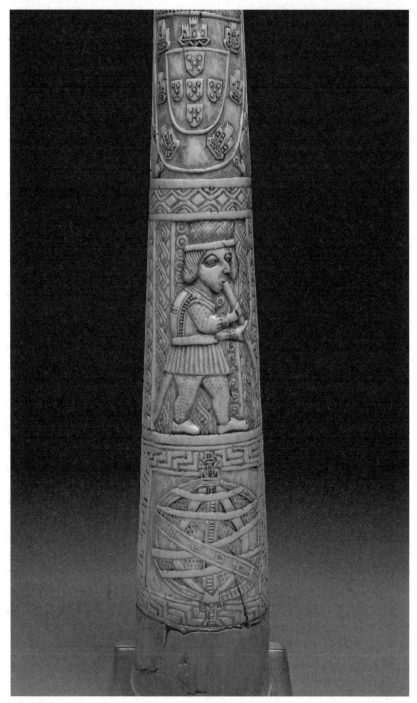

FIGURE 2.5 Common Knowledge. Images highlighting the intertropical situation of Portugal's empire were characteristic of Manueline architecture. An armillary sphere (bottom) and the coat of arms of the Portuguese House of Aviz (top) adorn an olifant made by craftsmen in Benin. Ivory objects like this horn from ca. 1525 were commissioned and purchased from West African artisans by Iberian travelers beginning in the late fifteenth century.

intertropical world of which that region was a part, and in which a growing number of Iberian and other European travelers lived, sailed, fell ill, and healed or died.

I have argued that the proliferation of Senegambian exchanges detailed by Carney and Rosomoff began as a consequence of the uncertainties that attended the earliest direct and sustained coastal interactions between European and African traders scattered beyond the Senegal, along the Upper and Lower Guinea coasts. I have also argued that those uncertainties had been in the making for over a half a century. Beginning in the 1450s, among sailors, merchants, courtly patrons, prospectors, and cosmographers, a shift is perspective had taken place in which at least one corner of the dreaded torrid zone had been found to be not only habitable but, in fact, densely inhabited, and brimming with an unanticipated profusion of plants and animals. Observers found, too, that contrary to the assurances of the Prester John legend and of Hippocratic environmentalism, the verdure and abundance of the Gulf of Guinea could not be taken as guarantees of the region's good health.

That did not mean that the West African experience and the interpretive and therapeutic uncertainties that it engendered were immediately taken to be generalizable across the entirety of the intertropical world. To the contrary: rather than a single global geographical space characterized everywhere by environmental and epidemiological coherence, it remained instead, to use Dennis Cosgrove's evocative phrase, "a place ... made up of places."[73]

Yet if omnipresent fevers belied the promise of heath in a particular region of sub-Saharan Africa, the uncertainty they engendered about the reliability of the Hippocratic framework did suggest the possibility of a link between fevers and verdant overseas locations generally.

A set of longstanding Scholastic debates gave that uncertainty more precise geographical focus. When João de Barros wrote of flaming swords and deadly fevers, it was not just a reference to West African geography but to the potential dangers of the very intertropical world that a growing number of Portuguese now inhabited. His imagery was biblical – a reference to the flaming sword of the Cherubim, the angel of the book of Genesis who guarded the earthly paradise from those unworthy of passage.[74] His use of the phrase was more than poetic license. The image

---

[73] Denis Cosgrove, "Tropic and Tropicality," in *Tropical Visions in an Age of Empire*, eds. Felix Driver and Luciana Martins (Chicago: University of Chicago Press, 2005), 216.

[74] *The Bible*, Genesis 3: 24 (KJV).

had become a standard, indeed ubiquitous, element in Scholastic arguments about a question that, as I have argued, now lay at the heart of the West African conundrum: the possibility of verdant nature in the very depths of the torrid zone. [75] As Alessandro Scafi has demonstrated, between the middle of the twelfth century and the end of the thirteenth century, a number of commentators had already put paradise somewhere along the equinoctial line.[76] Well aware of the basic contradiction – for how could the earthly paradise lay in a region scorched by the sun – thirteenth-century commentators were compelled to explain their positions. Some like Thomas Aquinas had sided with Aristotle in the view that the torrid zone was universally scorched, bleak, and impassible, that all who tried to cross it would burn in the attempt, and that therefore the southern temperate zone was, and would remain, simply inaccessible to humanity. If the mythical garden lay within the torrid zone, reasoned Aquinas, it could only be because of some kind of exceptional geography: it must either have sat atop a tall mountain or alongside a sprawling body of water – either of which might cool the air. But other commentators, including Aquinas's teacher in Paris, Albertus Magnus, took inspiration from Ptolemy. Unlike Aristotle, Ptolemy had drawn finer distinctions among regions within the torrid zone – distinctions based on details about the seasonal transit of the sun. He had claimed that the climate at the equator itself was in fact more temperate than at either of the tropics, which meant that the equinoctial region could easily accommodate the profuse nature and healthful climate of a terrestrial paradise.[77]

---

[75] Barros could have plucked the image from any one of a number of Scholastic texts. He may have been making a reference directly to the bishop of Seville. Along with a substantial corpus of medical texts, Isidore's *Etymologiae* had circulated for centuries within Portugal even before the founding of the University of Lisbon in 1290. The Alcobaça scriptorium housed at least one full copy. Written in a thirteenth-century hand, its cursive marginalia marked the passage of generations of readers from the fourteenth to the sixteenth centuries. The *Orto do esposo*, which was composed at Alcobaça, cited this text; it may have been a reference to this very manuscript. See references to the holdings of the scriptorium in BNP, Res., cod. 189, ff. 208–209; and Thomas L. Amos, *The Fundo Alcobaça of the Biblioteca Nacional, Lisbon*, 3 vols., (Collegeville, MN: Hill Monastic Manuscripts Library, 1988), vol. 3, 236. See also Bertil Maler, ed., *Orto do esposo* (Rio de Janeiro: Ministério da Educação e Cultura and the Instituto Nacional do Livro, 1956), 14–16.

[76] Scafi, *Mapping Paradise*, 172–179; Delumeau, *History of Paradise*, 83–96.

[77] This, he reasoned was because of the motion of the sun: it was virtually still over the tropics for two months as the solstice came and went, but always passed very quickly over the equator. Scafi, *Mapping Paradise*, 160–183. Wey Gómez, *Tropics of Empire*, 231–291 discusses the position of Albertus in detail.

For those inclined to side with Ptolemy, the possibility that the earthly paradise lay along the equinoctial line was a rather unproblematic proposition. But for those philosophers who sided with Aristotle, the figure of the Cherubim and the flaming sword had become a way to reconcile the existence of an equatorial Eden with the apparent fact of intertropical uninhabitability. Theirs was a figurative reading of the Biblical passage, in which the flaming sword was the equatorial heat itself.[78]

If most thirteenth-century commentators conceded that their claims were necessarily speculative, that was not the case for fifteenth-century Portuguese seafarers. Unlike his Scholastic predecessors, for Barros the geography was hardly speculative at all and the flaming sword reference was more pointed. When he invoked the image, he made one novel emendation: Barros stressed "deadly fevers." Not only had the opposing positions staked out by Aristotle and Ptolemy proven categorically untenable, but the actual bodily agent of death had become known. The natural world between the northern and southern tropics was potentially everywhere lush and abundant. It was also potentially ridden with fever.

As Portuguese observers settled across the intertropical world, they would find themselves confronted with similarly verdant and wondrous places. They would have to interrogate the perceived health of those places and, where and when fevers and other diseases erupted, they would need to account for them and treat the bodies that suffered them. Whether verdure and fever reigned together – and how to explain such a phenomenon – would remain open questions.

[78] Scafi, *Mapping Paradise*, 174.

PART II

THE INDIAN OCEAN WORLD, 1500–1600

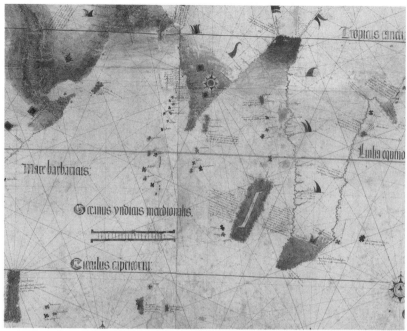

FIGURE 3.1 Imperial Aspirations. Coastal encounters in Asia were made manifest in pilots' charts, travel accounts, and illustrations of various kinds. The collection and collation of such diverse reportage enabled the creation of synthetic atlases in Lisbon. Here the accumulated information about Indian Ocean Asia, extensive already in 1502, reflected the intensity of metropolitan interest. Detail of South and Southeast Asia from the Cantino Atlas.

© Getty Images.

3

Itineraries and Inventories

Only time uncovers the truth of things.
Letter of Tomé Pires to Manuel I[1]

NO BELLS TO HONOR THE DEAD

Of the five India-bound ships that set sail from Lisbon to Goa in the spring of 1530, one fell behind and then disappeared somewhere in the Indian Ocean, finally slipping within sight of the Malabar Coast in late October, some five weeks after its companion vessels had made port. The figure the lost ship cut against the South Indian horizon was, for at least one contemporary, "haunting." It appeared "all but abandoned" as its torn sails whipped uncontrollably "first in one direction and then another," heaving the wooden vessel "wherever the wind might take it." Left to the whims of wind and sea, the ship had veered far to the south of its intended port. A Portuguese armada patrolling the Malabar Coast intercepted it. On board, the living were found strewn across the deck, "wailing softly [and] crying out to God for mercy." A mysterious affliction left them too weak to stand. It was rumored that among the stricken passengers were Pêro Lopes de Sampaio and António de Macedo. Sampaio was to fill his appointment as the new Captain of Goa; Macedo was to become Judge General, the superior Crown magistrate for all of Portuguese Asia. The patrolling ships managed to convey the survivors to

[1] ANTT, CC, pt. 1, mç. 19, n. 102, f. 4.

a hospital in nearby Cannanore where, one by one, they died – the would-be officials among them – of some mysterious illness.[2]

Goa was the heart of Portugal's Asian trade empire – capital of what the Portuguese called the *Estado da Índia*.[3] A collection of low-lying islands along the coastal plain of western India, Goa was cordoned off from the interior by the high peaks of the Sahyadris, part of the Western Ghats, whose streams drained into to the Mondovi and Zuari rivers and fed Goa's extensive wetlands. Among the Konkani villagers who farmed rice in its estuaries there was a belief that none other than Vishnu himself had reclaimed Goa from the seas.[4] And indeed, the struggle for life at the mercy of a bountiful but unrelenting natural world would plague Goa under the Portuguese.

This was the city that in 1538 became the permanent home of Garcia de Orta.[5] A physician with connections to the royal household of João III and an appointment as lecturer in natural philosophy at Lisbon's university, Orta sailed to India on the ship *Rainha* in 1534. He did so as the personal physician to Martim Afonso de Sousa, an energetic but controversial figure who would become the twelfth governor (1542–1545) of the Estado da Índia. Sousa had proven himself a valuable asset to D. João III in Brazil a couple of years earlier. Besides ridding (albeit temporarily) the South American littoral of French interlopers, Sousa championed the development of one of its earliest successful sugar plantations.[6] Having

[2] Correia, *Lendas*, vol. 3, 384–385. I say rumor because, whether or not he was aboard the ship that inspired this passage, António de Macedo did indeed become *ouvidor-geral*. Whoever the dying officials were, Macedo was not among them.

[3] On this typology of early modern empires, see Michael Adas and Hugh Cagle, "Age of Settlement and Colonization, 1500–1900," in *The Ashgate Research Companion to Modern Imperial Histories*, eds. Philippa Levine and John Marriott (Burlington, VT: Ashgate, 2012), 41–73.

[4] Alice Cabral Caldeira Santiago Faria, "Understanding Pangim as a Transformed Landscape," in *Histories from the Sea*, eds. Francisco José Gomes Caramelo et al. (New Delhi: Jawaharlal Nehru University, 2009), 93.

[5] The original was published as Garcia d'Orta, *Coloquios dos simples, e drogas e cousas medicinais da India, e assi dalgũas frutas achadas nella onde se tratam algũas cousas tocantes amediçina, pratica, e outras cousas boas, pera saber cõpostos pello Doutor garcia dorta: fisico del Rey nosso senhor, vistos pello muyto Reverendo senhor, ho liçenciado Alexos diaz: falcam desembargador da casa da supricaçã inquisidor nestas partes* (Goa: João de Endem, 1563). Here I work from Garcia da Orta, *Colóquios dos simples e drogas da Índia*, edited by Conde de Ficalho (2 vols., Lisbon, 1895). Henceforth *Colóquios*. In the text I use the modern form of the physician's name following the Biblioteca Nacional de Portugal, hence: "Garcia de Orta."

[6] Stuart B. Schwartz, *Sugar Plantations in the Formation of Brazilian Society: Bahia, 1550–1835* (New York: Cambridge University Press, 1985), 16–17.

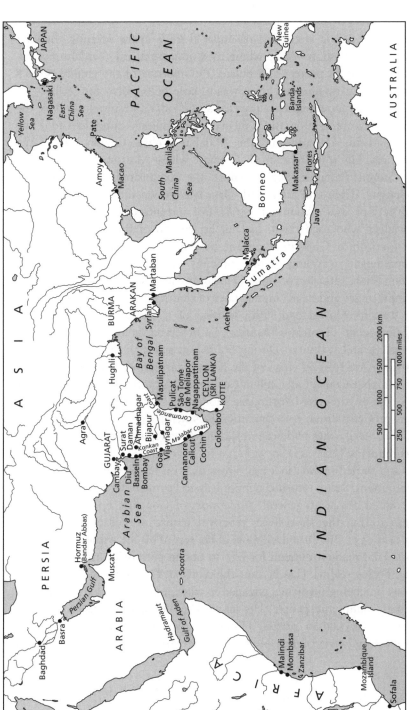

MAP 3.1 Portuguese Settlements and Principal Ports of Trade in Asia. Adapted by David Cox from Bethencourt and Curto, eds., *Portuguese Oceanic Expansion*, xx.

proven his skill in strengthening imperial trade in the Atlantic, the king dispatched Sousa to Asia, where as Captain-general (*capitão-mor do mar*), he was to protect and bolster the interests of the empire. Orta's first charge as an imperial agent was to keep Sousa alive and well.

In Sousa's company, Orta traveled along India's western littoral for the next four years. Diplomatic maneuvers and military campaigns took the physician to Ahmadnagar, the Malabar Coast, Ceylon, and Cape Comorin. His travels began in Gujarat, where Martim Afonso backed the Sultan Bahadur Shah against the expansionist Mughal ruler Humayun. Then and afterward, Orta was drawn into contact with the enormity of South Asian *materia medica* and into conversation with the specialists who used them. In Diu, he learned of the thriving trade in turbith from a Gujarati merchant (*vania*) and a Hindu herbalist.[7] In Ahmadnagar, traveling in the company of the physicians of Burhan Nizam Shah, Orta learned that spikenard was harvested from the banks of the Ganges and heard mythic tales of that river's curative power.[8] On his way to Ahmedabad, Orta learned of a treatment for dysentery: Muslim *unani* physicians (*hakims*), he observed, favoured a concoction of opium and walnuts.[9] During Sousa's attack against the Zamorin of Calicut, Orta took in views of the pepper, cardamom, and other flora of the Malabar Coast. Later still in Ceylon, as Sousa pressed the Kotte ruler to secure an attempted Portuguese monopoly on cinnamon, Orta learned that, properly dried, true cinnamon was neither gray nor dark but vermillion, "as if ashes had been mixed in red wine, with the red of the wine predominant."[10]

Orta settled in Goa in 1538. From then on his travels were brief and intermittent. Sousa returned temporarily to Portugal. Orta would later be appointed physician-general (*físico-mor*) of Goa first under Sousa and again during the short-lived viceroyal tenure of Pedro Mascarenhas (1554–1555). But Orta lived most of the rest of his life without an official post. That made it difficult for him to obtain permission to journey into neighboring realms. Goa became the center of Orta's world. There he set about practicing medicine, engaged in trade, and assembled a collection of both plants and people. His network of contacts – a varied lot that included Abyssinian priests, Hindu *vaidyas* (specialists of ayurveda), Javanese midwives (*daias*) and Konkani servants – spanned Indian Ocean

---

[7] Orta, *Colóquios*, vol. 2, 329–330.   [8] Ibid., vol. 2, 291–297.
[9] Ibid., vol. 2, 15–18.   [10] Ibid., vol. 1, 212, 201–217.

Asia. Through them, that world found its way into the anterooms, corridors, cabinets, and kitchen of the Orta household. [11]

That cast of characters and the knowledge they helped create also populated Orta's book. The *Colóquios dos simples e drogas e cousas medicinais da Índia* – loosely but not inaccurately understood as a natural history and guide to South Asian *materia medica* – brought all of Orta's learning, travel, observation, and experience together. [12] It combined information he collected from rulers, merchants, soldiers, and even traitors of the Portuguese state, together with that of vaidyas, hakims, market vendors, craftsmen, and members of his own household – exchanges that took the form of shipboard chatter, marketplace gossip, bedside consultations, casual household conversations, and rare audiences with powerful leaders. Ships, markets, households, and royal courts all became settings for the exchange of the rather specialized natural knowledge that helped sustain Portugal's empire. Printed in Goa in 1563, the *Colóquios* was one of the first books published in the colonial city. The press that printed it was the only one permitted to operate anywhere in Portugal's overseas dominions in the period – a measure of the importance of Goa to the Portuguese Crown and of the value of Orta's *Colóquios* to the inhabitants of Portuguese Goa.

As an inventory of some of the drugs and spices available in South Asia – and of the unfamiliar nature of the Indian Ocean world more generally – the *Colóquios* has become a touchstone for the participation of Portugal and its empire in the cultural and intellectual transformations sweeping sixteenth- and seventeenth-century Europe. From numerous studies, a collage of overlapping portraits of the book and its author have

---

[11] Orta's movements and associations are traceable only through the *Colóquios* and a handful of documents from Goa. Useful examinations of Orta's life, work, and travels include the essays in Palmira Fontes da Costa, ed., *Medicine, Trade and Empire: Garcia de Orta's Colloquies on the Simples and Drugs of India (1563) in Context* (Burlington, VT: Ashgate, 2015); Teresa Nobre de Carvalho, *Os desafios de Garcia de Orta. Colóquios dos Simples e Drogas da Índia* (Lisbon: Esfera do Caos, 2015); Conde de Ficalho, *Garcia da Orta e o seu tempo* (Lisbon: Imprensa Nacional, 1886); and Augusto da Silva Carvalho, "Garcia d'Orta. Comemoração do quarto centenário da sua partida para a India em 12 de Março de 1534," *Revista da Universidade de Coimbra*, 12 (1934): 130–133. Still useful is Jaime Walter, "Garcia de Orta: Relance da sua vida," *Revista da Junta de Investigações do Ultramar* 11 (1963): 619–622.

[12] More on the variety of informants and eyewitnesses on which Orta relied to write the *Colóquios*, is found in Rui Loureiro, "Information Networks in the *Estado da Índia*, a Case Study: Was Garcia de Orta the Organizer of the *Codex Casanatense* 1889?," *Anais de História de Alem-Mar* 13 (2012): 41–73.

emerged.[13] Because Orta combined philology with an empiricism of natural particulars in an attempt to identify familiar and unfamiliar drugs and spices, and because he readily challenged the claims of ancient and medieval authorities (Dioscorides, Avicenna, and many others) on the identities and qualities of numerous plants, Orta has often been portrayed as a Renaissance humanist.[14] His careful descriptions of plants and animals combined with his penchant for testing drugs both old and new on his own patients have seemed to some as evidence of an experimental program, which has led to claims that Orta was a Portuguese progenitor of a scientific revolution.[15] Historians of colonialism have seen in his ostensibly pioneering epistemology the stirrings of European scientific and technical superiority, and eventual global hegemony – a story in which Orta has been cast as a pioneer of tropical medicine.[16]

Along with these images has emerged one in which Orta plays a rather different part. Because his was a natural history underwritten by the convergence in Goa of the many overlapping networks of commerce, medicine, knowledge, and *naturalia*, Orta has also been portrayed as a stealthy, culturally ambidextrous intermediary between mutually distinct

---

[13] On the historiography of science and medicine in Portugal's early modern empire more generally, see Palmira Fontes da Costa and Henrique Leitão, "Portuguese Imperial Science, 1450–1800: An Historiographical Review," in *Science in the Spanish and Portuguese Empires, 1400–1800*, eds. Daniela Bleichmar, Paula de Vos, Kristin Huffine, and Kevin Sheehan (Stanford, CA: Stanford University Press, 2009), 35–53.

[14] Ogilvie, *Science of Describing*, 243–248; Daston and Park, *Wonders*, 148–155; and most recently Ines G. Županov, "Garcia de Orta's *Colóquios*: Context and Afterlife of a Dialogue," in Costa, ed., *Medicine, Trade and Empire*, 49–65.

[15] Among the most full-throated of such arguments is Almeida, "Portugal and the Dawn of Modern Science"; and Onésimo Teotónio de Almeida, "Sobre a revolução da experiência no Portugal do século XVI: Na pista do conceito de 'Experiência a Madre das Cousas,'" in *Actas do Quinto Congresso da Associação Internacional de Lusitanistas*, ed. T. F. Earle (Coimbra: Associação Internacional de Lusitanistas, 1998), vol. 3, 1617–1625. See also Domingues, "Science and Technology in Portuguese Navigation"; and Harold J. Cook, "Trading in Medicinal Simples and Developing the New Science: de Orta and His Contemporaries," in Costa, ed., *Medicine Trade and Empire*, 129–146.

[16] M. N. Pearson, "The Thin End of the Wedge: Medical Relativities as a Paradigm of Early Modern Indian-European Relations," *Modern Asian Studies* 29 (1995): 141–170; Fernando A. R. Nogueira, "Garcia de Orta, Physician and Scientific Researcher," in *The Great Maritime Discoveries and World Health*, eds. Mário Gomes Marques and John Cule (Lisbon: Escola Nacional de Saúde Pública, 1991), 227–236; Louis H. Roddis, "Garcia da Orta: the First European Writer on Tropical Medicine and a Pioneer in Pharmacognosy," *Annals of Medical History*, New Series 1/2 (1929): 198–207; and D. V. S. Reddy, "Garcia da Orta: His Learned Work 'Coloquios dos Simples e Drogas he Cousas Medicinais da India,' the First Medical Book to Be Printed in India, Published in Goa in 1563," *Annals of Medical History*, Third Series 1/6 (1939): 544–545.

worlds, one European, the other Indian. In this light, his *Colóquios* has appeared as a vehicle for the transmission of an Asian, Indian, or otherwise thoroughly indigenous form of curative knowledge.[17]

In this and the next two chapters, I test these claims. I contend that the text was not simply an extension of early modern Portuguese (or more broadly Iberian or European) interests and priorities. Nor was it a vessel for the straightforward communication of South Asian therapeutic expertise. Instead, the *Colóquios* belongs to the bustle, possibility, and uncertainty of life in mid-sixteenth-century Goa – a world rich with commercial and curative possibility but also riven with economic and epidemiological uncertainty.

I argue that the *Colóquios* spoke primarily to the interests and concerns of the Lusophone community of Goa but that it was relevant to Portuguese-speaking traders throughout the Indian Ocean world and beyond.[18] The book was part and parcel of a distinctive culture of natural inquiry that emerged in Goa and that was suffused with the twin concerns of enhancing both personal health and financial wellbeing – of surviving seasonal, torrential storms and profiting from the profusion of tradable nature, both of which, together, characterized Goa.

The imperial interests institutionalized in the Estado da Índia in the form of garrisoned trading outposts spread across the Indian Ocean and island Southeast Asia did pattern Orta's work. In important ways, it responded to the possibilities and limitations of the Estado. It was not however bound by the Estado. The formal networks of Portugal's empire and the networks that sustained Orta's investigative and curative endeavours did not map onto one another. Crown interests and the priorities of the Estado da Índia were not necessarily Orta's interests and priorities. And although his *Colóquios* remains the best-known example of natural inquiry to have come out of Portugal's empire in Asia, Orta was not the first or only Portuguese naturalist to attempt to sort out the cryptic identities, origins, and uses of Asian *naturalia*. Rather, his work built on

[17] Grove, *Green Imperialism*, ch. 2; and Timothy D. Walker, "Acquisition and Circulation of Medical Knowledge within the Early Modern Portuguese Colonial Empire," in *Science in the Spanish and Portuguese Empires*, eds. Daniela Bleichmar, Paula de Vos, Kristin Huffine, and Kevin Sheehan (Stanford, CA: Stanford University Press, 2008), 247–270. For a more detailed exploration of the issue, see Ângela Barreto Xavier and Ines G. Županov, *Catholic Orientalism: Portuguese Empire, Indian Knowledge, 16th to 18th Centuries* (New Delhi: Oxford University Press, 2014).

[18] Palmira Fontes da Costa comes to a similar conclusion in "Geographical expansion and the reconfiguration of medical authority: Garcia de Orta's *Colloquios on the Simples and Drugs of India* (1563)," *Studies in History and Philosophy of Science* 43 (2012): 74–81.

that of others, and especially of two well-connected apothecaries. Their work helped establish a range of questions and answers that would frame Orta's subsequent investigations of nature, and they helped create the imperial geography that Orta would refer to throughout the *Colóquios*.

Orta's predecessors never conceived of their work as addressed to the peculiarities of a globalized inter-tropical environment. Orta would not do so either. To understand Orta's work is to set aside narratives of European transformation and the modernist concerns that anchor them; it is to encounter Goa as Orta did, to peer over his shoulder as he read and wrote, and ultimately to see, feel, touch, and taste the drugs and spices that were the objects of his inquiry.

Before the Portuguese captured Goa in 1510, it was not a particularly notable port of trade. Diu and Cambay lay in Gujarat to Goa's north and formed a commercial axis that linked Malacca in the east to Hormuz and Aden in the west. Calicut and Cochin lay at the heart of the pepper trade on the Malabar Coast to Goa's south. When the Portuguese first sighted its harbors, Goa was a tributary of the sultanate of Bijapur – a principality only recently carved from the larger Bahmani kingdom that ruled over much of the Deccan Plateau. Like their former Bahmani rulers, Yusuf Adil Shah and his successors in Bijapur traced their linguistic, cultural, and intellectual roots to the Persians, Turks, and Arabs across the sea. Bijapur (as would the other sultanates of the Deccan) maintained ties that spanned the Indian Ocean world.[19] In Goa, a small but thriving community of financiers, merchants, and traders – both Hindu and Muslim – carried a brisk maritime trade principally in Arabian horses but also in taffeta and satin woven further inland.[20]

Such a cosmopolitan entrepôt with safe harbors, lucrative commercial ties, and minimal defenses was, from the point of view of Portuguese

[19] Richard M. Eaton, *A Social History of the Deccan, 1300–1761: Eight Indian Lives* (New York: Cambridge University Press, 2005), 33–104; S. M. Ikram, *Muslim Civilization in India* (New York: Columbia University Press, 1964), 107–121; João Manuel Pacheco de Figueiredo, "Goa Pré-Portuguesa," *Studia* 12 (1963): 243–259. The priority given to this inheritance did not go unchallenged. With the disintegration of the Delhi sultanate, the Bahmani kingdom and the smaller principalities that were carved from it sponsored the translation of ancient Sanskrit texts into the local vernacular. And though Persian may have remained for a time the language of the court, the arts and sciences flourished as well in Sanskrit and, in Bijapur, state records were kept in Marathi, the language of the Hindu ministers who produced them. Eaton, *Social History*, 60–61; Ikram, *Muslim Civilization*, 118–119.

[20] Ashin Das Gupta, "Indian Merchants and Trade in the Indian Ocean," in *The World of the Indian Ocean Merchant, 1500–1800* (New Delhi: Oxford University Press, 2001), 59–87; M. N. Pearson, *Merchants and Rulers in Gujarat: The Response to the Portuguese in the Sixteenth Century* (Berkeley, CA: University of California Press, 1976), 7–29; Eaton, *Social History*, 59–60, 74–75.

raiders, an ideal target. On the advice of the Goan privateer and sometime trader Timmayya, the recently-appointed governor of Portuguese Asia, Afonso de Albuquerque, took the city in 1510.[21] In 1515 Goa replaced Cochin as the Asian terminus of the Lisbon voyages, and in 1532 it became the administrative capital of Portugal's thin but sprawling seaborne empire in Asia. The Estado da Índia consisted of factories and defensive fortifications at or near key ports of trade spread from Sofala in East Africa to Macau in southern China. The commercial wealth generated by the Estado substantially underwrote Portugal's entire empire until it was eclipsed by Brazil and the Atlantic in the middle of the next century.[22]

Crown commercial policies in Asia targeted pepper, cinnamon, and a handful of other spices and were initially designed to allow the Portuguese to monopolize access to them and control their distribution westward. In practice – and notwithstanding the tremendous revenue they generated for Portugal's counting house – the results of these policies were decidedly mixed. Control was elusive. Albuquerque and his successors often failed to secure anything more than intermittent seaborne commercial primacy – and that along none but a handful of routes west of Cape Comorin.[23]

As it turned out, exclusive control was not only impossible but unnecessary and even counterproductive. Profitable commerce both for metropolitan Portugal and for private Portuguese and other European traders owed itself to the persistence and vitality of intra-Asian networks of exchange.[24] Albuquerque appreciated that fact even in 1510. Soon

[21] Timmayya's was a strategic move for he was then in the employ of Vijayanagar. On this and for a detailed account of Portugal's empire in Asia, see Bailey W. Diffey and George D. Winius, *Foundations of the Portuguese Empire, 1415–1580* (Minneapolis, MN: University of Minnesota Press, 1977), 250–251.

[22] Some qualification is necessary: Portuguese revenues in Asia derived from both the Estado (which was a vehicle for accumulating commodities in Asia for sale in Europe) and duties and profits from intra-Asian trade. Jorge M. Pedreira, "Costs and Financial Trends, 1415–1822," in Bethencourt and Curto, eds., *Portuguese Oceanic Expansion*, especially 58.

[23] A detailed discussion of Crown policies is of course not my intention, but it should be noted that individual spices were subject to different rules and regulations, all of which changed with time. On the accommodations worked out see Sanjay Subrahmanyam, *The Portuguese Empire in Asia* (New York: Norton, 1993), 66–78; Pearson, *Merchants and Rulers*, 39–56 and 98–99. For a detailed discussion on trade in particular spices see M. A. P. Meilink-Roelofsz, *Asian Trade and European Influence in the Indonesian Archipelago between about 1500 and about 1630* (The Hague: Martinus Nijhoff, 1962).

[24] The effect of Portuguese involvement was not to displace preexisting networks but often to reorient them. Sanjay Subrahmanyam, *The Political Economy of Commerce: Southern India, 1500–1650* (New York: Cambridge University Press, 1990). An alternative perspective is Pearson, *Merchants and Rulers*.

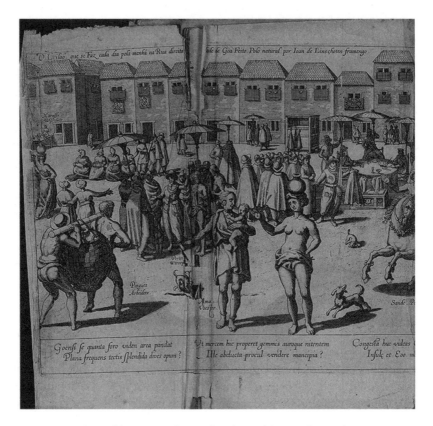

FIGURE 3.2 Assembling Asia. The marketplace of Goa as depicted in Jan Huygen van Linschoten, *Histoire de la navigatione de Jan Huygen van Linschoten aux Indes Orientales* (Amsterdam: Jan Evertz Cloppenburgh, 1619).
Courtesy of the Biblioteca Nacional de Portugal.

after having taken Goa, he marched with interpreters through its streets insisting, "in both Portuguese and in the language of Kanara," that "no merchant, be they foreign or domestic, should leave [but] should open their shops and continue to sell their merchandise in peace."[25]

If Goa was the heart of Portugal's empire in Asia; its lifeblood was the bustling commerce in the products of nature (this corporeal metaphor would be current in Goa by the latter half of the sixteenth century).[26] Along Rua Direita, Goa's bustling main thoroughfare, finely-coiffed

[25] Barros, *Da Ásia*, "Decada Segunda," pt. 1. bk. 5, ch. 3: 465–466.
[26] Souse, *Oriente Conquistado*, vol. 1, 36.

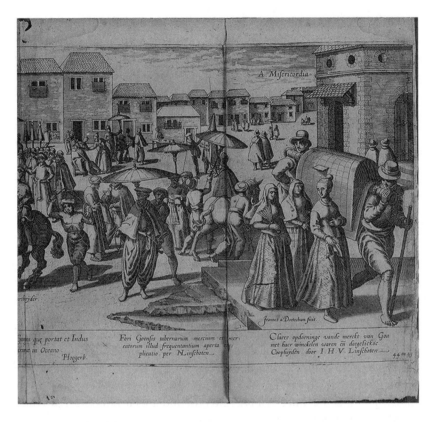

FIGURE 3.2 *(cont.)*

residents surveyed a pageant of fine linens, fruits, roots, leaves, seeds, saps, gums, minerals, and precious stones. Thinly curled sleeves of cinnamon from Ceylon; richly scented cloves from the volcanic soils of Ternate and Tidore; nutmeg and its brilliant red tendrils of mace from the Banda Islands; stacks of white sandalwood from Timor and Makassar; camphor from Borneo; musk from Pegu and northern China; white and black benzoin from Palembang (on Sumatra) and Siam; pearls from Bahrain; diamonds from the Deccan: these were only a fraction of the *naturalia* that were trundled back and forth across Goa's wharves and filled its crowded markets (Figure 3.2).[27]

---

[27] Meilink-Roelofsz, *Asian Trade*. See also A. J. R. Russell-Wood, *The Portuguese Empire, 1415–1808: A World on the Move* (Baltimore, MD: Johns Hopkins University Press, 1992), 126–128.

Abundance, mediated exchange, and the production of wealth were only part of the story. Goa's relationship with the natural world was more troubled – its survival more tenuous – than the history of Portuguese commercial expansion and intra-Asian imperial competition might suggest. What nature gave in abundance it could reclaim in torrential fits and widespread contagion. The environmental and epidemiological consequences of Portuguese colonialism in Goa would prove dramatic.

All seaborne trade across the Indian Ocean was timed to coincide with the Asian monsoons. The dry winds descending from the northeast each winter posed little hazard for Goa as they pushed the spice- and drug-laden Portuguese fleets homeward across the Indian Ocean, past the Cape of Good Hope, and out into the South Atlantic. Trouble came between May and September, when the southwest monsoons carried ships eastward from Africa, the Red Sea, and the Persian Gulf to Gujarat, the Konkan and Malabar Coasts, and Malacca. Inbound fleets faced crippling winds, torrential rains, and thunderous waves in a churning sea. It was one of these storms that split the fleet of 1530, that all but destroyed its lagging vessel, and that drained the life of two colonial officials.

And yet, despite their hazards, monsoons were the chief engines of extended seaborne exchange across Indian Ocean Asia. Pilots of all nations had no choice but to harness their ships to the capricious power of these seasonal storms. For the Portuguese, the eastward crossing was a source of immense uncertainty. Entry of Indian harbors was carefully timed with the end of the monsoons – and with little room for error. The force of mid-season gales was so great that it threatened to drive ships aground; crossing too late in the season or too cautiously risked losing the wind altogether and foundering in a listless sea.

For the passengers and crew who lived to see Goa (and in some years perhaps only half of them did[28]), they would have recognized in the city itself something of the storm-stricken ship that had brought them there. The summer monsoons beat upon the whitewashed walls of Goa's convents, colleges, and churches so violently that façades were shorn of paint and left raw in their wake.[29] When Goa's swollen rivers overflowed, whole parts of the city flooded. Water rushed into the streets, pooled,

---

[28] M. N. Pearson, *The Portuguese in India* (New York: Cambridge University Press, 1987), 93.

[29] Heldar Carita, *Palácios de Goa*, 2nd ed. (Lisbon: Quetzal Editores, 1996), 52–53; and Heta Pandit, *Hidden Hands: Masters Builders of Goa* (Goa: Heritage Network, 2003), 7–12, 35–39, 85–94.

and made even main thoroughfares impassable.[30] New arrivals, sick and dying, crowded into Goa's hospitals. The substantial medical infrastructure of Portugal's Asian capital – by 1550, Goa had no fewer than four hospitals[31] – swelled to capacity and then burst. The city's narrow alleys became makeshift shelters – the dank and fetid abode of last resort for many Portuguese immigrants. The vast majority of Portuguese and other Catholics who came to Goa were poor men, often single, and when the time came they would be summoned to join one of the royal garrisons that helped make up the Estado da Índia or serve aboard Portuguese fighting ships. Until then – and apart from the royal hospital meant to keep them alive – there were no formal arrangements to feed and house them. Many deserted.

Humanity itself flooded seasonally into and out of the capital of Portuguese Asia. In 1540, Goa had an urban population of around twenty thousand residents. By 1580 that number had nearly tripled. As many as two thousand Portuguese left Iberia each year to cast their lot with the trade in Asia. But, like so many ailing mariners, many refused to stay. The combination of intermarriage (which Albuquerque had originally encouraged) and the prospects of lucrative private trade (which lured so many Portuguese in the first place) brought migrants to other ports, often in the Bay of Bengal. By 1600, tens of thousands of Portuguese and other Europeans had disembarked in Goa and spread across the Indian Ocean world.[32] A diaspora of European traders took shape beyond Goa's

---

[30] Boxer, *Portuguese Seaborne Empire*, 297–298.

[31] These were the *Hospital Real* founded by Afonso de Albuquerque in 1511 (run by the Jesuits beginning in 1579 as the *Hospital do Espírito Santo* and, after their expulsion in 1759, run by the colonial state under the name *Hospital Real Militar*); the *Hospital da Misericórdia* (also referred to as the *Hospital de Todos-os-Santos*), which had opened by 1526 and was intended to serve the poor; the *Hospital de São Lazaro* (a leprosarium), which was in existence by 1530; and the Jesuit-run hospital for the poor, the *Hospital dos Pobres* that had opened by 1546. Significantly, by the 1631, at least one other hospital, the *Hospital da Nossa Senora da Piedade* (also run by the Misericórdia) was in operation. The relevant literature here tends to be synoptic and somewhat cursory rather than extensive and detailed, and, because of periodic changes in the names and administration of these institutions, conflicting accounts abound. Compare, for example, Fátima da Silva Gracias, *Health and Hygiene in Colonial Goa, 1510–1961* (New Delhi: Concept Publishing, 1994), 118–138; and Timothy D. Walker "Stocking Colonial Pharmacies: Commerce in South Asian Indigenous Medicines from Their Native Sources in the Portuguese Estado da Índia," in *Networks in the First Global Age, 1400–1800*, ed. Rila Mukherjee (New Delhi: Primus Books, 2011), 113–136.

[32] Malyn Newitt, *A History of Portuguese Overseas Expansion, 1400–1668* (New York: Routledge, 2005), 108; Pearson, *Portuguese in India*, 93 and 134–137. Pearson notes that Goa was a medium sized city at best by Asian standards.

legal and ecclesiastical reach. For the Éstado, the seasonal ebb and flow of Catholic migrants compounded a persistent shortage of personnel.[33]

Goa in autumn was damp, crowded, diseased, and unstable. Fevers and dysentery were endemic when the Portuguese took the city in 1510.[34] Albuquerque wrote to Manuel I to urge caution in the region, warning him that a year in Goa consumed "between six and seven hundred men ... [who] die of illness" (*doenças*). In hindsight, that was probably a fair estimate. Near the end of the century in the 1580s, Jan Huyghen van Linschoten (initially, in 1583, in the employ of the new Archbishop of Goa) offered a similar figure of five hundred men annually.[35] As the sixteenth century wore on, the health of Goa worsened. The numbers of dead recorded by Goa's Royal Hospital early the next century increased to over eight hundred men per year.[36] Not even the highest ranks of Portuguese colonial officialdom were safe. Afonso de Albuquerque succumbed to dysentery near the end of his governorship in the fall of 1515; nine years later fever claimed the life of Vasco da Gama, the Portuguese "discoverer" who had returned to fill his tenure as viceroy.[37]

An epidemic of dysentery swept through the city as early as 1536.[38] But it was in the 1540s, with successive waves of Portuguese settlement, and as Goa's epidemiological landscape was transformed, that yearly epidemics grew noticeably worse. In 1543, a plague of deadly diarrhea

[33] Ficalho, *Garcia da Orta*, 151–153; C. R. Boxer, *The Portuguese Seaborne Empire, 1415–1825* (New York: Alfred A. Knopf, 1969), 297–298; Timothy J. Coates, *Convicts and Orphans: Forced and State-Sponsored Colonizers in the Portuguese Empire, 1550–1755* (Stanford, CA: Stanford University Press, 2001), 87–90. The Bay of Bengal became a veritable haven for renegades. See Sanjay Subrahmanyam, *Improvising Empire: Portuguese Trade and Settlement in the Bay of Bengal, 1500–1700* (Delhi: Oxford University Press, 1990).

[34] M. N. Pearson, "First Contacts between Indian and European Medical Systems: Goa in the Sixteenth Century," in *Warm Climates and Western Medicine*, ed. Arnold, 23–24; and Vítor de Albuquerque Freire da Silva, "O Hospital Real de Goa (1510–1610): Contribuição para o estudo da sua história e regimentos" (MA thesis, University of Lisbon, 1997), vol. 1, 92–96.

[35] Bulhão Pato, *Cartas de Afonso de Albuqerque seguidas de documentos que as elucidam* (Lisbon: Acadêmia Real das Ciências, 1898), vol. 2, 37; Jan Huygen van Linschoten, *The Voyages of John Huyghen van Linschoten to the East Indies*, 2 vols., eds. Arthur Coke Burnell and P. A. Tiele (London: Hakluyt Society, 1885), vol. 1, 237.

[36] Pearson, *Portuguese in India*, 93, notes that losses between 1604 and 1634 as recorded in the hospital records amounted to 25,000 men, or just over 833 fatalities per year.

[37] Correia, *Lendas*, vol. 2, 452–453. On da Gama's death and afterlives see Subrahmanyam, *The Career and Legend of Vasco da Gama* (New York: Cambridge University Press, 1997).

[38] Correia, *Lendas*, vol. 3, 703.

and fever – what may have been Portuguese Goa's first cholera epidemic – swept through the city. Orta called it "colerica passio," as it seemed the body was besieged by an excess or corruption of yellow bile (choler).[39]

Colerica passio was (and modern cholera remains) a swift killer.[40] So dire was the situation in the autumn of that year that Governor Sousa refused to allow the tolling of church bells to honor the dead: such frequent soundings would, he feared, turn anguish into panic and lead to rebellion.[41] Caught between the sea, the inland sierra, and the seasonal monsoons – on spits of land that only the might of a god could reclaim from the rush of coastal waters – Goa teetered precariously on the edge of debacle. By the 1560s, a seasonal pattern in the city's afflictions had become apparent: fevers struck in May and June before the inundating summer monsoons; dysenteries arrived each year in their wake, usually in October and November.[42] By the end of the century, these would be taken as the signal diseases of Portuguese Asia.[43]

FLUVIAL DISARRAY, MEDICAL EMERGENCY

Environmental and epidemiological transformations in Goa exacerbated these ills. But pervasive and recurrent illness did not prompt the kind confusion and speculation it had in West Africa. It did not lead to sweeping claims about the ill-health of the entire South Asian littoral, and it certainly did not give rise to claims of intertropical coherence.[44]

---

[39] Orta, *Colóquios*, vol. 1, 255, 261.

[40] Andrew S. Azman, Kara E. Rudolph, Derek A. T. Cummings, and Justin Lessler, "The incubation period of cholera: A systematic review," *Journal of Infection* 66 (2013): 432–438.

[41] Correia, *Lendas*, vol. 4, 288–289.

[42] Sousa, *Oriente Conquistado*, vol. 1, 39; Correia, *Lendas*, vol. 2, 453, states that a most common time to die was in the weeks just following the summer monsoons. This remains the pattern for seasonal shifts in malaria and cholera incidence in southern India; Mosquitos hatch over the late spring and summer before the arrival of the monsoons; while in the fall flood waters continue to pose challenges to sanitation efforts, circulating intestinal pathogens whose concentration in still water (pools, ponds, and tanks) grows as water evaporates. See Surinder M. Bhardwaj, "Disease Ecologies of South Asia," in *The Cambridge World History of Human Disease*, ed. Kenneth F. Kiple (New York: Cambridge University Press, 1993), 642–649.

[43] Linschoten, *Voyages*, vol. 1, 232–241.

[44] In fact, however, they did inspire often favorable comparisons with other locations in the empire. Sousa, *Oriente Conquistado*, vol. 1, 37–38, 838–841; *DI*, vol. 4, 703–705; Duarte Barbosa, *O Livro de Duarte Barbosa. Edição Crítica e Anotada*, 2 vols., ed. Maria Augusta da Veiga e Sousa (Lisbon: Instituto de Investigação Científica Tropical

Explanations for disease were rooted in the particulars of life in Goa, in local environmental factors, or in the regional monsoons.

Clergy and occasional European visitors would blame what they saw as the spiritual apathy and moral turpitude that were a consequence of Goa's commercial success. As one member of the Company of Jesus put it, "the greed of Goa increases in proportion to its wealth."[45] To those who were inclined to see them, symptoms of generalized moral failing were pervasive; observers pointed to the filth of the Konkani villagers, the seductions of single women (a story I take up in Chapter 5), and the tyranny of wealthy men over household servants and slaves.[46]

When it came to more material causes for what observers referred to as the "putrefaction" of the generally healthy air of Goa and of the Malabar Coast further south,[47] dead elephants were a favored culprit. Around midcentury, one of these hulking beasts had inconveniently managed to end its life in a lake in the province of Carambolim, just outside of Goa, corrupting the air and spreading putrescence into the heart of the city.[48]

Yet both of those lines of reasoning overlooked more fundamental changes to the colonial landscape. Disease environments are never static or inherent in a place itself but instead shift in time with changes in demography, culture, and politics. Although most environmental histories of European colonialism in the sixteenth century focus on the Americas,[49] the case of Goa suggests important Asian parallels. Whether or not the bloated corpse of a decaying pachyderm ever sank into the mud of a shallow lake on the outskirts of the city, the account of contamination in Carambolim is a clue to the ways that Portuguese colonialism in Goa led to fluvial disarray and medical emergency.

---

and the Comissão Nacional para as Comemorações dos Descobrimentos Portugueses, 1996), vol. 1, 92–100 and vol. 2, 391–393.

[45] Sousa, *Oriente Conquistado*, vol. 1, 43.

[46] José Wicki, "Duas relações sobre a situação da Índia portuguesa nos anos 1568 e 1569," *Studia* 8 (1961): 133–220; Ines G. Županov, "Drugs, health, bodies, and souls in the tropics: Medical experiments in sixteenth-century Portuguese India," *Indian Economic and Social History Review* 39 (2002): 1–43. Subrahmanyam, *Portuguese Empire*, ch. 4, cautions against an easy reading of the decline literature as a reflection of clerical anxieties rather than historical circumstances.

[47] Sousa, *Oriente Conquistado*, vol. 1, 838–841; Barbosa, *Livro de Duarte Barbosa*, vol. 2, 19–27, 51–55, 238–243, 278–295, and 391–393.

[48] Sousa, *Oriente Conquistado*, vol. 1, 39; Orta, *Colóquios*, vol. 1, 306–308.

[49] An exception is Faria, "Understanding Pangim," which focuses on the early seventeenth century.

The province of Carambolim was flanked on all sides by water and was filled with streams and pools of countless shapes and sizes. The lake in question could have been any number of these. According to the Jesuit chronicler Francisco de Sousa, the body of water in question was larger than most and lay just beyond the neighbourhood of Trindade. And, indeed, the feature must have been hard for any visitor to miss, for just such a lake in precisely that location appeared on countless sixteenth and seventeenth century maps of the city. In what is perhaps the best known of these – the late-sixteenth-century chorographic engraving from the Latin edition of Linschoten's *Itinerary* – the anonymous hydrographic entity looms over Goa, above and slightly to the left of the city center. It is labeled simply "the lake" (*a lagoa*) (Figure 3.3).

An enclosed body of water it was, but this was not a lake at all. It was a massive (and in this case largely natural) irrigation tank.[50] On closer inspection, the Linschoten illustration suggests as much. The hatching along the upper left edge, indicating an embankment, hints at the engineered character of the landscape. The reservoir was fed by a rivulet that the Portuguese referred to as the Rio de Santiago. Like so many other such reservoirs in the area, the one in Carambolim was managed by the *gauncars* of the province.[51] These high-caste village leaders were responsible for everything from paying taxes to maintain the temples and shrines of Carambolim's families. Supervising the reservoir and the agriculture it supported was an extension of those duties.[52]

Far from a marginal province (and quite apart from its tank), Carambolim was well known to Portuguese officials, and especially to Jesuits like the chronicler Sousa. The populous and fertile region sat upland from Goa, at the top of a gentle slope, in a shallow depression where a small valley narrows among low rising hills. The landscape here was ideal for a defensive fortification, which is just what Afonso de Albuquerque

---

[50] Today the northernmost remnant of it is known as Carambolim Lake.

[51] Carambolim and its "lake," were referenced repeatedly in both contemporary Portuguese and Konkani sources as a concern. See Gajanana Shantaram Sinai Ghantkar, *History of Goa through Gōykanadi Script* (Panaji: Prabhakar Bhide and Rajhauns Vitaran, 1993); and the documents collected in Boies Penrose, *Goa – Rainha do Oreinte* (Lisbon: Comissão Ultramarina, 1960).

[52] João Manuel Pacheco de Figueiredo, "Goa Pré-Portuguesa," *Studia*, 13/14 (1964): 107–117. On reservoirs and other regional waterworks see Kathleen D. Morrison, *Daroji Valley: Landscape History, Place, and the Making of a Dryland Reservoir* (New Delhi: Manohar, 2009), ch. 4; and M. A. Nayeem, *The Heritage of the Adil Shahis of Bijapur* (Hyderabad: Hyderabad Publishers, 2008), 227, 248–250.

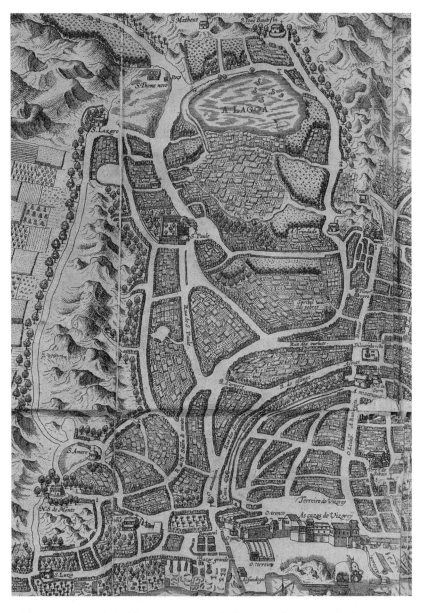

FIGURE 3.3 A Colonial Landscape. Detail of Goa and its environs from Jan
Huygen van Linschoten, Tertia pars Indiae Orientalis (Frankfurt: Matthias
Becker, 1601).
Courtesy of the Beinecke Rare Book and Manuscript Library, Yale University.

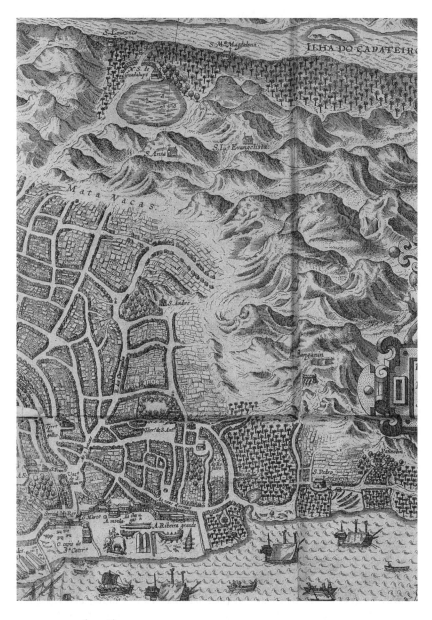

FIGURE 3.3 *(cont.)*

required be built there.[53] At the beginning of the 1540s, the size and wealth of Carambolim made it a target for the evangelical efforts of emboldened Catholic authorities. Carambolim had the largest Hindu temple on the island and, according to the Jesuit Luís Fróis, was "the largest and most noble *povoação* ... outside of the city [of Goa] itself."[54] In 1541, Goa's Vicar General Miguel Vaz ordered the temple destroyed and promptly replaced it with the church of São João Bautista (which Linschoten's engraver depicted just above the tank). Even so, by the end of 1559, Jesuit conversion campaigns had borne little fruit. "There was," by one estimate, "almost no one" among the villagers who had joined the Catholic fold.[55]

That did not, however, mean that missionary action and the destruction of their temples was having no effect at all on the people who lived in Carambolim. Quite the opposite: villagers were not converting, they were leaving. An exchange recorded by Jesuits there in 1560 explains why. That year, decades of evangelical activity and gradual depopulation culminated in a meeting of the remaining gauncars. At issue was whether they should collectively relocate the remaining communities to the region south of Goa, which was still part of Bijapur and where they hoped more tolerant Muslim rule might shield them from Jesuit incursions, or whether they should remain in Goa and submit to Jesuit tutelage. One of these gauncars – unnamed in the Jesuit source – cast his vote "to leave for the mainland with our families," in the belief that "it would be better to lose our property than to lose our souls [by converting to Catholicism]." Fourteen gauncars ultimately cast their lot with the Jesuits. An unknown number did not.[56]

Stark choices by Carambolim's gauncars about the moral and political fates of their communities bore directly on the health of Goa. For

[53] Barros, *Da Ásia*, "Decada Segunda," pt. 1, bk. 5, ch. 4; and [Anonymous], "Livro das Cidades, e Fortalezas, que a Coroa de Portugal tem nas Partes da Índia, e das Capitanias, e mais Cargos que Nelas ha e da Importancia Delles," *Studia* 6 (1960): 15–16.

[54] *DI*, vol. 4, 657.

[55] And, when they finally managed to recruit them, they never numbered more than "600 souls." *DI*, vol. 4, 645, n. 6, and 703. These and other tensions surrounding conversion are compellingly explored in Rowena Robinson, "Some Neglected Aspects of the Conversion of Goa: A Socio-Historical Perspective," in *Sociology of Religion in India*, ed. Rowena Robinson (New Delhi: Sage, 2004), 177–198.

[56] *DI*, vol. 4, 658–659. As Robinson, "Some Neglected Aspects," shows, it was a false choice as submission entailed embracing new inheritance laws that could lead to the dismemberment of village lands anyway, which was one reason some gauncars were angling to leave.

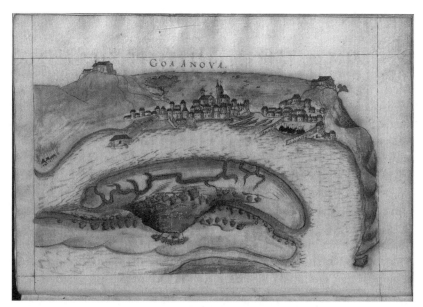

FIGURE 3.4 A Colonial Waterscape. The "lake" of Carambolim (above and to the left of Goa) as sketched by the Portuguese viceroy João de Castro. Courtesy of the Biblioteca Nacional de Portugal.

depopulation had left the reservoir in a state of disrepair. Here and perhaps elsewhere, colonization displaced Konkani communities whose wet-rice agriculture capitalized on the seasonal flooding caused by the summer monsoons. Village-based systems of tanks and irrigation works had begun to fail. In the wake of the monsoons, the "lake" had begun to overflow its embankment. On these occasions the road linking upland Carambolim with the city below could become a veritable river. That is precisely how it appeared in a sketch by D. João de Castro after he arrived in Goa in September of 1545 – just as that year's monsoon had begun to ebb and hence just as inland water levels would have been at their height (Figure 3.4).

When, early in the next century, Pedro de Resende depicted Goa for António Bocarro's survey of the Estado, the reservoir resembled not a confined lake but a sprawling canal that stretched far beyond the area of Trindade, narrowing as it came to within blocks of the dense Portuguese quarter, threatening even the chambers of the Misericôrdia.[57]

---

[57] António Bocarro, *O livro das plantas de todas as fortalezas, cidades, e povoações do Estado da Índia oriental*, 2 vols., ed. Isabel Cid (Lisbon: Casa da Moeda, 1992 [1635]).

PARTIAL PERSPECTIVES

The arrival of João de Castro in 1545 signalled the end of Martim Afonso's gubernatorial tenure (Castro replaced him and governed as viceroy of the Estado from 1545 to 1548). The years in which Martim Afonso governed were marked by more than just Konkani dissent, urban floods, and sweeping outbreaks of fever and dysentery. They coincided as well with the first years of a decade that was economically precarious not only for Goa but for the Estado da Índia more generally, as well as for private Portuguese traders throughout Indian Ocean Asia. In the early 1540s, famine had begun to plague the area stretching from the Red Sea to the Deccan. According to the chronicler Gaspar Correia, the situation in Coromandel was so dire that "almost the entire land was depopulated," while in the major Arabian ports, the cost of the rice staple jumped.[58] This shortfall was part and parcel of a broader economic downturn that embraced the entire region. No matter the reach, it dealt a severe blow to the economy of the Estado. Duties from two of its most important customs houses, Hormuz and Malacca, began to slacken in 1540, declined precipitously at mid-decade, and remained low as late as 1550.

To Sousa, an ambitious member of the service nobility who had helped salvage Portugal's Atlantic economy (his brother, Tomé de Sousa, soon to be Brazil's first governor), there was little time to waste. In one account, no sooner had he arrived in May of 1542 than he "ejected [his predecessor, D. Estêvão da Gama,] from his bed, without even allowing him time to don his shirt."[59] As it turned out, Sousa's policies would prove incendiary. His silencing of Goa's church bells and his fear of rebellion in the midst of an epidemic may have been rooted in matters not entirely medical.

During his three-year term, Sousa launched a series of controversial measures, which, if intended to make up for diminishing returns on trade duties, fell short of the mark. These included a stopgap effort to raid a Hindu temple in Kerala and the launch of an ill-fated expedition to the mythical "Island of Gold" (Ilha do Ouro), then believed to lie somewhere in the vicinity of Sumatra. The governor also instigated a series of attacks against the Mappilas – Malabari Muslim converts resident in Cannanore

---

[58] Correia, *Lendas*, vol. 4, 131–132; quoted in Subrahmanyam, *Portuguese Empire*, 94. But see also Ibid., *Portuguese Empire*, 92–96.

[59] Quoted from a contemporary source in Subrahmanyam, *Portuguese Empire*, 92.

and Cochin. The move abrogated a recent peace settlement and upset the thriving commerce between the Mappilas and many private Portuguese traders, *casados*, living up and down the Malabar Coast. Casados, many of whom came out to the Estado as unwed soldiers, had married and formed the core of a settled Portuguese presence in Goa, where they enjoyed privileges and protections as subjects of the Crown. Some of the most prosperous among them filled the ranks of Goa's municipal council, the *senado da câmara*, and of the prestigious lay brotherhood, the *Santa Casa da Misericórdia*. Through these two institutions, they dominated the local political affairs of Portuguese Goa. The casados, however, depended for their livelihood on commerce not plunder and Sousa's actions strained the very delicate relations upon which that trade depended. Many among the settled Portuguese community, moreover, saw Sousa's use of gubernatorial privilege as an abuse of power. The post of governor entailed the rights to a number of discretionary trading voyages. Sousa took full advantage of these but used his beneficence to reward them to none but a small coterie of family, friends, and allies. As if such exclusionary granting of privileges were not enough, he also used these voyages to gain access to spices, lac, and pepper in the Bay of Bengal – by now largely the de facto preserve of the casados. That, in particular, was an unpardonable offense. Contemporaries would remember Sousa as arrogant, corrupt, and unyielding and they complained about him bitterly – but often anonymously – in letters to Dom João III.[60]

Sousa may have incited particular hostility among casados, but rancor between casados and colonial officials was a permanent feature of the Estado.[61] The circumstances that greeted Sousa in 1542, and many of the tensions that began to mount soon thereafter, were not of his making

---

[60] Subrahmanyam, *Portuguese Empire*, 91–95.

[61] This division has continued to frame synthetic analyses of Portugal's empire in Asia since Boxer's foundational *Portuguese Seaborne Empire* and can be found in Pearson, *The Portuguese in India*; Subrahmanyam, *Portuguese Empire*; and Malyn Newitt, *Portuguese Overseas Expansion*. It should not, however, be drawn too firmly. Discord among officials and *casados* was as common as concerted action between them in pursuit of mutual interests. In the case of Goa and the western Indian littoral, see M. N. Pearson, *Coastal Western India: Studies from the Portuguese Records* (New Delhi: Concept Publishing Company, 1981), especially ch. 3 on "The Crowd in Portuguese India," 41–66; Isabel dos Guimarães Sá, *Quando o rico se faz pobre: misericórdias, caridade e poder no Império Português, 1500–1800* (Lisbon: Comissão Nacional para as Comemoracões dos Descobrimentos Portugueses, 1997); and the essays in Sanjay Subrahmanyam, ed., *Sinners and Saints: The Successors of Vasco da Gama* (Delhi: Oxford University Press, 1998).

alone. In terms of both its food supply and its finances, Goa met the economic straits of the 1540s with a resource deficit of its own. The gradual decay of Konkani rice fields and irrigation works – an upshot of Jesuit conversion campaigns and the relocation of Konkani peasants – caused not only flooding but put the staple in even shorter supply. And that put the Portuguese enclave increasingly at the mercy of its neighbours for rice imports.[62]

Goa's financial situation, meanwhile, mirrored that of the Estado. Formal transfer of the seat of colonial government from Cochin to Goa had taken place only ten years earlier, in 1532. By the time Sousa took charge, Goa's was the principal customs house for all of Portuguese Asia. Most of its revenue came from policing the seaboard, often forcing Indian shippers into port to pay duties. Law enforcement required ships, sailors, and supplies, as well as the constant re-provisioning of Goa's royal hospital – which not only tended to the needs of seamen and soldiers in the service of the Crown but coordinated the provision of *materia medica* to the city's other hospitals.[63] All of that, in turn, required resources that Goa – an island – could not raise by itself. The city needed a hinterland. Officials had had their eyes on the southerly, mainland province of Salsete, with its lush, fertile fields and abundant coconut palms – "the principal drug of that land" according to the Jesuit Francisco de Sousa – since 1510.[64] Whatever its precise boundaries were to be, a hinterland was essential for defence, the collection of rents, the shoring up Goa's food supply, and the harvest of medicine and raw materials (including timber for Goa's dockyards) and for the continued recruitment of a soldiery. Such a hinterland was not secured until 1545, when negotiations with the Bijapuri sultan Ibrahim Adil Shah gave the Portuguese lasting control over the neighbouring mainland territories of both Salsete and Bardes.[65]

So in 1543, when the bells of its cathedral fell silent, Goa was caught in something of a double bind – one financial, the other epidemiological. Financially the Portuguese were affected at two levels: the resources of the imperial state were strained but so too were those of Goa and its casados.

[62] Such as the traders at Basrur on the Kanara Coast south of Goa. See Subrahmanyam, *Political Economy*, 260–262.
[63] Walker, "Stocking Colonial Pharmacies."
[64] Barros, *Da Ásia*, "Decada Segunda," pt. 1, bk. 5, ch. 4; Sousa, *Oriente Conquistado*, 162–169.
[65] Newitt, *Portuguese Overseas Expansion*, 108–109. He reports that Goa's customs house accounted for a full 63 percent of the capital's revenue.

The epidemiological situation was, in part, an inescapable aspect of life in the area. But the demographic, hydrographic, and architectural shifts wrought by Portuguese settlement, together with the decline of wet-rice agricultural, exacerbated the threat of both hunger and disease. For Portuguese Goa to survive and remain profitable, its residents had to reckon with the natural world in a way that went beyond commerce – the buying and selling of pepper and spices – to attend to the management of health and hence to wield the curative power of nature.

Of course, it was during Sousa's tumultuous governorship, that Orta served his first term as physician-general. It was in the face of seasonal floods and crippling disease, economic uncertainty and financial decay, that Orta had formal responsibility for the health and wellbeing of Goa's inhabitants. Orta's investigative focus – on medicine and health as much as on trade routes and commerce – reflected the view from Goa. In this, the *Colóquios* amounted to a colonial perspective. But there were other points of view and alternate ways to balance the health of the colony and the wealth of the empire.

From the perspective of Lisbon, these problems looked somewhat different. Manuel I (1495–1521) and his successor João III (1521–1557) were more interested in a list of saleable commodities than in a compendium of sundry medicinal goods. Rather than a catalogue of *materia medica*, they sought and secured inventories of a narrow range of Asian plants, their origins, uses and prospective commercial values. For their own view of the imperial predicament, officials in Lisbon did not need reports from Goa. They had to look no further than the *terreiro do paço*, the royal courtyard that lay along the Tagus River. There, on the palace grounds in the middle of Lisbon was the Casa da Índia. The imperial institution presided over the city's wharves, receiving cargos from Portuguese ships newly returned from Cochin and later from Goa.

In the spring of 1519, in a fleet dispatched from Asia by the outgoing viceroy, Lopo Soares de Albergaria, came a cargo of cinnamon. The year before, Albergaria had managed to set up a fortified factory at Colombo. It was the first royal factory on Ceylon and this shipment of cinnamon was the first to be loaded and shipped by the Portuguese themselves directly from the island rather than purchased from middlemen on the Malabar Coast. The problem was that the Portuguese in Ceylon had little sense of what, exactly they were taking on. What were supposed to be the fine, aromatic, brown shavings bound for kitchens and apothecary cabinets in Lisbon, Seville, Antwerp and beyond, turned out to be but a worthless simulacrum of the real thing. Officers at the Casa da

Índia set the unidentifiable dregs ablaze.[66] Crown revenue literally went up in smoke. In fact, the burning of spices by officials at the Casa da Índia had become something of a seasonal ritual. The Portuguese humanist Damião de Góis, who spent part of his childhood in the royal household in these years, recalled near the end of his life the frequent sight and smell of these episodes as they played out in the imperial capital.[67]

Such scenes were the costly consequence of an unresolved problem of knowledge. And it was just such a problem of knowledge that affected trade in the Crown's most important commodity: pepper. Of the tiny dried berries that did more than any other product of nature (until sugar) to enrich royal coffers – there was immense confusion. Did black and white pepper come from the same plant? Were they of equal quality? Might one be sold more profitably than the other? Crown ministers and metropolitan apothecaries could only speculate – which they did with guidance from ancient and medieval authorities like Dioscorides and Isidore of Seville.[68] Yet even decades after the Portuguese first arrived in South Asia, Crown-appointed governors in Goa were still trying to puzzle out answers to these questions.

The problem of even definitively identifying – let alone acquiring – such valuables as cinnamon and pepper illustrates the distance – intellectual, even epistemic, no less than geographic – that separated European buyers and consumers from the Asian flora they so desired. Gathering specimens of nature from their source, it turned out, was different than acquiring them on the *praças* of Lisbon or even on the market in Cochin. The two endeavors, acquiring at the source and purchasing at the market, each required a different kind of knowledge. At the source it was not only a matter of discerning the fresh from the stale or spoiled. What was required was knowledge sufficient to allow a discerning buyer to distinguish between the thing itself and everything else that might look similar

---

[66] The document bearing the title "Emformação que me dey symão allũez buticayro mor del Rey noso sõr do naçymento de todelas droguas que vão pera o Reyno o quoal ha XXXIX anos q serue nestas partes da Imdia seu o ficio home gramdemente curyoso destas cousas" was first transcribed by Jaime Walter, "Simão Alvares e o seu rol das drogas da Índia," *Studia* 10 (1962): 136–149. Henceforth Walter, "Simão Alvares."

[67] Aubrey F. G. Bell, "Damião de Góis, a Portuguese Humanist," *Hispanic Review* 9 (1941): 244. Góis was a page between 1511 and 1523, at which time he left to serve João III at Portugal's factory in Antwerp.

[68] Stefan Halikowski-Smith, "Perceptions of Nature in Early Modern Portuguese India," *Itinerario* 31 (2007): 17–49.

(as with cinnamon), or the ability to identify a single thing even when it might be traded in multiple forms (as with pepper).

Imperial fortunes in Asia hung on answers to these kinds of questions, and yet it was precisely these kinds of questions that the institutions that constituted Portugal's empire in Asia were distinctly ill-suited to answer. The problem was the highly circumscribed character of the empire itself and its singularly commercial orientation. The predicament of metropolitan officials in the Casa da Índia and advisors to the Crown, no less than to newly-appointed officials in Goa, was that Portugal's network of garrisoned ports – the hallmark of the Estado begun by Albuquerque – was a purpose-built and distinctly coastal system. It was engineered to control maritime trade not to facilitate the investigation of nature. Small contingents of imperial officials generated records that could tell where, in what volume, and for what price the things of nature moved from point to coastal point. Once the vast Asian continental interior was in question, however, the imperial system had little to offer.

What the Crown and its agents needed was an inventory of nature that could make their Asian empire legible so that what was known among those Portuguese with long experience in Asia was known equally well not only to Crown-appointed officials in Goa but also to the Portuguese king and his advisors in Lisbon. And to do that they needed someone who could work at the margins of the official system in order to generate knowledge of the world beyond it. Properly undertaken, the project would render plants and information about them communicable across regions where the Portuguese settled, worked, and traded, and therefore also fell ill and healed, or died. It would make the names of things in Lisbon correspond to the names of things in Goa, Diu, and beyond – wherever the networks of the Portuguese empire stretched. This was not a project to turn what is often termed "local knowledge" into "global knowledge" but to convert local names in Malabar, Gujarat, or the Deccan into the local names known among the Portuguese, be they in Malacca, Mozambique, Bahia, or Pernambuco.[69]

Though propelled by the circumstances in Goa, Orta's *Colóquios* would enact just such a translation. Orta used the contacts enabled by the Portuguese empire to enhance not its grasp but its intellectual reach. In this, he was not alone. In fact, much of that work had already been done. Beginning in 1515, the Crown had begun to seek out expertise on matters

---

[69] Latour, *Science in Action*, especially 157–215; Raj, *Relocating Modern Science*; Roberts, "Situating Science."

of marketable nature and, when it did so, it turned not to physicians like
Orta but to the apothecaries Tomé Pires and Simão Álvares. Pires and
Álvares were part of the first generation of medical specialists to inhabit
the multiplying minor medical posts that helped constitute the empire. In
that way, they were among its commonest agents. They inventoried Asian
nature long before the *Colóquios* was ever printed. Both apothecaries
wrote in direct response to itemized inquiries from the Crown and the
Casa da Índia. Pires compiled a list of profitably traded drugs, spices, and
other natural commodities for Manuel I in 1516. Álvares sent a similar
list to João III in 1548. It was Álvares, not Orta, who resolved the
confusion over cinnamon and it was Álvares, too, who would debate
Orta on the true identity of pepper. Yet, unlike Orta, their positions
within – and apparent dependence upon – royal patronage deeply influenced the substance of their work, which reflected an almost single-
minded preoccupation with metropolitan wealth rather than the health
of colonial Goa. Their lists focused almost exclusively on the names,
descriptions, and origins of various plants, whose medicinal qualities
generally went unnoted.[70]

CARTOGRAPHIES OF NATURAL HISTORY

Those two lists – by Pires in 1516 and by Álvares in 1548 – were
foundational in the construction of an imperial archive of natural history.
Because they were written in response to formal inquiries, they are clues
not only to what officials did and did not yet know about their far-flung
trading empire, but also to what official did and did not think was worth
knowing. Because they were separated by some three decades, they are a
fair index of how those things changed over time in the years preceding
Orta's work. They reveal some of the techniques by which the natural
world of Indian Ocean Asia was rendered legible well before Orta
attempted to do so. And their work set precedents for Orta's own. Their
lists of drugs from India grappled with some of the questions about both
epistemology and plant identities that Orta would have to take up later in
the *Colóquios*. Problems that they seemed to have settled Orta could often
leave aside; questions they left open Orta would attempt to resolve.

---

[70] ANTT, CC, pt. 1, mç. 19, n. 102, f. 4. Based on evidence from a later period, Walker,
"Stocking Colonial Pharmacies," suggests this was a much broader and longer-lived
pattern.

Pires and Álvares also helped to craft a new cartographic imagination. Their lists were at once inventories of Asian nature and guides to Asian geography. It was not an accident. To render accounts of nature authored in Goa intelligible to readers in faraway Lisbon, Pires and Álvares both found that they had to make Asia visible for metropolitan officials who would rarely see it for themselves. Their inventories of Asian drugs helped to consolidate a lexicon of place names, a set of spatial relationships, and a distribution of both human communities and profitably traded nature that would constitute a shared knowledge about the Indian Ocean world. Their investigative and literary labour conjured in words a geography that maps had yet scarcely managed to do. Portugal's empire in Asia depended on a vision that situated the Estado da Índia within an emerging metropolitan vision of nature globally – a cartographic vision recognizable to private traders, royal factors, and Crown advisors alike. This, too, was Orta's inheritance.

Pires sailed east with impeccable connections both to the royal household of Manuel I and the Casa da Índia. He and D. Manuel had grown up together. His father had been the private apothecary of D. Manuel's predecessor, João II, and Pires himself had worked in the same capacity for D. Manuel's son and successor, the future João III. With the support of Jorge de Vasconcellos, then a minister of the Casa da Índia, and with the encouragement of Manuel I's personal physician, one Diogo Lopes, the king dispatched Pires to Cochin, where he arrived in 1512 with a letter in hand, appointing him to the first factorship available. Albuquerque dispatched him immediately to Malacca, then the recently acquired redoubt on what was, for the Portuguese, the very edge of the known world. There, between 1512 and 1516, Pires spent three productive years.[71] After his arrival, D. Manuel addressed to him a letter asking for details on some twenty-five plants associated with the easternmost reaches of the Mediterranean – items that the king and his ministers thought might have their origins somewhere in the Indian Ocean basin or perhaps elsewhere further east. Pires was to identify each item with as much certainty as possible and determine where each originated. Judging by the contents of Pires's list – which included rhubarb, amber, and lapis lazuli – the king's request was born of commercial interest more than curiosity. Pires dutifully explained which of these things were "valuable

---

[71] Armando Cortesão, ed., *Suma Oriental of Tomé Pires and the Book of Francisco Rodrigues*, 2 vols. (London: Hakluyt Society), vol. 1, xxii–xxiii.

merchandise" and which were of such little value they ought to be "tossed into the sea."[72]

Ensconced in the Strait of Malacca, Pires could not have been better placed to respond to Manuel I's inquiry. It was in the long narrow maw of that Strait that a profusion of *naturalia* converged – streaming down out of the Bay of Bengal to the northwest and from the South China Sea to the east. It was precisely that geography that presented a problem. In 1512, no one among the Portuguese knew much about it. The Southeast Asian coastline, at least as far as Sumatra, had been tentatively traced onto maps, which circulated in Lisbon within the guarded halls of the Casa da Índia. They were later destroyed in the famous Lisbon earthquake of 1755. But Alberto Cantino, a spy in the employ of the Duke of Ferrara, smuggled a copy of the composite atlas out of the city in 1502.[73] The Cantino planisphere silently discloses what imperial officials did and did not know about the geography of Indian Ocean Asia. That vast labyrinth of islands and inlets to Malacca's east had yet to make their mark on the cartographic imagination of Manuel I and his ministers. Sumatra was there, visible across the strait from the royal factory, but the Sunda Islands were not. The "oceanus yndiais meredionalis" was all but blank, its empty space broken only by navigational lines charting little more than the extent of Portuguese ambitions.

For Pires that was no small problem. Manuel I had asked him to determine the origins of various plants. But how could he possibly assign individual plants to particular places when all that lay before him was undifferentiated space? Pires had first to fill in the map before he could situate plants within it. As even the Cantino atlas testified, meaningfully defining places meant more than demarcating territory. Places were defined according to the human, physical, and natural geography that distinguished one place from another.[74]

They were defined, in other words, by what they contained. To constitute a place in the imperial imagination, Pires had to compile details that facilitated such distinctions. This could include notes on such things as local material culture or spiritual life – the stuff that made for what

---

[72] ANTT, CC, pt. 1, mç.19, n. 102, f. 1.

[73] Alfred Pinheiro Marques, *Origem e Desenvolvimento da Cartografia Portuguesa na época dos Descobrimentos* (Lisbon: Imprensa Nacional-Casa da Moeda, 1987), 142–143.

[74] On these elements as tools of early modern place-making, see Barbara Mundy, *The Mapping of New Spain: Indigenous Cartography and the Maps of the Relaciones Geográficas* (Chicago: University of Chicago Press, 1996), especially 20–23.

Anthony Pagden identified as the "origins of comparative ethnology."[75] It might include depictions or verbal descriptions of prominent geological formations – the Cantino map plotted the location of Serra Leoa with an escarpment in the shape of a towering stone lion. Defining a place might also entail an account of the flora and fauna found to characterize it – plants and animals described or visually depicted even if they had not yet been named and thereby inserted into an expanding Portuguese lexicon. Hence the Cantino planisphere marked what was to become Portuguese America with a flock of colorful birds.[76]

In similar fashion, Pires crafted his account of Asian flora for Manuel I. As of the date he signed it, 27 January 1516, Pires had not yet traveled beyond the Strait. So he collected the necessary details from the sailors, traders, and other travelers who came and went in Malacca. Few Portuguese were among them in this early period but Francisco Rodrigues was. Rodrigues was a pilot in the small fleet dispatched eastward from Malacca in November of 1511 by Albuquerque in the wake of his successful invasion that August. The fleet piloted by Rodrigues was the first of the Portuguese to make the run and by the time it returned to Malacca in December of 1512, Pires was there to inventory its cargo and gather any details that Rodrigues had to offer.[77] It was a fortuitous meeting, for the pilot was also handy with a pen. And if Rodrigues knew of the close relationship between Pires and Manuel I then he probably also shared with him a set of elaborate illustrations that he would later dedicate to the king. Rodrigues's drawings captured precisely the kinds of details that could find their way onto the imperial map: depictions of the architecture, prominent flora, and coastal topography of the Lesser Sunda Islands (Figure 3.5).

As Albuquerque wrote to Manuel I in the months leading up to his Malacca invasion, these kinds of illustrations were instrumental to the emerging empire, as they would allow the king, "to truly see ... the course your ships must take to the Clove Islands, ... and the islands of Java and Banda, of nutmeg and maces[.]"[78]And indeed Rodrigues's book,

---

[75] Pagden, *The Fall of Natural Man*, 10–26.

[76] Bird's and their colorful feathers commonly stood for the Americas according to Alessandra Russo, "Cortés's objects and the idea of New Spain: Inventories as spatial narratives," *Journal of the History of Collections* 23 (2011): 229–252.

[77] Cortesão, ed., *Suma Oriental*, lxxviii–xcvi.

[78] Quoted in Cortesão, ed., *Suma Oriental*, lxxviii–lxxix, from an unspecified source. For a more sustained discussion of the kinds of translation at stake, see Michael Wintroub,

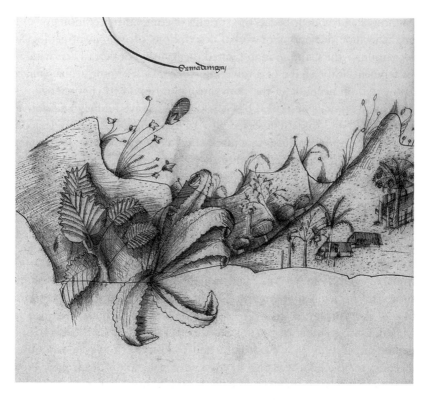

FIGURE 3.5 Word, Image, Empire. An ensemble of sketches by the pilot
Francisco Rodrigues from the *Livro de Francisco* Rodrigues.
Courtesy of the Bibliothèque de l'Assemblée Nationale, Paris.

with its nautical rules, maps, and panoramic drawings, soon made its
way to Lisbon.[79]

With these kinds of accounts to hand, Pires wrote a list that simultaneously conjured a geography and succinctly located within it the flora of
interest to D. Manuel. This involved a bit of linguistic finesse. What Pires
knew of Southeast Asian geography was now considerably more detailed
than what his sovereign knew. So every explanation had to be moored to
known places and practices. When he wrote, for example, that the highly

"The Translations of a Humanist Ship Captain: Jean Parmentier's 1529 Voyage to
   Sumatra," *Renaissance Quarterly* 68 (2015): 98–132.

[79] Cortesão, ed., *Suma Oriental*, xcv. See more recently José Manuel Garcia, *O livro de
   Francisco Rodrigues: O primeiro atlas do mundo moderno* (Porto: Editora da Universidade do Porto, 2008).

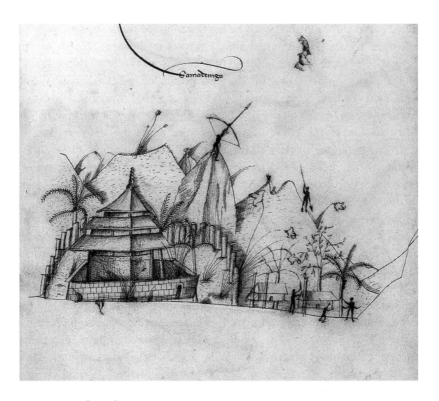

FIGURE 3.5 (*cont.*)

valued cebulic myrobalan[80] came from "Bengal, Malacca, and Borneo," he took care to weave a cartographic tapestry that located these seemingly arcane and unfamiliar places according to more familiar ones, which he used as points of orientation: "Bengal borders on Orissa on one side and Arakan on the other. Malacca [borders] on Kedah on one side and Pahang on the other. Borneo are islands [*sic*] two hundred leagues east of Malacca. These islands have much gold, edible camphor, and these myrobalans."[81] Taken alone, these references were incomplete. Did D. Manuel or the ministers of the Casa da Índia understand the whereabouts of Orissa, Arakan, Kedah, or Pahang? Probably not by this entry

[80] Myrobalan refers to a variety of plumb-like fruits that were introduced into the *materia medica* of Western Christendom by Islamic authors around the early eleventh century. See Efraim Lev and Zohar Amar, *Practical* Materia Medica *of the Medieval Eastern Mediterranean According to the Cairo Genizah* (Boston, MA: Brill, 2008), 218–221.

[81] ANTT, CC, pt. 1, mç. 19, n. 102, f. 2v.

alone – but Pires clarified each in his coverage of other things. So in his entry on incense, Pires noted that Orissa lay "between Narsinga and Bengal."[82] Hence between these two entries alone, officials in Lisbon could make some sense of this profusion of place names: Orissa separated Bengal from Narsinga (Viijayanagar), which lay next to Malabar. The entire chain of unfamiliar places was anchored by the Malabar Coast. He knew Manuel I could locate the lengthy Malabar Coast easily enough. After all, in 1516 that was still where the Estado's administrative heart of Cochin was and where nearly all of the empire's pepper left port for Lisbon. Pires used this technique in almost every entry on his list, steadily, if tediously, constructing an intelligible geography within which to place the things of nature that most interested Manuel I and his circle. Often the entries linked not only drugs and places, but also people and uses: inhabitants of Borneo not only possessed cebulic myrobalan but camphor of such quality that they could eat it directly.

For Pires, talking about plants and (where possible) their uses meant talking about places and the peoples who inhabited them. This kind of overlapping of concerns was part and parcel of a tradition of travel writing and map making that linked Herodotus and Marco Polo to the earliest Portuguese accounts of West Africa, Vijayanagar, and, later, South America. The tradition led to the production of ornately and colourfully illustrated maps by countless sixteenth-century European cartographers. It was not a Portuguese innovation.[83] But wielding it in order to fashion a focused account of commodifiable flora from the unfamiliar islands east of Malacca was a step compelled by the peculiar challenges that Pires faced in the early years of the Estado.

Thirty years later, Álvares faced the opposite problem. The Portuguese had been embroiled in trade disputes in the Moluccas since the 1520s.[84] By the late 1540s, accounts of the region's politics, commerce, and geography had established a shared lexicon of peoples and places to which officials in Lisbon and correspondents throughout the Estado could refer. Malacca itself, the site of much of Pires's inquiries, had meanwhile become something of a geopolitical fulcrum.[85] Álvares had seen all of these seminal perspectival shifts take shape. He was a career functionary

---

[82] ANTT, CC, pt. 1, mç. 19, n. 102, f. 2.

[83] Margaret T. Hodgen, *Early Anthropology in the Sixteenth and Seventeenth Centuries* (Philadelphia, PA: University of Pennsylvania Press, 1964); Rubiés, *Travel and Ethnology*; Davies, *Renaissance Ethnography*.

[84] Roelofsz, *Asian Trade*, 153–172.   [85] Subrahmanyam, *Improvising Empire*, xiii–xix.

who spent most of his life on the Malabar Coast. His early service was undistinguished and he rose only slowly to the pinnacle of colonial medical officialdom. He had come to Asia in 1509, when the Estado was in its infancy, when Cochin was its administrative center, and when plans to capture Goa had scarcely been hatched. By the 1510s he had managed to distinguish himself from among growing number of Portuguese apothecaries then plying their trade and trafficking their expertise on the Indian littoral. Not only was Álvares the apothecary called upon to settle the cinnamon question in the 1510s, but when D. João de Castro replaced Martim Afonso de Sousa as the head of the Estado da Índia in 1545, he chose Álvares as his personal apothecary. Castro's family ranked among the upper nobility of the Portuguese court and the viceroy would go down in the history of Portuguese Asia as, among other things, the illustrious conqueror of Diu. It was during one of a series of pitched battles for that lucrative Gujarati port city, when Álvares jumped into the fray to care for wounded men, that he earned a glowing commendation from the viceroy. Castro soon assigned to Álvares the task of clarifying the origins of the whole gamut of commodities then traded on the royal account.

Rather than situate a limited range of *naturalia* within a makeshift geography crafted from disparate elements, Álvares had to place an expanding number of natural things into an extensive and largely familiar geography. He relied upon this shared cartographic understanding when he organized his list to João III. Like Pires, the Strait of Malacca remained the pivotal point of orientation and Álvares began his account of Asian *naturalia* with the items known to come "by way of Malacca" – that is, from everywhere east of the Strait.[86] The entry was subdivided so that items were discussed according to their place of origin moving from east to west, beginning with the camphor that came from China and ending with the cubebs from Java. Having dispensed with the flora of the region beyond the Strait, Álvares then moved on to that which originated in the Bay of Bengal, which spread out northwest of Malacca. Next came the drugs of the Malabar Coast to Goa's south, followed by those of the Canara Coast between Goa and Cambay. Álvares closed with a discussion of the Arabian ports of Hormuz and then Aden. And just as he had handled the region east of Malacca, so too within each of these other regions as well: Álvares tacked slowly from east to west, steering the

---

[86] Walter, "Simão Alvares," 140.

royal imagination from port to port describing each specimen of nature in its turn according to its understood place of origin. The account of nature that began with Chinese camphor thus ended with the rhubarb taken by Khorsani traders to Hormuz.

Álvares had created a map in the form of a list. He could do it thanks to the inventory of nature and places inaugurated by Pires and his contacts. But, like any other map, the list reflected as well the extent and limitations of the Estado da Índia. If the Portuguese now had ports that fanned out across the Indonesian archipelago, they had made little headway in China or beyond the Strait of Hormuz. In consequence, several items resisted such easy geographic compartmentalization. The origins of a certain salt that came to Hormuz from either "Persia" or "Mecca,"[87] simply could not be pinned down.

That was one of a number of issues that, decades earlier, Pires had not been able to resolve. On these, Álvares's contribution was most substantial. The identification of a medicinal substance called "liquid storax," for one, proved especially problematic. To D. Manuel's inquiry about it decades before, Pires had replied bluntly, "I do not know what liquid storax is ... nor did the apothecaries with whom I studied." Pires noted that what passed under that name in metropolitan Portugal was a substance that arrived by way of Venice. He explained that to the learned men (*doutores*) of Iberia liquid storax was thought to be a medicinal simple – a single substance derived from a single plant or mineral. But based on his limited sojourn in the Indian Ocean, Pires had been given to understand that what was traded under that name in Aden was made of ingredients that included "yeast, honey, and oil" – a concoction, he pointed out, which was "good merchandise here [in Cochin], and valuable."[88]

In liquid storax, in other words, Pires was confronted with what might have been two very different substances traded under the exact same name. Were they the same? It was possible but not certain enough for Pires to stake a claim to it. Pires committed himself only to the suggestion that what was meant by liquid storax depended on where one was – a single name that could attached to multiple things. The references to Venice and Aden were important. It was the closest to certitude that Pires was able to get: if the drug could not be identified with certainty, then at least it could be anchored to peoples and places that were. The question of

---

[87] Walter, "Simão Alvares," 146.   [88] ANTT, CC, pt. 1, mç. 19, n. 102, 4.

liquid storax was therefore an open one when Álvares was asked to submit a report to João III. For Álvares, this liquid storax was composed of several different substances, the principal of which was called "aguyla," though "no one knows the truth of its origins."[89] In a way, Álvares was right. Aguyla could be bought in Malacca even before the Portuguese took it. And a succession of Portuguese accounts penned both before and long after Álvares compiled his list placed the origins of this scented wood everywhere from Ceylon to the Malay peninsula and Siam. They found it as far away as Japan.[90] Countless Portuguese had enough experience with the intra-Asian trade in this wood to make a claim; no one could really be sure of the truth.

It was in precisely this way that, over time and as the imperial archive expanded, an imperial system designed to facilitate trade permitted limited investigative activity. Although a definite answer to the mystery of aguyla proved elusive, the space for uncertainty narrowed. Questions, though unresolved, became more specific. Indeed, the identity of liquid storax as a compound rather than a simple was itself an instance of the ways in which the commercial networks converging on Goa and Malacca permitted the clarification of questions about widely-traded but, to many Portuguese newcomers, still cryptic commodities.

The confusion caused by divergent claims about potentially distinct substances traded under the same name was one of the central problems that Orta would have to resolve in the *Colóquios*. Orta, however, was a physician. He had philological training that enabled him to grapple with this and other problems in ways that apothecaries such as Pires and Álvares could not. By combing through the work of Dioscorides and Avicenna, Orta was able to identify the aguyla of Álvares, and therefore the liquid storax of Pires, with a plant he referred to as "aguila brava," and that came, so he claimed, from beyond the Ganges River.[91]

In this way, the work of Pires and Álvares helped establish some of the questions and answers on which Orta could build in his own investigations. In their installment of a shared catalog of plants and place names,

[89] Walter, "Simão Alvares," 141–142.
[90] Sebastião Rodolfo Dalgado, ed., *Glossário Luso-Asiático*, 2 vols. (Hamburg: Helmut Buske Verlag, 1982 [Coimbra, 1919–1921]) vol. 1, 17–18; William Roxburgh, "Aquilaria," *The Transactions of the Linnean Society of London* 21 (1855): 206.
[91] This according to the entry for "Agallochum," in the version of Dioscorides by Jean Ruel, which Orta references repeatedly throughout the *Colóquios*: Ioanne Ruello, *Pedanii Dioscoridis Anazarbei: De Medica Materia Libri Sex* (Basel: n.p., 1542), bk. 1, ch. 21: 22; Orta, *Colóquios*, vol. 2, 47–67.

the work of Pires and Álvares before him, and therefore a whole gamut of seamen like Rodrigues, established a more nuanced common geography to which the Crown and its agents, and colonial naturalists like Orta, could refer. Orta's remark that pepper was spread from Malacca, Martaban, Java, and Pegu represented the articulation of an established fact that would have been unthinkable without the investigative work of those before him.

The efforts of successive generations of naturalists spread across the Estado da Índia had generated not only a shared cartographic imagination, they had also helped make particular plants and animals stand in not only for discrete places but broad regions. Coconut palms and elephants became iconic of Indian Ocean Asia. Rodrigues sketched coconut palms in his voyage through island Southeast Asia, all the way to Sumbawa (just west of Timor). The Jesuit Francisco de Sousa pointed out that they were the "principal drug of the land" in Carambolim and Salsete south of Goa.[92] One of his Jesuit colleagues would pen a treatise dedicated entirely to the cultivation of the tree.[93] According to Orta, the Greeks knew nothing about the plant and medieval Arab scholars knew precious little more. From his South Asian itinerary, Orta had learned a good deal. The coconut palm yielded sweeteners and spirits and rigging for ships; it could be used as a purgative, a pain reliever, and an antidote for poisons. It was, as Orta admiringly wrote, a source of "many things necessary for life."[94] Elephants, as Orta took great care to point out in the *Colóqiuos*, were beasts of very particular kinds of burden, and especially so in India. Their ostensible loyalty, intelligence, and strength made them useful on the battlefield, where they served as both mobile fortifications and hulking foot soldiers, and in Goa's dockyard, where they hauled the massive timbers of teak harvested from Goa's hinterland for shipbuilding and repair.[95] Along the Konkan and Malabar coasts, elephants were so

---

[92] Sousa, *Oriente Conquistado*, 162–169.

[93] *Arte Palmarica escrita por um Padre da Companhia de Jesus* (Nova Goa: Imprensa Nacional, 1918).

[94] Orta, *Colóquios*, vol. 1, 233–253.

[95] Orta, *Colóquios*, vol. 1, 303–324. Teak, at the time an abundant hardwood, was especially sought after for ship construction in part because its resin forestalled the rusting of iron nails. See K. M. Mathew, *History of the Portuguese Navigation in India* (Delhi: Mittal Publications, 1988), ch. 11.

prized locally and such an object of fascination among Portuguese that they were given as endowments to houses of worship.[96]

It was in these localized and highly particularistic ways that both the coconut palm and the elephant made their appearances in the text of Cristovão da Costa's *Tractado de las Drogas, y medicinas de las Indias Orientales*, a Spanish study of the plants and animals of the East Indies printed in Burgos in 1578 and heavily based on Orta's *Colóquios*. Among the woodcuts that populated Costa's text were two of the elephant. In one, the exotic flora and exotic fauna so characteristic of Costa's "East Indies" were assembled into this single image in which the creature nestles up to a coconut palm (Figure 3.6).

Coconut palms and elephants each had particular and regionally varied uses. But, both separately and together, they had by the late sixteenth century come to stand in, as Costa put it, for "all of the rest of the medicines, plants, birds, and animals that there are in these parts," that is: the Indian Ocean world that was so desirable a destination for Costa and so many others before and after him.[97]

EPISTEMOLOGIES OF THE PEPPER TRADE

Pires, Álvares, and Orta were part of a cross-generational intellectual community. But important differences distinguished the way they carried out their work. A midcentury debate over pepper dramatized those differences, highlighting the relative importance of such things as networks, textual authority, and empiricism in investigative endeavors across generations of Portuguese naturalists in the Indian Ocean world.

---

[96] Artur Teoodoro de Matos, ed., *Documentos Remetidos da Índia ou Livros das Monções (1625–1736)*, 2 vols. (Lisbon: Academia das Ciências, 1999–2001), vol. 1, doc. 93 and doc. 470; Fernão Lopes de Castanheda, *História do descobrimento e conquista da Índia pelos portugueses*, 2 vols. (Porto: Lello and Irmão, 1979), vol. 1, 463.

[97] Cristovão da Costa, [Cristobal Acosta] *Tractado de las Drogas, y medicinas de las Indias Orientales, con sus Plantas debuxadas al biuo por Christoual Acosta medico y cirujano que las vio ocularmente* (Burgos: Martin de Victoria, 1578), 295, 281–295. See also the discussion in BNP Res. Cod. 414: "História de serviços com martírio de Luís Monteiro Coutinho, Goa 1615," and especially the watercolor illustration that appears around f. 23v–24, which was created by the mathematician Manuel Godinho de Herédia. On the emergence of this metropolitan vision, see also the discussion in Amélia Polónia, "Global Interactions: Representations of the East and the Far East in Portugal in the Sixteenth Century," in Rila Mukherjee, *Networks in the First Global Age, 1400–1800* (New Delhi: Primus Books, 2011), 263–301.

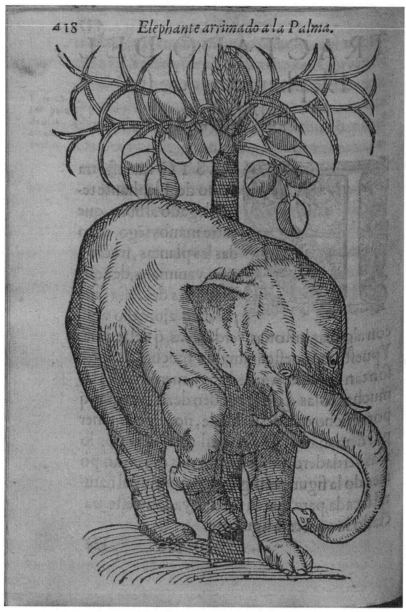

FIGURE 3.6 Emblems of Asia. The coconut palm and the elephant from
Christovão da Costa, Tractado Delas Drogas, y medicinas de las Indias Orientales
(Burgos: Martín de Victoria, 1578).
Courtesy of the Biblioteca Nacional de Portugal.

Orta never met Tomé Pires. But by the time Sousa appointed Orta physician-general of Goa, Álvares had been living in the city for almost a decade. It was Álvares who resolved the earlier confusion surrounding cinnamon. In the midst of a financial crisis, when the governor sought clarification on the nature of pepper, it was to both Orta and Álvares that he turned. The substance of their exchange can be summed up easily: Orta and Álvares – the physician and the apothecary – disagreed. Orta, citing Dioscorides, Pliny, Galen, Isidore of Seville and, "all the Arabs," argued that pepper was of two kinds – one black, the other white – and that the two varieties came from different trees. He insisted that many Portuguese who were "not very curious" could not tell the difference between them but that Indians along the Malabar Coast certainly could. At this, Álvares scoffed. He insisted that Orta was mistaken and to prove the point, Álvares explained what had happened on his return voyage to Lisbon in the spring of 1530.[98] He was traveling with a cargo of pepper when, somewhere off the coast of Mozambique, the ship began to take on water. The fleet dropped anchor at Mozambique Island, where the pepper was transferred to a seaworthy vessel. Álvares, explained that while he was handling the pepper he saw that corns of what at first looked like black pepper began to shed their outer covering to reveal a white rind. Álvares took this as evidence that black and white pepper were indeed the same thing.[99] Orta heard him out but promptly objected. He pointed out that in such a large cargo of black pepper, one was sure to find occasional traces of the white kind. But he reasoned that if white pepper were merely black pepper that had shed its covering because of the jostling and rubbing of transit, then the white pepper first found at Mozambique would have multiplied by the time it reached the Casa da Índia. Indeed, officials at the *Casa* would have found themselves inundated with white pepper when they had expected black. And, so argued Orta, that was not what happened.[100]

Sousa, having heard the exchange, had no idea whom to believe. Orta's deductive reasoning was as impeccable as the list of ancient authorities he cited to support it. But the evidence of experience mustered by Álvares was just as compelling. For his part, Álvares readily conceded his initial faith in the wisdom of the ancients. He explained that while in Cochin he had heard the scribes of the raja suggest that the two varieties of pepper

---

[98] Orta, *Colóquios*, vol. 2, 248 provides the physician's explanation and his account of Alvares's reply.

[99] Walter, "Simão Alvares," 143.   [100] Orta, *Colóquios*, vol. 2, 248.

were one and the same but had thought it preposterous because it ran
"counter to what the ancient authors had written." It was only after he
had handled "with my own hands" some two or three *arrateis* of pepper
that Álvares was compelled to change his mind.[101]

On the face of it, the decision that confronted Sousa is precisely the one
familiar to students of Iberian science who have attempted to chart
relationships between early modern encounters, imperial exigencies, and
metropolitan epistemic transformations – in some cases arguing that
Spanish and Portuguese endeavors abroad ushered in the modern epistemological era characterized by a deep concern with and respect
for the kind of empiricism that would later underwrite Baconian
experimentalism.[102] From this perspective, the governor stood at an
epochal precipice where two distinct and even mutually exclusive
world-historical eras collided. Sousa might side with Orta and the long-
established tradition of textual exegesis. Or he might follow Álvares and
align himself with the empiricism so often taken as the harbinger of a
scientific modernity.

The governor did not see his choice in these terms at all. As Orta
recorded in the *Colóquios*, Sousa wrote to the king of Cochin for advice
and received in return a small sack of white pepper, along with a cursory
note stating that "he [the king] had many trees of the white kind in his
territory [of Cochin]."[103] For the governor, the issue was not an epistemological one – at least not in the sense that it pitted textual authority
against that of experience. It was instead about how an individual's
claims might best be substantiated – regardless of the *kind* of evidence
deployed. And the truth about nature – be it built upon the weighty edifice
of ancient wisdom or the fleeting evidence of experience – was constituted
by the agreement of opinions among members of the broader networks to
which Sousa, Orta, and Álvares had ready access.

Witnesses and corroborating testimony were instrumental in constitut-
ing the truth about nature. Each in his own way recognized this point.
Sousa and Orta had insinuated themselves as best they could into intra-
Asian networks. Sousa was at the time on good terms with the leaders of
Cochin. Orta's particular expertise in the ancient Greek and medieval Arab

---

[101] Walter, "Simão Alvares," 142.

[102] Cañizares-Esguerra, "Iberian Science." See also Almeida, "Portugal and the Dawn of
       Modern Science"; Domingues, "Science and Technology"; and Barrera-Osorio, *Experi-
       encing Nature.*

[103] Orta, *Colóquios*, vol. 2, 248.

medical traditions provided common intellectual ground for his exchanges with Arab physicians at the courts of Bahadur Shah and Burhan Nizam Shah. Their medical learning was grounded in many of the same texts and they could readily refer to and discuss the same passages. It was in that way that Orta's professional training would ultimately distinguish his techniques of knowledge production from those of his apothecary colleague: that background sustained the personal affiliations that constituted a network to which Álvares was not privy. Álvares knew just as well how important personal affiliations were in the certification of natural knowledge. Back on Mozambique Island in 1530, with white and black peppercorns working themselves through his hands as if in a sieve, the very first thing Álvares claimed to have done was to gather corroborating witnesses. He immediately reported his findings to the treasurer and the fleet captain. And once he arrived to Portugal, it was to a select group of physicians and apothecaries that he submitted his opinion and the evidence for it – with the official standing of his witnesses in all likelihood lending weight to his testimony.[104] It was to the primacy of such networks for the production of knowledge that Costa had in mind when, at the end of his *Tractado*, he noted that Orta knew what he did of "the elephants and medicinal drugs of these parts" not only because of his curiosity and diligence but by virtue of "his relations with other people."[105]

I have argued that generations of Portuguese naturalists in Indian Ocean Asia built on the work of one another – in the questions they asked, the answers they gave, and the spatial imagination they created and made use of – so that a knowledge of Asian nature would be intelligible to audiences a world away. I have shown that the medical and commercial challenges of expansion and settlement had – over the course of the sixteenth century – given rise to multiple, although never entirely distinct or mutually exclusive, intellectual networks and investigative interests. Portugal's empire in Asia enabled – in fact depended upon – the production and accumulation of natural knowledge mobilized by those networks long before Garcia de Orta sailed from Lisbon. Natural inquiry was the work not only of Martim Afonso de Sousa's personal physician. It was also the work of apothecaries like Pires and Álvares and of pilots like Rodrigues.

Alessandra Russo has shown how commercial, craft, and epistolary networks turned brightly colored plumage into a metonym for the

---

[104] Walter, "Simão Alvares," 143.   [105] Costa, *Tractado*, 295.

Americas in the early sixteenth century.[106] Successive efforts to make sense of the creatures that circulated in and around Goa had similar effects. Elephants and coconut palms came in the same period to stand in for the Indian Ocean world.

As the case of pepper suggests, successive generations of naturalists could find themselves not only at odds with one another but with the arguments of modern historians about the nature of their work. What is immediately clear from the pepper debate is that while Orta has so often been cast as the forward-looking protagonist in a whiggish drama of epistemic transformation, it was the apothecary Álvares who insisted on the primacy of his own bodily engagement with the objects in question as a source of certain truth on such fundamental questions of nature as the relationship between black and white pepper. As important: at issue in the question over pepper were not so much the distinct and mutually exclusive epistemologies of a physician and an apothecary but the distinct networks of affiliation in which they were insinuated.

As I will explore in the next chapter, Orta did indeed practice a particular kind of innovative empiricism. But it did not amount to the elaboration of a novel philosophical program. His was an empiricism tempered by the realities of trade in the Indian Ocean world, a way of knowing that was never entirely at ease with the evidence of the senses, and that was always informed by the authority of ancient texts. His was, I will argue, an intellectual program far removed even from that of his best-known reader and translator, the Flemish naturalist Carolus Clusius. If Orta's study of the drug traffic coursing through Goa was never merely a reflection of the interests and outlooks of metropolitan officials, neither was it simply an instantiation of humanist inquiry in a sixteenth-century Republic of Letters.

Before turning to an exploration of the *Colóquios*, it is worth taking one last look at the experiences of the apothecaries Pires and Álvares. For in Goa, as at the courts of Europe,[107] patronage had its traps. On this point, too, the experiences of Pires and Álvares are instructive. After three very productive years in Malacca, Pires had expected to return to Lisbon and was on his way there when, during a layover in Cochin, he was appointed as an ambassador to the Chinese emperor. He could hardly say no. But the embassy was disastrous. Pires, an apothecary of the royal

---

[106] Russo, "Cortés's objects."

[107] Mario Biagioli, *Galileo, Courtier: The Practice of Science in the Culture of Absolutism* (Chicago, IL: Chicago University Press, 1993).

court, a masterful bureaucrat, skilled collector of information, and a loyal servant, wound up in shackles in a prison in Canton, accused of espionage. Rumor had it that he died in prison, although years later a Portuguese adventurer in Canton met a young woman claiming to be his daughter.[108]

It was the favor of the viceroy João de Castro that spelled the downfall of Álvares. The apothecary was an assiduous keeper of accounts. In his letter of 1548, he reported that D. João's factor in Bassein was defrauding him.[109] Rooting out swindlers, however, turned friends and colleagues into enemies. When Álvares inspected the Portuguese factories of the Malabar Coast as apothecary general, he was greeted with hostility and resentment. Despite his expertise, Álvares was a pariah, bereft of all credibility beyond official circles. His letter to João III inventorying the drugs of Asia emphasized his isolation, poverty, and his long and arduous work in the service of the Crown.[110] Certainly he was posturing before his royal benefactor. But it also seems the aging Álvares had neither the means nor (anymore) the local relations to support himself. His life and livelihood now depended heavily on royal patronage and on the thin twine of relations linking Goa to Lisbon. He disappeared without a trace after his missive of 1548.

The prospect of a similar fate would always hang over Orta and his work. The culture of inquiry that took shape in Goa was one that only uneasily embraced South Asian *materia medica* and the curative knowledges of its diverse practitioners. That is the subject of Chapter 5.

---

[108] This remarkable story is sketched out in Cortesão, ed., *Suma Oriental*, xviii–lxiii.

[109] Walter, "Simão Alvares," 149. The issue reported by Alvares seems to be that the royal factor in Bassein was charging the Crown for turbith purchased from Mangalor at market price when, according to Alvares, it could be harvested in the hinterland of Bassein for less. The king, Alvares suggested, should only have to pay the laborers. The factor, whom Alvares does not name, knew this and carried it out but continued to charge the inflated price. Hence the factor was essentially stealing money from the royal account.

[110] Walter, "Simão Alvares," 139–140, 149.

4

Drug Traffic

I do not doubt that if someone who had a good knowledge of the matter of simples, with good principles of philosophy and medicine, came here, he would greatly advance medicine. And an artist who knew well how to draw and paint plants might offer such delight with their representation; because the great degree of originality in this area is unimaginable[.]

Letter from Filippo Sassetti to Francesco I, the Grand[1]

LOST IN TRANSLATION

Knowledge travels and is changed in the process. Orta first published the *Colóquios* in Goa, on India's Konkan Coast, in April of 1563. Much like the drugs and spices it detailed, the book became an item of global exchange. Copies were in Lisbon by the following January. A Latin edition prepared by the Flemish naturalist Carolus Clusius appeared some three years later, in 1567, at the Frankfurt book fair, under the title *Aromatum et simplicium aliquot medicamentorum apud Indos nascentium historia.*[2] Across Western Christendom, amid a culture increasingly interested in novelties, wonders, and exotica of many kinds, Orta's book found a wide and diverse readership (Figure 4.1).[3]

---

[1] Translated by Lawrence Venuti and quoted in John M. de Figueiredo, "Ayurvedic Medicine in Goa according to European Sources in the Sixteenth and Seventeenth Centuries," *Bulletin of the History of Medicine* 58 (1984): 228–229.

[2] Carolus Clusius, *Aromatum et simplicium aliquot medicamentorum apud Indos nascentium historia* (Frankfurt: Christopher Plantin, 1567). Henceforth *Aromatum et simplicium.*

[3] On the interest in wonders and exotica in this period see Daston and Park, *Wonders,* 135–172; and the essays collected in Pamela H. Smith and Paula Findlen, *Merchants and Marvels: Commerce, Science, and Art in Early Modern Europe* (New York: Routledge,

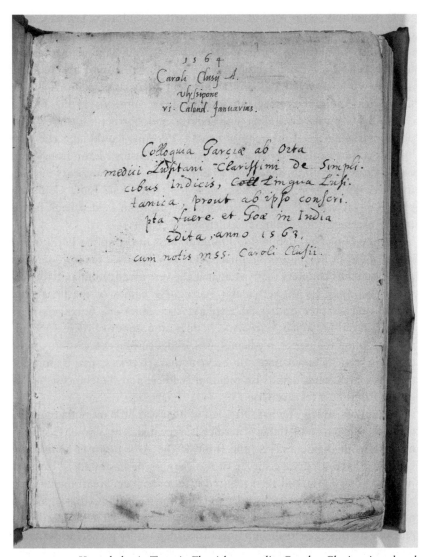

FIGURE 4.1 Knowledge in Transit. Flemish naturalist Carolus Clusius signed and dated his copy of Garcia de Orta's Colóquios dos simples e drogas e coisas medicinais da Índia (Goa: João de Endem, 1563), January 6, 1564.
Reproduced by permission of the Syndics of Cambridge University Library.

2002). For a discussion of the intra-European circulation of the Portuguese edition, see Teresa Nobre de Carvalho, "A Behind-the-Scenes Glimpse into the Princeps Edition of *Colóquios dos simples* (Goa, 1563)," *Early Science and Medicines* 21 (2016): 232–251.

Through this Latin version, countless artists, sculptors, printers, merchants, and many others who made up the increasingly heterogeneous community of naturalists in late-sixteenth-century Europe gained access to the work of a Portuguese physician and the expertise of his collaborators a world away. Latin and subsequent vernacular editions of the *Colóquios* found their way into the hands of surgeons at the French court, the libraries of Italian universities, and northern Europe's first physic garden at the University of Leiden. Versions would later travel to Spain's colonies on the far side of the Atlantic. Clusius's Latin translation of the *Colóquios* established Orta as Europe's best contemporary authority on Asian *materia medica*.[4] In 1620, the Dutch East India Company physician Jacobus Bontius carried Orta's work from Leiden back to the Indian Ocean world, testing and revising its claims.[5]

Yet the book that debuted in Frankfurt was not simply a Latin translation of Orta's Portuguese original. Orta had composed the *Colóquios* as a dialogue. His chapters – fifty-nine in all – were arranged in alphabetical order according to the vernacular Portuguese names of the flora (and fauna: one chapter addressed elephants) in question. Some chapters covered several plants at once. And besides an account of these – including their humoral aspect, medicinal uses, and a careful description – most chapters also included notes on current market prices, major ports of trade for each item, details on regional politics, and the choicest bits of gossip from the streets of Goa.

To Clusius, much of what Orta had written was little more than useless verbiage – a litany of things "needlessly repeated," he wrote, "as often happens with dialogues." At the front of the *Aromatum et simplicium* Clusius offered a cursory survey of the changes he had made: "I passed [the text] into Latin and then reduced it to a summary, rearranging each chapter into a more agreeable order and rejecting some things that seemed to me to be unnecessary."[6] This, however, was an understatement. Clusius replaced the dialogue form with unadorned, expository prose. He did away with the original alphabetical order of the chapters and rearranged them instead into two distinct "books." The first covered more familiar *naturalia* like aloe and rhubarb; the second included such things as neem and jackfruit,

[4] Ogilvie, *Science of Describing*, 60.
[5] Carvalho, "Garcia d'Orta"; Ambroise Paré, *The Apologie and Treatise of Ambroise Paré, Containing the Voyages made into Divers Places with many of his writings upon Surgery*, ed. Geoffrey Keynes (London: Falcon Educational Books, 1951 [ca. 1564]), 198–200; Cook, *Matters of Exchange*, 118, 191–207.
[6] Clusius, *Aromatum et simplicium*, 5.

which were unknown in ancient sources and often unfamiliar to Clusius and his contemporaries. Both sections and their respective chapters were clearly set out in a table of contents; specific details were indexed by chapter and page number at the back of the book. Clusius expunged countless details about town life and trade routes in Goa. Most of the characters that enriched the fifty-nine dialogues of the *Colóquios* were cut from the *Aromatum et simplicium*. In their stead, Clusius introduced some dozen woodcuts, "procured [in an effort] to describe as well as possible the drugs" in question.[7]

In circulation, the *Colóqiuos* had been transformed. Clusius had not only rendered Orta's Portuguese into Latin, he had reenacted some of the work of collecting, selecting, organizing, and representing that Orta had already carried out (Figure 4.2).

The changes might have seemed quotidian and unremarkable to the readers of the *Aromatum et simplicium*; they were, after all, part and parcel of the work of editing in early modern Europe.[8] The differences in their work might also be interpreted as an effect of the generational shifts in the study of nature and the presentation of natural knowledge. Orta was considerably older than Clusius. By the time Orta was appointed to a natural philosophy lectureship in Lisbon in 1530, having finished his studies at Salamanca and then at Alcalá de Henares, Clusius was still a young boy at his parents' home in Artois, just south of Antwerp. The study of nature and the conventions which governed the presentation of natural knowledge in March of 1534 – when Orta boarded the ship *Rainha* to sail for Goa – differed in important ways from those which Clusius would consider over thirty years later, when a trip through Iberia (he traveled in the employ of the young Jacob Fugger) brought him to Lisbon and into possession of Orta's book.[9] In the intervening decades, the methods employed in the study of nature, the symbolic meaning of natural objects, the uses to which they were put, and the conventions that governed the textual presentation of natural knowledge had all become more diverse.[10]

---

[7] Clusius, *Aromatum et simplicium*, 7.

[8] I thank Peter Burke for reminding me of this important detail. For more on traditions of editing, see Ann Blair, *Too Much to Know: Managing Scholarly Information before the Modern Age* (New Haven, CT: Yale University Press, 2010), 173–229.

[9] Cook, *Matters of Exchange*, 85; Orta left for Goa on March 12. These and other details can be found in Walter, "Garcia de Orta"; and in the essays in Costa, ed., *Medicine, Trade and Empire*.

[10] Ogilvie, *Science of Describing*; Smith and Findlen, eds., *Merchants and Marvels*; Daniela Bleichmar and Peter C. Mancall, eds., *Collecting Across Cultures: Material Exchanges in the Early Modern Atlantic World* (Philadelphia, PA: University of Pennsylvania Press, 2013).

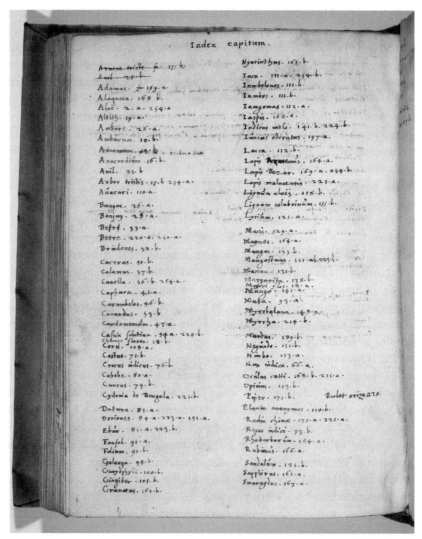

FIGURE 4.2 The Process of Translation. Flemish Naturalist Carolus Clusius's handwritten index of Orta's *Colóquios*.
Reproduced by permission of the Syndics of Cambridge University Library.

Yet the changes were more than an inconsequential aspect of the circulation of natural knowledge. So much was clear to both authors. Orta was deeply aware that his own project differed substantially even from those of his contemporaries back in Europe – among them Niccolò Leoniceno, Leonhart Fuchs, Jean de Ruelle, and Pietro Mattioli – whose works he had not only read but frequently cited. At the beginning of the *Colóquios* Orta confessed to readers his worry that "some day this little book may be printed [merely] to make a joke of me, or to expose my poor reasoning."[11] Clusius, though critical, never actually ridiculed Orta. When he wrote of the changes he had made to Orta's book, he pointed out that "our author [Garcia de Orta] had his reasons" for crafting the *Colóquios* in the way that he did.[12] What those were, Clusius could not have known and did not speculate.[13]

In their substance, the differences between the *Colóquios* and the *Aromatum et simplicium* reflected the interests, preferences, and perspectives that distinguished the culture of inquiry of northern Europe from that of colonial Goa. They are measures of just how different the practices of natural inquiry actually were in the worlds inhabited by the two naturalists. These worlds were not mutually exclusive – quite the contrary. Natural history was a humanist invention, and both Orta and Clusius were familiar with its conventions.[14] They shared a fundamental sense of what kinds of information were appropriate to the production of natural knowledge, of what sorts of details were required to produce an accurate inventory of nature. Both the *Colóquios* and the *Aromatum et simplicium* evinced the common intellectual framework of their authors – one heavily influenced by their humanist medical education and modeled on the work of Dioscorides. To each plant, the first century Greek physician devoted one chapter. And within each chapter he followed the same general format: he began with the name of a plant, offered details about its habitat, appearance, medicinal properties and proper uses, discussed harvesting and storage, the identification of false or adulterated specimens, and closed with such details as veterinary or non-medical uses.[15] Published studies of nature for most of the sixteenth century – including both the *Colóquios* and the *Aromatum et simplicium* – were generally concerned with securing this kind of knowledge about the natural world. But what was to be studied, how it was to be studied, and how knowledge produced through that study was to be represented

---

[11] Orta, *Colóquios*, vol. 1, 23.   [12] Clusius, *Aromatum et simplicium*, 5.

[13] Clusius, *Aromatum et simplicium*, 7.

[14] On this invention and the culture of natural history as practiced by Clusius and his circle see Ogilvie, *Science of Describing*.

[15] Robert T. Gunther, ed., *The Greek Herbal of Dioscorides*, trans. John B. Goodyear (New York: Hafner Publishing Company, 1968 [1934]); John M. Riddle, *Dioscorides on Pharmacy and Medicine* (Austin, TX: University of Texas Press, 1985), 25–93.

on the page were shaped as well by time, place, and circumstance. The project of natural history was variable, its forms multiple.[16]

If Clusius's representational conventions responded to the interests and concerns of his discursive community, and if his decisions reflected the perspectives and preferences of that community, so too did those of Garcia de Orta. From the techniques by which he produced knowledge about nature to the ways he decided to present that knowledge in the *Colóquios*, Orta's work was improvised in response to the distinctive circumstances that obtained in Goa between his arrival to India in 1534 and the printing of his book in 1563. The size, shape, content, and organization of the *Colóquios* are clues to the culture of inquiry that had come to characterize Goa by the middle decades of the sixteenth century.

LANGUAGE, NOVELTY, AND GLOBAL ORDER

Orta and Clusius shared not only a common intellectual ancestry but a culture of Renaissance humanism that privileged Latin as a vehicle for learned discourse. A thorough grounding in Latin had become essential to the study of nature in Europe in part because it was the language of university instruction. When in the late fifteenth century scholars and physicians sought to reform medical curricula by improving the instructional texts upon which they were based, Latin remained the language of learned discourse. As the practice of nature moved beyond the purview of learned medicine, its community of practitioners expanded to include lawyers, theologians, ministers, and professors in other fields, as well as merchants, apothecaries, artisans, printers, and a range of literate craftsmen. A command of Latin became an important social and cultural marker for naturalists. It signified community membership. It gave personal letters an added patina of intimacy and publications an enhanced veneer of authority. Among this eclectic assortment of participants, interests in nature ranged widely from a concern for medicine, a fascination with the exotic, and an appreciation of the aesthetics of nature, to the use of nature as a tool for self-fashioning through public display, for the purposes gifting and patronage, or for trade and profit. Their varied contributions to the study of nature were not always accorded equal authority. But fluency in Latin granted naturalists from diverse backgrounds access to a community within which the social hierarchies often

---

[16] Foundational here is N. Jardine, J. A. Secord, and E. C. Spary, eds., *Cultures of Natural History* (New York: Cambridge University Press, 1996).

associated with the life of the mind could be temporarily suspended.[17] When Clusius wrote that his Latinized version of the *Colóquios* was meant to allow others to "enjoy the utility of this book," it was this motley assortment of people and priorities that he had in mind.[18]

In an important way, Orta was at once part of that world and yet removed from it. He had been educated in Latin in the late 1510s and early 1520s, just in time to study from the first generation of revised medical books produced by Niccolò Leoniceno and his students in Ferrara. The *Colóquios* was – at least in part – his answer to the urgings of the Sienese physician and professor of medicine, Pietro Andrea Mattioli, and the inquiries of Tomás Rodrigues, Orta's friend and a physician of the royal court in Lisbon. Mattioli, a controversial and cantankerous figure, was best known for his commentary on Dioscorides, which, after its publication in Venice in 1555, became the most widely used textbook on *materia medica* in late-sixteenth century Europe.[19] Mattioli had written to Rodrigues in Lisbon, insisting that the Portuguese physician and his colleagues capitalize on their access to the flood of Asian *naturalia* streaming in from across the seas in order to clarify some of the confusion surrounding the drugs of antiquity. Rodrigues thought the suggestion a good one. But he believed that Orta, at work in Goa, was best positioned to carry it out.[20]

That did not, however, mean that Orta began his investigations with the Paduan professor's concerns in mind or that the interests of his friends and colleagues in Lisbon were the same as his own in Goa. If, as I argued in the last chapter, Orta was not simply an intermediary between communities of European and Asian physicians and naturalists,[21] neither was his project simply a Renaissance humanist one. Orta's chosen language of exposition, and his sense of which naturalia were most deserving of inquiry and discussion, were determined by the idiosyncratic priorities of the physician in Goa and the culture of inquiry that obtained there. The same was true for the way in which Orta decided to arrange material within his book. Differences in the ways in which Orta and Clusius ordered material on the page reflected differences in priorities, perspectives, and ultimately in the ways in which naturalists imagined the globe.

[17] Ogilvie, *Science of Describing*, 54–58 and 87–138.

[18] Clusius, *Aromatum et simplicium*, 5.   [19] Ogilvie, *Science of Describing*, 59, 190, 201.

[20] Orta, *Colóquios*, vol. 1, 216.

[21] Pearson, "Thin End of the Wedge," 141–170; and Grove, *Green Imperialism*, ch. 2.

The use of Latin may have served his European contemporaries well. But Orta participated in exchanges among many communities of diverse and dispersed origins. His work demanded a different linguistic tack. Latin, so characteristic of humanism elsewhere in Europe, had a checkered history in Portugal. Even as the House of Avis encouraged intellectual and artistic ties between Lisbon, Antwerp, and Rome, the use of Latin met with impassioned resistance – even satire. After the first volume of his *Décadas* came to print detailing the West African voyages, João de Barros wrote the *Diálogo em louvor da nossa linguagem* (*Dialogue in Esteem of Our [Portuguese] Language*), extolling Portuguese as a language of learning and refinement.[22] His contemporary, the novelist Jorge Ferreira de Vasconcellos, lampooned his Lusophone countrymen who preferred the humanist's Latin – in one of his novels parodying their cultural preferences with a pedantic Coimbra student who insisted on the use of Latin even in love-making.[23] Across Portuguese Asia, among Goa's *casados* no less than among private traders spread across the Bay of Bengal, and those scattered more widely across island Southeast Asia, Orta's discursive community was one in which university-trained physicians numbered few among the preponderance of apothecaries, merchants, and traders who, if they had a choice at all, preferred Portuguese to Latin. Those two factors – the limited embrace of Latin as the language of learned discourse in Portugal and colonial intellectual communities in Goa and beyond that were far more conversant in Portuguese than Latin – combined to make the vernacular an asset. Use of the vernacular did not threaten Orta's credibility. It enhanced it.[24]

There were other linguistic concerns too. A true accounting of nature and access to its curative potential required the very language, Arabic, that Orta's contemporaries in Europe roundly condemned. Prominent naturalists like Leoniceno, Fuchs or Mattioli blamed medieval Arab and Persian authors for what they saw as the barbaric translation of ancient

---

[22] João de Barros, *Diálogo em louvor da nossa linguagem* (Lisbon: Ludovico Rodrigues, 1540). His work, and this perspective, were echoed some decades later by Pedro de Magalhães Gândavo, *Regras que ensinam a maneira de screver a ortographia da língua Portuguesa, com um Diálogo que adiante se segue em defenão da mesma língua* (Lisbon, 1574).

[23] Anson C. Piper, "Jorge Ferreira de Vasconcellos: Defender of the Portuguese Vernacular," *Hispania* 37 (1954): 400–405.

[24] Leonard Y. Andaya, "The Portuguese Tribe in the Malay-Indonesian Archipelago in the Seventeenth and Eighteenth Centuries," in *The Portuguese Tribe and the Pacific*, eds. Francis A. Dutra and João Camilo dos Santos (Santa Barbara, CA: Center for Portuguese Studies at the University of California at Santa Barbara, 1995), 129–148.

texts and the introduction of countless errors. As Leoniceno pointedly wrote, the authors of foundational Arabic texts, and especially Avicenna, were but "cruel tyrant[s]" followed by slavish dilettantes. Orta was sympathetic to many of the criticisms by his humanist colleagues; the sloppy transcription and inattentive editing of earlier generations was indeed a cause of confusion. But Orta was impatient with careless accusations. On the question of Arabic texts and their authors, he did not mince words. It was Leoniceno and "so many other modern writers" who were wrong. They may "say so many vile things of the Arabs," but "the faults are their own [rather than of the Arab and Persian physicians whom they accuse]." Amid the wide-ranging and unfamiliar flora and fauna of Asia, with access (albeit heavily mediated, as I argued in the last chapter) to the drugs that had been the concern of Greek, Arab, and Persian physicians for centuries, and faced with the prominence of Arab merchants and the pervasive use of Arabic as the language of trade throughout Indian Ocean Asia, the expertise of Arab and Persian authors and their Arabic language texts were indispensable. "To speak the truth," Orta concluded, "the Arabs ... deserve our praise not our scorn."[25] The centrality of Arabic not only shaped Orta's citation strategies, they made the language itself into a crucial epistemic tool. Rather than refer to translations and commentaries of Dioscorides to correct the claims of Arabic texts, Orta often performed the operation in reverse.[26] The terminology from Arabic texts could be far more reliable guides to nature in the Indian Ocean.[27]

Like language, the organizational strategies chosen by Orta and Clusius were meant to address the specific concerns of their respective communities. Particularly for Clusius this meant distinguishing between what was new in accounts of the world overseas from what was not – separating the ordinary from the exotic. Most studies highlight the importance of overseas encounters in the Americas in generating this preoccupation. I argued in Chapter 2 that earlier West African encounters had already begun to propel such a shift. As Brian Ogilvie has shown, so too did encounters within Europe. The realization, initially among medical humanists, that their own hinterlands in Basel or Bordeaux were rife with

---

[25] For Leoniceno on Avicenna, see Ogilvie, *Science of Describing*, 131. For Orta on Leoniceno, see the *Colóquios*, vol. 1, 193–194.

[26] See for example his discussion of myrobalan in, Orta, *Colóquios*, vol. 2, 151–160.

[27] On the dynamics of translation from Greek to Arabic, see Ahmed Ragab, "'In a Clear Arab Tongue': Arabic and the Making of a Science-Language Regime," *Isis* 108 (2017): 612–620.

flora that looked nothing like the descriptions left by Dioscorides (who, after all, had worked only in the Mediterranean basin) meant that, in botanical terms and from the perspective of those immersed in the pages of Dioscorides's *De materia medica*, the world north of the Alps was something of a new world too.[28]

It was this preoccupation with the new – inspired by widespread encounters in the Old World and the New – that prompted the most fundamental change that Clusius made as he transformed the *Colóquios* into the *Aromatum et simplicium*. In rearranging the contents of the former into the two constituent books of the latter, he separated out the familiar in book one from the novel and the exotic, which he collected into book two. In the back half of the *Aromatum et simplicium*, the unanticipated encounters with jackfruit or mangos that played out initially in the markets of Goa were recapitulated on the page for naturalists in Leiden or Paris who were unable to venture quite so far afield.[29]

By contrast, the *Colóquios* was not a book meant to seduce the imaginations of faraway European readers. And novelty was marginal to Orta's project. His alphabetical organization was not designed to draw attention to the new. Things such as lychees, neem, and *negundo* that were unknown to European readers were spread out, isolated, and buried amid other all-too-familiar and lucrative commodities like pepper, cinnamon, and cloves.

If the two physicians ordered their books differently, it was because they ordered their worlds differently too. From the perspective of Clusius and so many of his readers, there was nothing at all incongruous about grouping flora from South Asia together with the plants of South America. Novelties came from both regions and it was the interest in novelty that subsumed, even elided, regional specificity. In book two of the *Aromatum et simplicium*, the vast – and internally diverse – material, therapeutic, and botanical worlds encompassed by Iberian empires in Asia and the Americas were brought together – scarcely pages, and sometimes even paragraphs, apart. The interpersonal and textual mediations that permitted plants and paraphernalia collected globally to mingle just pages away from one another

---

[28] Ogilvie, *Science of Describing*, especially 133–137. See also Alix Cooper, *Inventing the Indigenous: Local Knowledge and Natural History in Early Modern Europe* (New York: Cambridge University Press, 2007).

[29] Despite the tremendous merits of Ogilvie's, *Science of Describing*, well attested in the notes of this and other chapters, his attempts to assimilate travels to Lapland with the biological, cultural, and geographic disorientations attendant on global sea travel are something of a stretch.

also enabled a particular way of conceiving of global geography. Clusius collapsed the vast and highly differentiated colonial worlds encompassed by Iberian empires in Asia and the Americas into the global, non-Eruopean world he termed "the Indies." In the *Aromatum et simplicium*, this confla-tion of East and West, and the compression of globally dispersed human and natural geographies, materialized most thoroughly in four simple woodcut illustrations. Ensconced in the middle of the second book were two strings of decorative beads. These adorned indigenous bodies observed not by Orta among Konkani townspeople or Gujarati courtiers in South Asia but by the French Franciscan priest André Thevet among the Tupi-nambá on the edge of Guanabara Bay (modern Rio de Janeiro) in South America.[30] Such arrangements – the rigid separation of the familiar from the novel and the collapsing of Portuguese and Spanish colonial worlds in Asia and the Americas into "the Indies" – were anathema to Orta's project.

Orta crafted his book so that it spoke directly to the concerns of a dispersed community of imperial and intra-Asian traders whose interest in the natural world could be charted along the twin axes of commerce and practical medicine. If the *Colóquios* were going to be of use to learned physicians, apothecaries, merchants and traders, and to Goa's Lusophone householders more generally – that is, if it were going to serve the needs of the widest possible range of interests among Portuguese-speakers caught in the throes of Portuguese imperialism in Asia – Orta had to be careful not to tailor his book too neatly to the concerns of any single one of those groups. That demanded an order of exposition rather different from the one that Clusius would choose later. If Orta had wanted to emphasize the causes of disease, he might have organized the *Colóquios* around various illnesses that the Portuguese confronted. He could have drawn on his formal training in the humoral theory of the Galenic corpus and loaded key chapters with extensive and rather precise elaborations on the humoral character of each plant, filling the pages of the *Colóquios* with ruminations about the bodily effects of the pronounced seasonal changes

---

[30] Clusius, *Aromatum et simplicium*, 229–230. Thevet was in Brazil between November 1555 to January 1556. The combination of their work was aided no doubt by the fact that the printer, Christopher Plantin, also printed Thevet's *Singularitez de la France Antarctique, autrement nommee Amerique, & de plusieurs terres & isles decouvertes de nostre temps* (Paris: Christopher Plantin, 1558). Indeed, Plantin may well have insisted on reusing some of that material so that Clusius's book would be more marketable. However, according to Florike Egmond, "Figuring Exotic Nature in Sixteenth-Century Europe: Garcia de Orta and Carolus Clusius," in Costa, ed., *Medicine, Trade, and Empire*, 183, the inclusion of images was at Clusius's insistence.

in local climate (as others would soon do in the Atlantic).[31] But Orta did not. Had he wanted the text to be of greatest value to the Crown or to merchants, apothecaries, and traders in royal employ, Orta might have followed the examples of Pires or Álvares and focused solely on the provenance of the drugs and spices in question.[32]

Orta, however, chose the organizational device that reflected the single most common concern to each of these groups: plants. Chapters organized alphabetically according to the common, vernacular (Portuguese) name for each plant in question not only adhered to the long-standing herbal tradition associated with (and, among humanists, authorized by) Dioscorides, it also made the *Colóquios* an imminently flexible guide to Asian *naturalia*.

Rather than a notional "Indies," it was the expansive but tightly intertwined world of Asia, with its dense maritime networks manifest in the crates and barrels that lined the wharves of Goa, that bounded and centered the spatial framework in the *Colóquios*. Intentionally conflating the things of Asia with those America would have been unthinkable. Rather than the homogenizing view of a Flemish naturalist – and certainly in contrast to a perspective that would situate Goa at the ostensible periphery of an expansive and interconnected world system centered in Europe – the world of the *Colóquios* was one in which Asia generally, and Goa in particular was at the center. For Orta it was in Goa that the health of a colony, the commerce of far-flung Lusophone communities, and his credibility as a physician and naturalist were all on the line. In the *Colóquios*, Orta portrayed India not simply as a point of origin for ships bound for western Christendom but as a destination – one in which bezoars from Spanish America, books from the Levant, and rhubarb from China, all converged. Clusius's spatial imagination assimilated disparate parts of the overseas world and collapsed them into so many points of origin for things exotic.[33] Orta's was based on the itineraries of Asian networks of exchange.

EMPIRICISM BY THE BOOK

For both Orta and Clusius, the evidence of the senses was integral to natural inquiry. But viewing them both as part of a single, coherent

---

[31] See Chapter 6.
[32] See, for example, Barbosa, *Livro*. On the apothecaries Tomé Pires and Simão Álvares, see Chapter 3.
[33] A habit of geographical thinking that, many decades later, became widespread in northern Europe, according to Schmidt, *Inventing Exoticism*.

tradition of natural history in which first-hand, somatic encounters with nature were increasingly accorded epistemic primacy over the authoritative claims of writers from the Greek, Roman, and Islamic worlds over-states the case.[34] The authority afforded to the evidence of experience not only changed – in both degree and kind – in tandem with generational shifts in the study of nature within Europe during the two naturalists' lives, but it, too, was an expression of the distinct concerns and the particular interpretive challenges they faced. For Orta these grew from encounters textual, experiential, and cross-cultural alike.

For Orta, books anchored inquiry into the identity, essence, and medical uses of a plant wherever possible. Hence, Orta did not need to experience camphor to know with unwavering certainty that it was cold and dry in the third degree. Avicenna had said so and for Orta that was enough.[35] This did not mean that sensory experience had no place at all. Quite the contrary: the evidence of the senses frequently served Orta as confirmation of textual determinations. Hence, when it came to the question of whether the *altith* of Avicenna, the *laserpicium* of Galen, and the *imgara* of the Hindus were all the same thing as the asafetida of Orta's countrymen, Orta confirmed that they were by using the tools of philology first and only then buttressing his conclusion by noting that they all shared "the absolute worst smell in all the world."[36]

As these claims suggest, the textual corpus that Orta relied upon did authorize an epistemology of the senses. But it was a narrow and conservative one that allocated epistemic primacy in characteristic ways. Physical attributes – the size, shape, colour, appearance and arrangement of a plant's constituent parts – were particularly dubious. These were among the things that Aristotle had termed "accidents." No certain knowledge could be based on them. The evidence of touch, taste, and smell, however, provided clues to the essential qualities of a plant, and those in turn revealed its curative uses. As Orta put it, "qualities proceed from the species."[37] Touch, taste, and smell revealed qualities "proper" to each plant. When properly understood and judiciously mustered as evidence, "one need not worry of being fooled" by the evidence the provided.[38]

There was nothing novel about this epistemology. Orta's description of camphor – that it was cold and dry in the third degree – hints at its

---

[34] As in Almeida, "Portugal and the Dawn of Modern Science"; and Almeida, "Sobre a revolução da experiência." But see Ogilvie, *Science of Describing*, especially 87–100.
[35] Orta, *Colóquios*, vol. 1, 160.   [36] Orta, *Colóquios*, vol. 1, 80, 75–87.
[37] Orta, *Colóquios*, vol. 1, 158.   [38] Orta, *Colóquios*, vol. 1, 160.

provenance. It was a thoroughly Galenic view of plants and their curative properties. Much like the vision of the humoral body, which now underwrote learned medicine (and which was acquired through careful study of any one of the new editions of the Galenic corpus[39]), every item of nature possessed essential qualities that could be plotted along the twin axes that spanned from hot to cold in one direction, and from moist to dry in the other.

Whenever possible Orta adhered to this view of nature and its qualities to confirm the identity of plants, to determine their medicinal uses, and to explain their action upon the ailing body. The influence of this Galenic framework over the *Colóquios* was pronounced. When it came to questions about the identity and classification of *materia medica*, the overlapping claims of a text and the narrowly authorized evidence of the senses easily trumped the particulars of nature. So, for example, never mind that black and white pepper looked so different and were produced, as Orta believed, by different trees. They both burned the tongue, confirming what was already written about them: the precious item was hot and dry in the third degree. For the purposes of preparing a medicinal recipe, the two were virtually interchangeable.[40]

With the qualities of plants like camphor, asafoetida, and black and white pepper so precisely described and set out in a book, there should have been little disagreement over their identities, qualities, and uses. Their taste, smell, and other essential qualities had been recorded by ancient and medieval authors; they could be identified, sorted, and put to use with ease. But in practice, as Orta well knew, things were not so straightforward. With his attention trained on the Arabic corpus, Orta found that even as Rasis had agreed with Avicenna that the gum of camphor was cool in the third degree, the two men were still at odds over whether it was moist (as Rasis had argued) or dry (which was Avicenna's position). In cases like these, textual authority was again primary and decisive. Orta trained his powers of discernment not upon natural particulars but upon the weight of accumulated judgement. The careful compilation of opinions, rather than a closer inspection of nature, could lead the diligent researcher to a defensible answer. In this case, since

---

[39] The literature here is immense but for a survey on the distribution of Galenic texts in sixteenth-century Europe, on the one hand, and on Galenism among Portuguese physicians in this period, on the other; see Ian Maclean, *Learning and the Marketplace: Essays in the History of the Early Modern Book* (Leiden: Brill, 2009), chs 4 and 13, respectively.

[40] Orta, *Colóquios*, vol. 2, 246–247.

"most if not all" subsequent authors had agreed with the Avicenna, Orta felt confident that he could do so as well.[41]

What Orta found increasingly disturbing was that disagreement on matters of touch, taste, and smell characterized a proliferating number of things. Some of these were of little consequence. On one occasion, the taste of a watermelon put Orta and Antonia, one of his Konkani servants, at odds. She assured him that the strange looking fruit with the marbled green rind and brilliant red flesh was "quite good." Orta, having tried it, was repulsed. It had "the taste of mud" he wrote. Why had they disagreed? For Orta the answer was simple: the young woman had spoken "according to her taste."[42]

Alone, this incident of gustatory dissent might have seemed immaterial to the production of natural knowledge. But that was neither the first nor the last time that Orta found himself at odds with his South Asian contemporaries.[43] The contemptible melon was not just a marginal case. It was emblematic of a much more profound problem – one that portended therapeutic catastrophe were the plant in question a prized medicament and were the qualities at issue the very vegetable essence that indicated its humoral aspect and curative use. At issue was not the appeal of a particular drug or spice to any individual person but the commensurability of accumulated sense experiences among the range of specialists in Goa who claimed expertise in the arts of preserving health and prolonging life.

In the cosmopolitan milieu of Goa – in which midwives, apothecaries, hakims, vaidyas, and many others participated in colonial natural inquiry and curative care – even the qualities and uses of pepper were matters of debate. While Orta and his medieval Muslim predecessors agreed that pepper was hot, the Hindu vaidyas in Goa insisted rather the reverse. The said pepper was cold. Orta thought the opinion rather absurd, "something to laugh at," and wrote smugly that "one need not prove that a flame is hot; one knows it simply because it burns."[44]

But the laughter rang hollow. That even highly regarded authors might come to contradictory conclusions about the qualities of the same plant seemed to suggest that claims about the identity and uses of individual plants based on such encounters were highly dubious. Orta finally had to concede. The truth, he wrote in a more sober passage, is that "one finds most appealing the smells to which one is accustomed."[45] Given not only

[41] Orta, *Colóquios*, vol. 1, 160.   [42] Orta, *Colóquios*, vol. 2, 133.

[43] Orta, *Colóquios*, vol. 1, 75–87.   [44] Orta, *Colóquios*, vol. 2, 249.

[45] Orta, *Colóquios*, vol. 1, 80.

his disappointing encounter with watermelon but the longstanding disagreement surrounding camphor, Orta might have added taste and touch as well. Rather than yielding universally recognizable qualities, sensory evidence – much like gustatory preferences – were culturally bound. Increasingly it seemed to Orta that, in at least some cases, what were supposed to have been the facts of nature were little more than culturally rooted matters of opinion.

When textual claims seemed contradictory or otherwise dubious, the investigator needed recourse to some other kind of evidence. Orta turned to a plant's physical attributes. The observable, outward appearances of a plant, in addition to its inner, essential qualities and textual claims about it, became indispensable to the study of nature.

When both the scholarly claims of old and the assessments of touch, taste, and smell so plainly variable, Orta did not abandon his texts and senses. He reallocated epistemic primacy among them. When attempts to assess inherent, inward qualities failed to yield certainty, only then did Orta emphasize the importance of a plant's outward features. Only in these rather specific situations did physical features and the sense of sight become proportionally more important. Hence when he and the apothecary Álvares disagreed over the question of pepper (whether white and black pepper were different kinds produced by different plants), Orta's answer (yes on both counts) hinged first on textual authority, secondarily on subtly different smells, and then finally on the subtly different shapes of the stems, leaves, and berries themselves.[46]

That was how Orta used the evidence of the senses. His was a recursive empiricism – one that first looked to confirm what was already known, shuttling back and forth between textual claims and long-authorized forms of somatic encounter.[47] It was an empiricism still bridled to deductive reasoning and leveraged to confirm the claims of the texts of old. It was, in short, an empiricism by the book. It took seriously both textual

---

[46] See my discussion of the "Epistemologies of the Pepper Trade" in Chapter 3; and Orta, *Colóquios*, vol. 2, 240–250.

[47] On what I have termed here and elsewhere "recursive empiricism," see Cagle, "Cultures of Inquiry, Myths of Empire: Natural History in Colonial Goa," in *Medicine, Trade and Empire*, ed. Costa, 107–128. Although inspired by different circumstances Ann Blair identifies a similar technique in *The Theater of Nature: Jean Bodin and Renaissance Science* (Princeton, NJ: Princeton University Press, 1997), ch. 3. See also Daston and Park, *Wonders*, 135–146; and Pamela H. Smith, *The Body of the Artisan: Art and Experience in the Scientific Revolution* (Chicago, IL: University of Chicago Press, 2004).

authority and the evidence of the senses. When necessary, it took an expanded view of the value of the visible, physical attributes that natural philosophy looked upon with deep scepticism. Still, taken alone, neither category of evidence was sufficient for the production of certainty. But together they offered a legitimate basis for a correct accounting of nature.

Of course, Orta's networks were commercial networks. In transit, all properties susceptible to the senses could not only change but change markedly.

GLOBAL TRADE AND THE LIMITS OF EXPERIENCE

Global networks packed Goa's markets with objects from around the world. Africa, the Americas, and Europe were all simultaneously (if unevenly) brought into view along Goa's streets and in its market stalls. Strolling along Rua Direita, Orta could compare coconut palms from the Maldives and the Malabar Coast, the quality of pearls from India and Peru, and the price of myrrh in China and Malacca.[48] Yet even if Goa were a center of discernment and calculation, it was still only a single point in a global network. That, in turn, posed significant investigative challenges. Historians have often argued that global commerce generated a surge of appreciation for sensory experience as an authoritative source of knowledge about nature. The silk merchant, the apothecary, and the collector of rarities all had much to gain from a discerning hand, a cultivated palate, and a careful eye. Touch, taste, sight, and smell – the evidence of the senses – constituted a way of objective knowing that divorced the thing in question from either intuition or received wisdom.[49]

Orta was inclined to agree. As he saw it, the circuits of exchange that were the very sinews of Portugal's empire could take on special significance in the cataloguing of nature and its uses:

Now that the sea routes are better known, and [now] that there are more ships [that sail] so often to Portugal [and] to other parts of the West, we ought not wonder that, at much less cost, there are so many more [drugs and simples] – and without their being falsified. And we buy these medicines more cheaply in this place, where they grow better [because the land] is better suited to produce them.[50]

---

[48] Orta, *Colóquios*, vol. 1, 236–237; vol. 2, 120–121, 352.
[49] Here I work from the discussion in Cook, *Matters of Exchange*, especially ch. 1. Other examples include the essays in Smith and Findlen, eds., *Merchants and Marvels*.
[50] Orta, *Colóquios*, vol. 2, 292.

For Orta, in other words, the advantage of Portugal's imperial commercial system was not simply that it offered "the West" a cheaper and more stable supply of commoditized nature from the fertile lands of Asia, but that, once they were part of the imperial commercial system, plants, medicines, and sundry other products of nature could no longer be manipulated, adulterated, substituted (one thing for another) or otherwise "falsified." Imperial commerce, with its unified shipping network and systematic record-keeping rendered all manner of *naturalia* stable. Their observable qualities, their uses, their very identities could thereby be fixed.

Both density and predictability (there were "*so many more* ... [and] *without their being falsified*") were critical attributes of this idealized imperial system of circulation. As long as the empire could channel to and from Goa specimens that had not been "falsified" or otherwise manipulated prior to entry into the imperial circuits of exchange, then they may safely have been assumed to be no more and no less than what was claimed of them. In similar fashion, when Orta attached names and qualities to things of nature, the stability of those associations was secure beyond Goa to the extent that the network that circulated them remained intact.[51] The identities and qualities that Orta affixed to plants in the *Colóquios* and the circulatory streams that brought plant matter under Orta's purview in the first place – and which thereby made the book possible – were mutually reinforcing. Orta's text and the commercial streams that enabled it reinforced one another in a tautological loop that sustained both survival and profitable trade in the capital of Portugal's empire in Asia.

But the *Colóquios* reveals a much more complex relationship between commerce and science, and a much more multifaceted history of epistemic transformation. Networks of empire were always bounded and those boundaries had further implications for the place of sensory experience in the making of natural knowledge. The stabilizing potential that derived from the density and predictability of an imperial system of exchange was always mitigated in practice by its inescapably segmented character and its consequently limited reach. Well before most products of nature were at his disposal, they had been collected, sifted, sorted, selected, rejected, and otherwise submitted to regimes of accumulation and order of which most Portuguese – Orta included – had limited knowledge and little or no influence.

---

[51] Here of course, I am referring to the notion of "immutable mobiles" developed in Latour, *Science in Action*, 223–228.

Of this, the camphor trade was emblematic. Camphor came to the ports of western India from Borneo and China. Used to treat burns and cure insomnia, it was a drug derived from the desiccated gum of certain resinous trees – usually from branches cleaved from the trunk. The slim branches of camphor themselves could be purchased outright, which according to Orta is how the apothecaries in Goa often bought it. Portions of the ready-made drug were also traded. These came in an assortment of sizes, appearances, and qualities. Upon receiving a shipment of prepared camphor, vanias used copper sieves of varying weaves in order to sort the drug into four groups based on size. What vanias labeled their categories, Orta did not say. The Portuguese chose *cabeça* (head) as the name of the largest of these and *pé* (foot) to refer to the most diminutive – about the size of a grain of rice.[52]

Goa's merchants then subdivided each of these sizes of camphor into categories based on qualities discernible by their colour. The best and most expensive, but also the scarcest, were large masses almost entirely white in colour. But camphor bruised easily. In transit most pieces of camphor sustained the hard knocks and exposure to moisture that gave them a vermillion hue and often streaks and stains of black. These were the middling variety. The worst, what Orta referred to as the "dregs," were all black.[53] By the time camphor arrived to markets in Goa or Cambay, where Orta discussed it with the Hindu merchants who had befriended him, camphor the drug bore no resemblance whatsoever to camphor in its vegetable form – those slender, woody branches.

In a way, that sieve used to sort ready-made camphor marked nothing less than the boundary – the outermost limit – of Portugal's empire in Asia. It was a stark reminder to Orta that he was one receiver among many in one of numerous locations within the broader system of intra-Asian, and ultimately global, commerce. If commerce helped naturalists like Orta resolve problems of knowledge, it helped produced them just as readily.

In so many other ways, too, nature tended to change in transit. Even commoditized, plant matter in particular had life cycles of its own – quite

---

[52] In the identification of camphor, I have relied on Ficalho's notes in Orta, *Colóquios*, vol. 1, 162–171; and Markham, trans., *Colloquies*, 88, n.4. According to Ficalho, the camphor ostensibly from China is the product of *Laurus Camphora* (sic) (Linn.). According to Markham, the camphor of Borneo and Sumatra is the product of *Dryobalanops aromatica*, which is *D. camphora* (Colebrook) and that of Formosa is from *Camphora officinarum* (Linn).

[53] Orta, *Colóquios*, vol. 1, 153.

apart from those which carried it from germination to fruit-bearing maturity. Consequently, as Orta found, commercial networks provided for variety far more easily than they could be used to identify with certainty the things in transit and to know their culinary and curative qualities. Thanks to the very networks upon which Orta, Goa, intra-Asian trade, and Portugal's empire all depended, the identification of valuable commodities and the description of indispensable medicinal plants always involved a great deal of uncertainty.

If, as with pepper and camphor alike, the bumps and bruises of sea travel changed their outward appearance, and if, as with caphor, changes in appearance were partly a consequence of the manipulations required to transform plant matter into medicinal simples, it was also true that regional variations in the techniques of preservation could give the same medicinal simples radically different appearances, tastes, and smells. That, too, made *materia medica* harder to identify. So, for example, Orta noted that the asafetida, that came to Goa from Gujarat was a slightly opaque, brown gum that was firm but brittle; the same simple from the Arabian port of Hormuz came preserved in "the blood of a young bull" and wrapped in a clumpy earthen coating.[54]

Divergent appearances might also be the result of intentional deception. In Orta's experience, commerce – especially over long distances and across multiple points of exchange – inevitably led to adulteration and falsification. In the *Colóquios*, Orta rarely missed an opportunity to point this out and regularly commented on how merchants were unscrupulous in their commercial dealings.[55] On this count, Orta charged no single group more frequently than his own countrymen. A common mercantile vocation among New and Old Christians as part of a diasporic Portuguese "nation" may have enabled a unified sense of identity and sustained relationships of trust that underwrote global trade,[56] but Orta did not see it that way at all. Neither the physician nor any other Portuguese traders had access to the points of origin of all the plants that concerned them, and even if they could control the trade in any one of these things over the entirety of its journey into his hands, Orta had no reason to believe they would transport it, along with any information about it, any more

---

[54] Orta, *Colóquios*, vol. 1, 82.   [55] Orta, *Colóquios*, vol. 1, 154–155.

[56] Daviken Studnicki-Gizbert, *A Nation Upon the Ocean Sea: Portugal's Atlantic Diaspora and the Crisis of the Spanish Empire, 1492–1640* (New York: Oxford University Press, 2007).

reliably than any other trading group in the Indian Ocean world.[57] The process of exchange entailed an ill-defined but nevertheless seemingly inevitable succession of transformations regardless of who transported it.

An emphasis on particulars and evaluations of worth based on subtle observable distinctions may have provided common ground upon which merchants, traders, physicians, and apothecaries could meet. But the profit-generating practices of the merchant and trader rarely inspired the trust of those intent on establishing certain knowledge of nature. When it came to the deceptive manipulation of commodified nature, "one sees all manner of things," cautioned Orta, and one must be prepared for them whether in the production of natural knowledge or in the pursuit of profitable "speculation."[58]

Because the reliability of the networks, of informants, of the identity and quality of the *naturalia* themselves all remained major problems, Orta had to devise an epistemology that embraced the widest possible range evidence. Since so many items had been identified and described on the printed page, texts were indispensable. But they were also incomplete and inaccurate, possibly underwritten by little more than opinion, and therefore, on their own, generally dubious. The evidence of the senses, narrowly authorized by the intellectual culture in which Orta had originally been schooled, took on proportionally greater importance. It also took on a new kind of importance. In the case of textual accounts that seemed plainly untrue, text and experience could be deployed in tandem. But which *kinds* of somatic impressions were most important were still at issue. Appearances were accidents. Only taste, touch, and smell, disciplined by the humoralist claims of the textual tradition, could yield knowledge about the inherent curative properties of a plant. The networks of trade in Indian Ocean Asia reinforced this epistemological hierarchy of the senses, for the networks on which Orta relied tended so often to distort physical appearances. Taste, touch, and smell remained indispensable tools for the identification and description of nature. Yet, because transit often changed these qualities too, and because, anyway, descriptive consensus in textual sources seemed so often elusive, physical appearance were a necessary epistemic tool.

Finally, if commerce propelled particular kinds of epistemological innovation, it was also true that the epistemic resources of old – those fragile, bound volumes of print and manuscript – could be leveraged to

---

[57] Orta, *Colóquios*, vol. 1, 151; and vol. 2, 248.   [58] Orta, *Colóquios*, vol. 1, 90.

resolve question that were narrowly commercial. One such question was the elusive port of origin for Chinese camphor. As anyone who traded in the drug well knew, there were two kinds of camphor. The best came from Borneo. The much inferior variety arrived from China. The problem was that no one seemed to know which of China's many ports conducted the trade.

Orta used humoral theory to resolve the question of camphor's commercial origin. Because the property of camphor was to evanesce, the best camphor could be identified by its strong and lasting scent. Conversely, bad camphor – often adulterated – could be assumed to break down more quickly and have a weaker scent. Smell could be used to distinguish between the superior camphor from Borneo and the inferior kind from China. That much was easy to deduce. But precisely which port in China dispatched the inferior camphor remained a mystery. Solving it meant combining the physician's humoral theory and the merchant's commercial savvy. When it came to the port of origin for Chinese camphor, Orta understood that there were two possibilities. Chinese camphor could ship from either Canton, where the Portuguese had a trading factory, or from a port he called "Chincheo," where they did not and which Orta understood to be much less frequented.[59] As far as Orta could discern, camphor did not come through the Portuguese factory at Canton. It was, however, through the port of Chincheo that merchants from Borneo traded. That meant ample opportunity for Chinese traders there to acquire and adulterate camphor before exporting it back overseas. Precisely how camphor might be adulterated at Chincheo – whether an ostensibly inferior Chinese camphor was combined with that from Borneo or whether the Borneo camphor itself was combined with such common adulterants as slivers of stone, raw poplar (*alambre*) gum, or even fine wood shavings ("farinha de um páo") to constitute the inferior variety – Orta did not know.[60] But on the basis of expectations born of humoral theory and on determinations based on known trade routes, Orta believed he had identified the geographical origins – if not the exact constitution – of Chinese camphor. It came, he claimed, from Chincheo.

Did such knowledge make it easier to turn a profit in the camphor trade? Maybe, but maybe not: for Orta it had real, but only limited (and

[59] Orta's "Chincheo" was probably Changchau in Fuhkien (now Fujian) province. See Henry Yule and Arthur Coke Burnell, *Hobson-Jobson: A Glossary of Anglo-Indian Words and Phrases* (London: J. Murray, 1886), 200–201.
[60] Orta, *Colóquios*, vol. 1, 154.

perhaps disappointing), practical value. With camphor and so many other *materia medica*, claims about ports of origin were used to establish prices. Camphor ostensibly from Borneo traded at a price that was many times higher than that from China. The difference was enough to lead less savvy traders to believe that price verified the origins and hence the quality of the drug in question. But price was an abstraction that could occlude a drug's real history. Orta's friend, a vania in Cambay heavily involved in the camphor trade, told him that when his stock of Bornean camphor ran low, he simply mixed it with a bit of that from China and then sold it as before – as if it had not been adulterated at all.[61]

THE POLITICS OF DEPICTION

It was hardly surprising that Clusius should have insisted that his *Aromatum et simplicium* include at least a few pictures.[62] By April 1563, when the first pages of the original *Colóquios* were printed and bound in Goa, serious books of natural history throughout Italy and northern Europe had begun to fill with often elaborate floral images. Illustration was a laborious and expensive business. It required a veritable contingent of specialists – from authors, proofers, and paper-makers to wood sculptors, painters, and printers. How images made their way into books was as variable as the reasons for their inclusion. But the process raised a host of questions that were of special concern to naturalists. Plants changed with the seasons. How best to depict them and what, exactly, deserved most elaboration – the roots, leaves, flowers, fruits – were thorny issues. By the time Clusius came into possession of Orta's *Colóquios* in January of 1564, those questions had led to the development of array of techniques. Across the middle decades of the sixteenth century, images were all the rage in serious publications on natural history.[63]

Ubiquitous they may have been, but pictures of plants had also proven deeply controversial. In the early 1530s, as Orta traveled the length of the Indian subcontinent, his counterparts in Italy and northern Europe hotly debated the use of illustrations in natural history texts. In 1542 one of

---

[61] Orta, *Colóquios*, vol. 1, 154–155.
[62] This is the interpretation of Egmond, "Figuring Exotic Nature," 183.
[63] Sachiko Kusukawa, "Illustrating Nature," in *Books and the Sciences in History*, eds. Marina Frasca-Spada and Nick Jardine (New York: Cambridge University Press, 2000), 90–113; Brian Ogilvie, "Image and Text in Natural History, 1500–1700," in *The Power of Images in Early Modern Science*, eds. Wolfgang Lefèvre et al. (Boston, MA: Birkhäuser Verlag, 2003), 141–166; and Ogilvie, *Science of Describing*, 34–37.

Clusius's elder colleagues, the German physician Leonhart Fuchs, published *De historia stirpium*. The event capped a decade of heated and even rancorous debate on the matter of pictures, with insults exchanged publicly and in print. Fuchs's book brimmed with elaborately detailed woodcuts. Fuchs himself oversaw their execution with great care and wrote pointedly on their importance. It had been Fuchs's longstanding contention that the way a plant looked was sufficient to allow the careful, disciplined observer to draw definitive distinctions between even very similar specimens. A plant, in other words, could be identified by its outward appearance. And once identified, its humoral complexion and curative attributes were assuredly known, because Dioscorides and Galen had recorded them. Over the centuries, repeated transcription and translation of their work had confused the relationship between names of plants and their corresponding descriptions and curative attributes. Comparing ancient descriptions with contemporary plants was, for Fuchs, the best way to sort out that confusion. In this way, mimetic depictions not only enabled Fuchs and his readers to identify plants but to know their medicinal uses. And that was the principal point of contention. Pictures, Fuchs's detractors argued, simply could not be used in that way because, as Aristotle had said, physical features were accidents and could not guarantee an inference of innate qualities. Only taste, touch, and smell could do that.[64]

Whether Orta knew about the controversy or not is an open question. But by the time he had the *Colóquios* prepared for publication he had acquired a copy of Fuchs's book. Orta cited it in his own chapters on spikenard and zedoary. To Orta, who in his own book often expressed a distinct appreciation for the visual,[65] the inclusion of illustrations in the *Colóquios* entailed two irresolvable problems. First, confronted with the transformations of objects in transit, Orta might well have asked what, precisely, he ought to depict – and what epistemic advantage a picture might be supposed to provide. Would it be more profitable to illustrate the branch of camphor itself or the life-saving medicament derived from it, which made it so valuable in the first place and which was perhaps just as commonly purchased from Goa's apothecaries? If the latter, could images

---

[64] Kusukawa, "Leonhart Fuchs," 403–427, but especially pp. 415–421.

[65] Orta, *Colóquios*, vol. 1, 260, praised the Chinese not only for their "subtle" skill at "buying and selling" but for their manual skill, and especially their refined print-making and painting capabilities. It was on the basis of such art, and especially of depictions of Ming scholars, that Orta formed his own high opinion of the wisdom of Chinese rule.

meaningfully convey the subtle differences between the darkened block of camphor, for example, and the dark brown bolus of asafetida gum?

If images were of dubious value, they were also dangerous. In Goa, the trouble surrounding the production of pictures had as much to do with the colonial politics of craftsmanship as with the epistemic claims inherent in the act of depiction. Goa was a vigorously, even violently, Catholic enclave.[66] Pictures may or may not have been taken to imply tendentious claims to authoritative knowledge about nature. But the act of producing them would certainly have suggested the patronage of – and close relationships with – native Konkani craftsmen. Portuguese regularly turned to Konkani and other South Asian artisans for the creation of decorative furniture (chests, caskets, cabinets), as well as religious icons.[67] Those collaborations did little to distinguish Goa from Portuguese trading communities elsewhere in the Indian Ocean or in East and West Africa.[68] Nor would they distinguish the Portuguese in Goa from their French or English counterparts in other parts of the subcontinent in the following centuries.[69] But in Goa, the patronage of native artisans for works pertaining to matters of faith – be it the painting of churches, the sculpting of statuary, or the creation of small religious objects – was viewed with suspicion. In 1588 it would be outlawed altogether.[70]

The close working relationships between an author and the coterie of craftsmen who were essential for the production and placement of mimetic depictions within a text were precisely the kinds of personal ties that would draw the attention of Goa's religious authorities. Patronage relationships, as with matters of food and dress, were a principal focus of invigilation for the Goan Inquisition. Patronage of non-Christian Konkani craftsmen suggested to the city's Catholic religious authorities a pernicious cultural affiliation that deserved censure, imprisonment, or worse. Orta, a New Christian who would repeatedly appear before the

---

[66] A. K. Priolkar, *The Goa Inquisition: Being a Quatercentenary Commemoration Study of the Inquisition in India* (Bombay: V.G. Moghe at the Bombay University Press, 1961); Paul Axelrod and Michelle A. Fuerch, "Flight of the Deities: Hindu Resistance in Portuguese Goa," *Modern Asian Studies* 30/2 (1996): 387–421; and Teotonio R. de Souza, "The Council of Trent (1545–1563): Its Reception in Portuguese India," in *Transcontinental Links in the History of Non-Western Christianity*, edited by Klaus Koschorke (Wiesbaden: Harrassowitz, 2002), 194–196.

[67] Luís de Moura Sobral, "The Expansion and the Arts: Transfers, Contaminations, Innovations," in *Portuguese Oceanic Expansion*, eds. Bethencourt and Curto, 404–416.

[68] Sobral, "The Expansion and the Arts," 390–428.

[69] Jasanoff, *Edge of Empire*; and Raj, *Relocating Modern Science*, especially 27–59.

[70] HAG, PAR, "Provisões a favor da Cristandade," ff. 53–54 and 94–95v.

Holy Office in Goa, was himself long an target of suspicion.[71] In the
Colóquios, he made plain that even when it came to procuring *materia
medica* from Goa's large indigenous quarter, it was not he but rather one
of his household servants, his "buyers," who actually made the trip.[72]
Images would have offered indisputable evidence for relationships that
Orta needed to deny. They entailed risks that were best not taken. For
Orta, words would suffice.[73]

Orta's was a science and a spatial framework crafted *in situ*. Both were
dependent upon cross-cultural collaborations and underwritten by networks of a distinctly commercial orientation in which the language of
exchange was more often Arabic or one of a number of South Asian
languages than Portuguese. The constellation of interests that underwrote
investigations of nature, the precise questions asked about nature, the
ways evidence was mustered to answer them, indeed the very definition of
evidence itself, and the way those answers were presented in print: these
were some of the ways in which the practice of natural history differed for
Orta and Clusius. For Orta, the conflation of East and West implicit in
exoticizing frameworks like "the Indies" – however much it titillated the
imaginations of narrowly-traveled naturalists in Europe – was of little use
for making sense of a wealthy, cosmopolitan, and interconnected world
of seaborne commerce and seasonal storms. The claims to truth about
nature conveyed in the *Colóquios* reflected in both their content and
organization the preoccupations of the ethnically and linguistically
diverse, geographically disparate participants in those networks. Taken
together, those circumstances helped constitute the culture of inquiry in
colonial Goa.

It was a culture of inquiry underwritten by commerce. But the relationship between trade and natural inquiry was a fraught one. Trade never
necessarily propelled an epistemological transformation that privileged
outward features over inward qualities and textual scholarship. Experience always worked in tandem with texts. No single kind of evidence
(textual or experiential) and certainly no single kind of experience (of
inner properties or outward appearances) was on its own sufficient to
bear the full burden of proof in the study of nature. As the extent and

---

[71] Carvalho, *Garcia d'Orta*, 32–63.   [72] Orta, *Colóquios*, vol. 2, 133.
[73] My characterization of Orta – his ostensible preference for illustration, which he articu-
lates only in prose in the *Colóquios*, and his simultaneous concern for its attendant risks –
may buttress the case made by Ruy Manuel Loureiro for Orta as the person responsible
for the illustrated but anonymously authored *Codex Casanatense 1889*. See Loureiro,
"Information Networks in the *Estado da Índia*."

credibility of the available textual record for any single item varied, and as the forms it might take in the markets of Goa multiplied, so the particular arrangements of proof for the claims concerning any one item in the *Colóquios* varied, too. And because some criteria became more valuable in the identification of certain plants but was of marginal utility for others, Orta's chapters took on a distinctly uneven and slightly disorganized quality. They were, however, underwritten by a highly functional, if also highly eclectic, approach to the production of natural knowledge.

This was not a revolutionary epistemology. It was, however, a workable one, and it was in this context that Orta used the term "experiment" (in archaic Portuguese, *esprimentar*). "Experiment" as Orta used it had a fairly wide array of meanings. It could connote experience, as in "to try," and this was principally how Orta used it. But he also employed the term to refer to chemical and mechanical manipulations of various objects of nature, as when he distilled waters of various plants. Occasionally he used it to suggest that he had or had not tried a particular remedy on a patient. For Orta, "experiment" *could* mean any of these things. It *could not*, however, be taken to imply that Orta had created a systematic experimental program. For there is no evidence either in the *Colóquios* or in any of the few documents left behind that suggest that Orta was engaged in the systematic production of probabilistic "matters of fact" through the application of technology to nature.[74] If "experiment" referred no more and no less than to a first-hand somatic encounter, it was by itself only half of Orta's epistemic toolkit. It was in marrying text with experience (rather than experiment) toward the production of certainty (rather than probability) that Orta understood the concept of "experiment" and ultimately sought to certify natural knowledge.[75]

Amid the vertiginous transformations inherent in practices of circulation – illustrations of nature in a book meant to provide certain knowledge made little sense. The uncertainties inherent in circulation made illustrations unworkable and perhaps irrelevant; the politics of craftsmanship made them dangerous. In the *Colóquios* and unlike in the *Aromatum et simplicium*, pictures were given no quarter.

---

[74] I have based my understanding of "matters of fact" on the rather specific use by Shapin and Schaffer in *Leviathan and the Air*. My contention on this point stands in sharp contrast with, for example, that of Almeida, "Portugal and the Dawn of Modern Science"; and Almeida, "Sobre a revolução da experiência."

[75] My argument for epistemological conservatism is similar to that of Paula Findlen, *Possessing Nature: Museums, Collecting, and Scientific Culture in Early Modern Italy* (Berkeley, CA: University of California Press, 1994), 57–70, 198–208.

Yet there was no escaping the expertise and technical skill of indigenous Goans. Even basic aspects of the publication of the *Colóquios* were probably handled by a skilled "Indian" who, according to one Jesuit, had "shown great knowledge of the process of printing" soon after Goa's press was up and running.[76] As it was printed in Goa in 1563, tensions surrounding precisely those aspects of life in the colonial city were coming to a head and would remain pervasive over the closing decades of the century.

The culture of inquiry that obtained in Goa was one that embraced South Asian *materia medica* and curative knowledge even as it wrestled with the indigenous social and religious significance of local therapeutics and the authority that Portuguese colonialism placed in the indigenous and *mestiço* women who were the healers of first resort for most householders in the colonial city. This was a culture in which secular and religious authorities participated. But they were never entirely at ease with it. A closer look at the intertwined anxieties of commerce and medicine in Goa help make sense of yet another aspect of the *Colóquios* – of not only what Orta included in the book but how he included it. When Clusius prepared the *Aromatum et simplicium*, he excised the anecdotes of life in Goa that Orta had seen fit to include. The *Colóquios* was packed with intrigue, rumor, and unsubstantiated gossip from Goa's busy streets. Why would a book devoted to telling the truth about nature mingle so many facts with so much fiction?

[76] *MB* vol. 5, 173, n. 40; and *DI* vol. 3, 514.

5

Facts and Fictions

I want no censure from a friar lest it come from the pulpit.
Garcia de Orta[1]

A TEMPLE ON THE MAINLAND

It was late in the summer of 1589 and the wind and rain of the summer
monsoons had begun their annual assault on Goa, bringing with them the
familiar depredations of this most uncertain of seasons. Throngs of idle
soldiers and seamen waited out the storms for their next assignment. The
city's main quarters had become damp and crowded. Many of Goa's
streets were flooded. Hospitals filled. The specter of disease loomed over
the city, enhanced no doubt by recollections of the dysentery epidemic
that had swept the island a year earlier.[2] The fleet due in from Lisbon had
by this time left Mozambique, pulled by the monsoon eastward across the
Indian Ocean, though when it might arrive – and in what condition – no
one could know. Anxiety ran high.

It was "principally at this time, awaiting the ships from the kingdom,"
wrote the Inquisitors Rui Sodrinho and Fray Thomas Pinto to Philip I,
that "depravity and disorder" too were at their height in Goa. Manuel de
Sousa Coutniho and Dona Ana Espanholim – the governor of all of
Portuguese Asia and his wife – had abandoned the sanctity of the island's
Catholic Church for the pagan succor of a Hindu shrine on the mainland,

[1] Orta, *Colóquios*, vol. 2, 54.
[2] Alberto C. Germano da Silva Correia, *La Vieille-Goa* (Bastorá: Tipografia Rangel, 1931),
268–307, lists the years of several outbreaks including this one.

where they "dealt in the mysticism of witchdoctors" (*feitiçeiros*), asking – as it turned out – for some measure of help or guidance or assurance in the midst of what they feared was an impending disaster. Sometime later, in the subdued calm of Goa's São Domingos monastery, Dona Ana confessed to Fray Thomas that she and her husband had wanted "to foresee the things to come" by interpreting "dreams" and to consult with the sorcerer, that he might "cast spells."[3] Stern and unforgiving, the Inquisitor Sodrinho had little tolerance for transgression – even when the life and livelihood of Portugal's Asian capital were at stake. In punishment, the governor's wife was levied a severe fine. But it was decided that Coutinho himself should plead for mercy in trial before the Inquisition. The Holy Office, however, along with other members of the clergy, had earned enemies among some of the city's most powerful casados. Since trying a *fidalgo* could only inflame tensions, the trial would take place not in Goa but Lisbon. And so it was that one of the most powerful Portuguese officials in Asia sailed from Goa in shame.[4]

Medicine was underwritten by assumptions about the relationship between nature and the human body, including conceptions of the occult forces of life and death, and was closely intertwined with religion.[5] In Goa, where survival so often hinged on the curative intervention of Hindu

[3] António Baião, ed., *A Inquisição de Goa: Correspondência dos inquisidores da Índia*, 2 vols. (Coimbra: Imprensa da Universidade, 1930), vol. 2, 127. The letter was written by Rui Sodrinho and Fr. Thomas Pinto from Goa, dated 20 of November 1589. Prohibitions against the practice of Hindu rituals in areas under ostensible Portuguese rule date from at least 1559. See the succession of regulations in HAG, PAR, "Provisões a favor da Cristandade," ff. 34–35v, 35v–36, 36v–37, and 65–67v.

[4] Baião, *Inquisição*, vol. 2, 127. See also Célia Cristina da Silva Tavares, "A Cristandade Insular: Jesuítas e Inquisidores em Goa (1540–1682)" (PhD diss., Universidade Federal Fluminense, 2002), 185–214.

[5] On perspectives common to Western Christendom generally, see John Henderson, *The Renaissance Hospital: Healing the Body and Healing the Soul* (New Haven, CT: Yale University Press, 2006); and for Portugal in particular see Iona McCleery, "Both 'Illness and temptation of the enemy': melancholy, the medieval patient and the writing of King Duarte of Portugal," *Journal of Medieval Iberian Studies* 1 (2009): 163–178; and my discussion of devotional literature on the eve of Vasco da Gama's 1498 landfall in Cagle, "Beyond the Senegal." Still useful is Oswei Temkin's discussion of the negotiations required to make Galenic medical theory and human physiology fit within a Christian frame in Temkin, *Galenism: Rise and Decline of a Medical Philosophy* (Ithaca, NY: Cornell University Press, 1973), 42–44, 73, 144–150. On Ayurveda, see Dagmar Wujastyk, "Healing and Medicine in Ayurveda and South Asia," in *Encyclopedia of Religion*, 2nd ed., ed. Lindsay Jones, 3852–3858 (New York: Macmillan, 2005); and A. L. Basham, "The Practice of Medicine in Ancient and Medieval India," in *Asian Medical Systems: A Comparative Study*, ed. Charles Leslie (Berkeley, CA: University of California Press, 1977), 18–43. Note that I do not discuss *unani* medicine, a form of humoral medicine

vaidyas, the practice of medicine was always pregnant with subversion. Secular and religious officials alike took an immediate interest in the activities of the colony's Hindu physicians. They distinguished Brahman priests (the feitiçeiro of the governor and his wife) from the vaidyas who focused on bodily illness.[6] But such distinctions were never drawn very sharply. Hindu priests and physicians alike, together with herbalists and midwives and many other medical specialists who practiced their craft in Goa, all seemed to represent a threat to the moral integrity of the Portuguese Catholic enclave. Efforts to curtail the primacy of Hindu physicians and other practitioners in Goa strengthened during the 1540s, just as the environmental and demographic transformations that accompanied Portuguese colonialism grew more acute. By the beginning of the seventeenth century the contest over medicine had become entwined in a power struggle among disparate colonial interests – a contest that pit the powerful Company of Jesus against members of Goa's municipal council, the senado da câmara, and the Santa Casa da Misericôrida confraternity (membership and familial affiliation in these two bodies often overlapped).[7] Vaidyas readily contested any assault on their clinical primacy in Goa. Portuguese officials never represented a united and sustained front, and countless members of the Portuguese settlement continued to prefer the work of vaidyas and other South Asian specialists to their countrymen or coreligionists.[8] But the contest was real and it was fought in terms that were both religious and more broadly cultural. At stake were both the orthodoxy of Catholicism in Goa and its Portuguese identity – one defined not only by religion but by personal networks of

based on the Arabic corpus, because the Portuguese were much less tolerant of its practitioners (*hakims*) in Goa. For a contemporary account of Islamic medicine see Pedro Teixera, *Relaciones del origen, descendencia y sucesion de los reyes de Persia, y de Hormuz, y de un viage hecho por el mismo autor desde la India Oriental hasta Italia por tierra* (Antwerp: n.p., 1660 [1610]), 175–182. Valuable modern studies include Seema Alavi, *Islam and Healing: Loss and Recovery of an Indo-Muslim Medical Tradition, 1600–1800* (New York: Palgrave, 2008); and Guy Attewell, *Refiguring Unani Tibb: Plural Healing in Late Colonial India* (Delhi: Orient Longman, 2007).

[6] HAG, PAR, "Provisões a favor da Cristandade," fls. 28v–29. Sumptuary laws ensured that by dress alone, Brahmins were easily identifiable to Portuguese authorities.

[7] C. R. Boxer, *Portuguese Society in the Tropics: The Municipal Councils of Goa, Macao, Bahia, and Luanda, 1510–1800* (Madison, WI: University of Wisconsin Press), 12–41; and Sá, *Quando o rico se faz pobre*.

[8] Walker, "Stocking Colonial Pharmacies"; Walker "Acquisition and Circulation"; Pearson, "Hindu Medical Practice"; Pearson, "First Contacts"; and John M. de Figueiredo, "Ayurvedic Medicine in Goa according to European Sources in the Sixteenth and Seventeenth Centuries," *Bulletin of the History of Medicine* 58 (1984): 228–229.

association, language, dress, food, medicine, and the gendered order of the colonial household.[9]

The practice of medicine in Portuguese Goa traversed fault lines that were at once cultural and political. Between 1510 and the early seventeenth century, all of Portuguese Goa was caught at the convergence of two simultaneous but contradictory processes: an increasing reliance on the curative expertise of South Asian specialists of many kinds and the imperative to constrain their influence. Long before Garcia de Orta filled his inkwell or organized his notes, the difference between traversing and transgressing those fault lines had become fluid and uncertain. Orta and his investigations were enabled by that uncertainty. His *Colóquios* – underwritten by the testimony of widely dispersed and diverse collaborators – was in many ways a reflection of it. But, as I noted in the last chapter, the tensions surrounding the practice of medicine and the pursuit of natural inquiry in Goa set limits on what could be said in print and how it could be said. In this context, the dialogic form itself would become a highly useful expository tool.

Vaidyas were prominent members of Goan society before the Portuguese arrived in 1510 and they kept up a flourishing practice in the city for decades thereafter. Their presence was embraced; their medical opinions were taken as authoritative. In the midst of the colerica passio epidemic of 1543, when governor Sousa took the last desperate measure of ordering an autopsy on one of the corpses of the recently deceased, he insisted that, "*all* men learned in the art of healing are asked to attend."[10] So lucrative was the business of medicine and so prosperous were Goa's Hindu physicians that they could afford to move along the streets in the high style characteristic of Portuguese colonial aristocracy – on horseback or in a palanquin, armed with saber and accompanied by a small retinue. By the middle of the sixteenth century, vaidyas had become the preferred healers of some of Portuguese Goa's most powerful secular and ecclesiastical officials, who according to Linschoten, "do put more trust in them … than in their own countrymen."[11] In the fall of 1589, the

---

[9] See the exploration of these themes in Ines G. Županov, *Missionary Tropics: The Catholic Frontier in India, 16th–17th Centuries* (Ann Arbor, MI: University of Michigan Press, 2005).

[10] Correia, *Lendas*, vol. 4, 288–289.

[11] HAG, PAR, "Provisões a favor da Cristandade," fls. 83–83v; and J. H. van Linschoten, *The Voyages of John Huyghen van Linschoten to the East Indies* (London: The Hakluyt Society, 1885), vol. 1, 230. See also Walker, "Stocking Colonial Pharmacies," 118.

heretical governor Coutinho had done no more than subscribe to what was by then a longstanding convention.

Precisely when vaidyas became inextricable members of Portuguese medical communities in Asia is difficult to pin down. Two of the earliest discussions of Portuguese medical affairs in Asia offer contradictory perspectives. One came at the end of Tomé Pires's 1516 list to Manuel I – in that bit of unsolicited pecuniary advice tucked gently, almost unnoticeably, into Pires's brief postscript. There the apothecary insisted that the only things in the way of medicine that need come from Lisbon were "turpentine, ceruse, verdigris (*azinhavre*), a little scammony, olive oil from Portugal, [and] mastic," for they were otherwise expensive and hard to find. "All [else] can be secured here ... [or prepared] with the things that exist here" and compound medicines in particular "can be prepared and dispensed ... [by] the [king's] apothecaries, surgeons, and physicians [spread across Portuguese Asia], for that is what they are paid to do."[12] Pires's sense of Portuguese medical affairs in Asia was clear enough: much Asian *materia medica* was not only familiar but fresh, abundant, and readily available and Portuguese specialists were sufficient in number to handle the needs of the Estado. But when in 1516, Pires wrote all this down, the extent of his Asian travel was limited to a pair of brief layovers in Cochin and a three-year term in Malacca. Given the extensive seaborne travel already undertaken by many of this country-men – men like the pilot Rodrigues – the opinion, though earnest, seems to have been based on little more than his own narrow experience.

For Afonso de Albuquerque – among the few Portuguese officials in Asia at the time with a tie to the court of Manuel I that was more direct that Pires's own – the view was altogether different. Having traipsed militantly from Hormuz to Malacca and back again, Albuquerque thought the Estado was much too thinly spread.[13] He had begun to take account both of the precise range of ailments that threatened to under-mine his work and the kinds of treatments that might mitigate Portuguese losses. "There are physicians [spread along the Malabar Coast], he explained to D. Manuel, "who cure in this way":

To those who are weak with fever, they give them meat to eat, and fish, and give them purgatives of fig seeds (*figueira de inferno*), or leaves, finely crushed, in a drink. If they suffer from dysentery (*camaras*) they are given fresh coconut water ... If the suffer from nausea (*arrebeça*) their heads are washed with cold

[12] ANTT, CC, pt. 1, mç. 19, n. 102, f. 4.
[13] Pato, *Cartas de Afonso de Albuquerque*, vol. 2, 37–38.

water to stop the vomiting. To those who are injured, they lance [the wound] with hot oil every day, thrice a day. For prolonged illnesses, the remedy . . . is a sojourn to their temples.[14]

For Albuquerque, Indian vaidyas and their curative techniques were not only effective, they buttressed imperial designs.[15] That he could detail specific treatments suggests that before he succumbed to fever in the fall of 1515, vaidyas had already become *de facto* members of Portuguese Goa's diversifying medical community – one in which the Portuguese apothecaries, surgeons, and physicians to which Pires referred perhaps only months later (Albuquerque's letter is undated) were already numerically and intellectually minor contributors.

The relative scarcity of Portuguese physicians was perhaps the most oft-cited justification for the embrace of Hindu physicians in Portuguese Goa. That, at least, was how Goa's viceroys and members of its senado da câmara presented their case to the Crown in intermittent requests for metropolitan physicians. And indeed, that too few metropolitan physicians were available to supply the growing needs of not only an expanding Christian community in Goa but throughout Portugal's empire in Asia is plain enough: the explanation was repeated with such consistency and accords so well with available information on the state of medical education in Portugal and throughout the empire that these claims were probably true: there *were* too few Portuguese physicians in the Estado to treat even the entire Christian community in Goa. On its own, need might explain why Portuguese settlers turned to vaidyas in particular moments of severe distress.[16]

Yet that explanation alone accounts for neither the credibility they were afforded by Portuguese settlers in Asia nor the authority they wielded in Goa. Ultimately it is unconvincing because of its unstated

[14] Afonso de Albuquerque, *Comentários do grande Afonso de Albuquerque, Capitão Geral que foi das Índias Orientais em tempo do muito poderoso Rey D. Manuel, o primeiro deste nome* (Coimbra: Imprensa da Universidade, 1922), 326.

[15] On Albuquerque as an agent of centralized power under the Crown and the architect of Portuguese India, see Subrahmanyam, *Portuguese Empire in Asia*, 67–69.

[16] Figueiredo, "Practice of Indian Medicine"; but see later and the discussion in Walker, "Acquisition and Circulation," 256. For a critical appraisal of the relationship between need and early modern medical innovation, see Joel Mokyr, "Induced Medical Innovation and Medical History: An Evolutionary Approach," *Journal of Evolutionary Economics* 8 (1998): 119–137. Estimates of the number of physicians that the Crown and his advisors deemed necessary can be taken from Pissurlencar, *Regimentos*, which outlines the allocation of funds for each outpost, including the fees of apothecaries, physicians, and surgeons, and the cost of upkeep for hospitals.

and specious assumptions about learned medicine anywhere in Europe at the time, and about the attitudes and expectations of would-be patients. Across Western Christendom, the authority of learned medicine was itself always tenuous. Often, and especially in Portugal, unless a city or town kept a physician under retainer, he could be hard to find. Those wishing to secure his expertise could paid dearly for it. Instead, and especially but by no means exclusively among the lower and middling orders, itinerant lay healers and the women of a household were the healers of first resort. Historians' reliance on the written record and on formal educational-cum-legal and occupational titles like physician, surgeon, or apothecary has only obscured that work.[17] Where the titles of surgeon and apothecary were concerned, those who claimed it may or may not have passed the formal examination and carried the license that Portuguese and other authorities increasingly required of them by the sixteenth century.[18] Their ranks could shade easily into the world of lay healers. Wise women and unlettered or semi-literate lay healers of many kinds were often cheaper and easier to find than physicians. And instead of an authority built of obscure knowledge vouchsafed by anonymous, bookish professors, the wisdom of lay healers and the efficacy of their cures were often vouchsafed by friends and kinsmen.[19]

In many parts of early modern Europe, much as in Europe's expanding colonies, the expertise of a physician – whose formal training was anyway only partly concerned with restoring health[20] – was a costly and often dubious luxury. Across early modern Europe but perhaps especially in

---

[17] Mary Fissell, "Introduction: Women, Health, and Healing in Early Modern Europe," *Bulletin of the History of Medicine* 82 (2008), 1–17.

[18] Laurinda Abreu, "A organização e regulação das *profissões médicas* no Portugal Moderno: entre as orientações da Coroa e os interesses privados," in *Arte Médica e Imagem do Corpo: De Hipócrates ao final do século XVIII*, eds. Adelino Cardoso, António Braz de Oliveira, and Manuel Silvério Marques (Lisbon: Biblioteca Nacional de Portugal, 2010), 97–122. Iona McCleery, "Medical Licensing in Late Medieval Portugal," in *Medicine and the Law in the Middle Ages*, eds. W. J. Turner and S. M. Butler (Leiden: Brill, 2014), 196–219; and Francis A. Dutra, "The Practice of Medicine in Early Modern Portugal: The Role and Social Status of the *Físico-mor* and the *Surgião-mor*," in *Libraries, History, Diplomacy, and the Performing Arts: Essays in Honor of Carleton Sprague Smith*, ed. Israel Katz (New York: Pendragon Press, 1991), 135–169.

[19] Monica Green, *Making Women's Medicine Masculine: The Rise of Male Authority in Pre-Modern Gynecology* (New York: Oxford University Press, 2008); Wear, *Knowledge and Practice*; Alisha Rankin, *Panaceia's Daughters: Noblewomen as Healers in Early Modern Germany* (Chicago, IL: University of Chicago Press, 2013).

[20] Cook, "The new philosophy and medicine."

Iberia by the middle of the sixteenth century, the ranks of those who performed restorative bodywork of all kinds included a varied cast of practitioners possessed of widely varied knowledges. In Lisbon, healers of African descent had become particularly common.[21] The prominence that they and other unlettered specialists enjoyed would by the middle of the seventeenth century become a source of deepening worry – professional and financial no less than medical – for metropolitan physicians (a story I take up in Chapter 8).

The diversity of curative knowledges available and actively accessed by Portuguese, other Europeans, and by Asian travelers alike in both Goa and beyond in the early sixteenth century was not the exception but the rule. That does not mean that Portuguese observers did not offer explanations for their particular curative choices. They did. In these, vaidyas figured prominently. Some Portuguese considered the work of Goa's vaidyas superior to their own because they were most familiar with locally available *materia medica*[22] (notwithstanding Pires's assertion that familiar medicinal flora were plentifully abundant). Some observers argued from the other side: it was not the medicines that were different so much as the illnesses of the region.[23] In the words of Duarte Barbosa, the "the *land* is unhealthy," as evidenced by its seasonal fevers, dysenteries, and bouts of colerica passio.[24] In short, local illnesses were understood to be different from those of Iberia and therefore local healers could best treat them. In a variant of both points of view, some Portuguese suggested that the most effective remedies for the ailments of any place were the plants that grew there – a common claim based partly on Hippocratic environmentalism and partly on the belief that their god located medicinal plants where the diseases they treated were likely to occur. In that case too, local healers were the preferred choice.[25]

[21] John Slater, Maríaluz López-Terrada, and José Pardo-Tomás, eds., *Medical Cultures of the Early Modern Spanish Empire* (New York: Routledge, 2014); Walker, *Doctors, Folk Medicine, and the Inquisition*; Sweet, *Domingos Álvares*.

[22] Linschoten, *Voyages*, vol. 1, 236; and Academia Real das Ciências, ed., "Breve relação das escrituras dos gentios da India Oriental e dos seus costumes," in *Collecção de notícias para a historia e geografia das nações ultramarinas, que vivem nos dominios portuguezes, ou lhes são vizinhas* (Lisbon: Typografia da Academia, 1812), 52–53.

[23] Dr. John Fryer, *A New Account of East India and Persia: Being Nine Years Travels, 1672–1681*, 2 vols. (New Delhi: Asian Educational Services, 1996 [facsimile of 1909–1915]), vol. 1, 180.

[24] Barbosa, *Livro*, vol. 1, 144. Italics added for emphasis.

[25] Correia, *Lendas*, vol. 3, 288; Surendranath Sen, ed., *Indian Travels of Thevenot and Careri: Being the Third Part of the Travels of M. de Thevenot into the Levant and the*

Contemporaries, in short, grounded their claims in one of three arguments: either Asian diseases were different or local plants worked best or both; vaidyas were believed to know more about disease or more about medicine or both. In any case, their knowledge was – in Goa at least – widely regarded as superior, their conclusions decisive. Just as the inhabitants of West Africa knew best how to survive fevers and dysentery in the Gulf of Guinea so, too, did vaidyas and other South Asian specialists know best how to keep well along the Konkan Coast.

Extant requests to the Crown for Portuguese physicians came from Goa only amid the worsening diseases and intensified religious conflicts of the 1540s. The widespread and pervasive reliance on vaidyas had begun to suggest to the growing contingent of missionaries and Church leaders the strength – among longstanding Catholics and new adherents alike – of an alternative cosmology and the allure of an alternate faith.[26] And the two were impossible to disentangle: Church attacks on the cultural edifice of Hinduism extended to the practice of medicine, opening the question not of the credibility of vaidyas' medical opinions or methods but about their authority – whether and to what extent they should be authorized to pronounce definitively on matters of health pertaining to the Christian community.[27] As religious tensions in Goa began to deepen, reliance on vaidyas became an increasingly contentious and divisive aspect of colonial life.

Under intensified scrutiny, the moral economy that bound physicians and patients broke down. As trust dissolved, feelings of vulnerability and suspicion took root.[28] The expulsion of Konkani villagers and attempts to extirpate Hindu rituals that began in the early 1540s, and which transformed local hydrography to the detriment of Portuguese Goa (see Chapter 3), were bolstered on June 10, 1568, with the proclamation of a new set of strictures decided on earlier that year at the meeting of the First Provincial Council. Among the measures announced by Goa's archbishop

---

Third Part of a Voyage Round the World by Dr. John Francis Gemelli Careri (New Delhi: National Archives of India, 1949), 162.

[26] In addition to the material referenced later, see Viceroy D. João de Castro's discussion of the destruction of Hindu temples in HAG, PAR, "Provisões a favor da Cristandade," fls. 73v–74v.

[27] A point addressed in Ines G. Županov, *Disputed Missions: Jesuit Experiments and Brahmanical Knowledge in Seventeenth-Century India* (New Delhi: Oxford University Press, 1999), ch. 1.

[28] On the centrality of trust in the historical practice of ayurveda, see Dagmar Wujastyk, *Well-Mannered Medicine: Medical Ethics and Etiquette in Classical Ayurveda* (New York: Oxford University Press, 2012), especially ch. 6.

Jorge Themudo and printed by Johan Endem (who had only just printed Orta's *Colóquios* a few years earlier) was a proscription of any medical treatment administered by non-Christian physicians on Christian patients.[29]

Reflective of the posture of the Church in Goa, which placed a great deal of stress on outward appearances – public displays of emotion and devotion rather than strict adherence to orthodoxy – the measure of 1568 was part of a wider set of proscriptions focused on associations and symbols of belonging: ritual, as well as dress, food, and other signifiers of personal association. Non-converts were to be separated from new adherents, whether at markets or in residential quarters of the city. Christians were not to patronize Hindu doctors, midwives, barbers, and artisans or other craftsmen. The death of the father was declared sufficient cause for forcing Hindu mothers to surrender their children to Christian families (and the same would happen in Brazil, as I discuss in Chapter 6). It was only following Xavier's example that Jesuit missionaries themselves donned locally made cotton garments instead of the black woolen robes they had brought with them.[30]

Clerical concern for medicine extended to the visibility of Hindu physicians in Goa's streets. Sensitivity to the symbolic meaning of a pervasive and authoritative non-Christian medical presence had a firm precedent. Only Portuguese physicians had ever been allowed to practice medicine in Goa's prestigious royal hospital. They may have been expert, but they were not to bear the imprimatur of an endorsement by the Catholic monarch. In 1572, at the urging of Goa's municipal council, then viceroy Barreto banned the use of palanquins and horses by vaidyas.[31] Barreto's own personal physician, however – himself a vaidya – was exempt from these measures.[32] And even if support for it among Goa's most prosperous and influential residents was sufficient to have the measure enacted, that was not enough to sustain the new law's enforcement. The divided opinions and limited achievements of Goa's councilors on this front only reflected wider opinion. Vaidyas remained credible, integral and, for many Christians in

[29] HAG, PAR, "Provisões a favor da Cristandade," fls. 74–75v, 83–83v, 91–92v; Teotonio R. de Souza, "The Council of Trent (1545–1563): Its Reception in Portuguese India," in Klaus Koschorke, ed., *Transcontinental Links in the History of Non-Western Christianity* (Wiesbaden: Harrassowitz Verlag, 2002), 194–196; and Županov, *Missiary Tropics*.

[30] Souza, "Council of Trent," 193–194.   [31] Figueiredo, "Ayurvedic Medicine," 228.

[32] Figueiredo, "Goa-Pré-Portuguesa," 162. Two years later he prohibited *vaidyas* from practicing in Goa altogether, with the exception of the one who served as his own personal physician. See HAG, PAR, "Provisões a favor da Cristandade," fls. 83–83v.

Goa, still authoritative on medical matters. As Linschoten observed during his stay in Goa between 1583 and 1589,

There are in Goa many heathen physicians which observe their gravities with hats carried over them for the sun, like the Portuguese, which no other heathens do, but only ambassadors, or some rich merchants. These heathen physicians do not only cure their own nations and countrymen but the Portuguese also, for the viceroy himself, the archbishop, and all the monks and friars do put more trust in them than in their own countrymen, whereby they get great store of money, and are much honoured and esteemed.[33]

Sumptuary laws aimed at physicians were reenacted again several decades later but with similar results.[34]

Just as aggressive efforts either to obscure or preclude the reliance of Portuguese Christians on Hindu physicians proved unsuccessful, any consensus among Portuguese religious and secular officials over how best to manage health in Goa remained elusive. The Jesuits, who were particular proponents of these efforts (it was after all Francis Xavier who began to champion the installation of the Inquisition in Goa almost immediately after his arrival), adopted a strategy of assimilation. If Hindu physicians were too knowledgeable to be displaced outright, Jesuit missionaries would learn what they knew. The Spanish traveler Pedro Teixeira observed during his visit to Goa at the end of the sixteenth century that "in India there are doctors which are called *pandytos* that are learned and good philosophers and I saw them on many occasions dispute with our theologians and doctors of the things of nature and they give a good account of it."[35] Pandits (Teixeira's "pandytos") were Hindu priests, not physicians, but such theatre, which was a common element in Jesuit conversion strategies,[36] included vaidyas, too. As Teixeira's remark suggests, it was a risky strategy: the better the "account" that pandits and vaidyas could give of nature, the weaker the Jesuit argument for their exclusion from medicine and the less traction the Jesuits' own more exclusionary curative work might have. Much to the consternation of Jesuit priests, Hindu physicians held their ground in

---

[33] Linschoten, *Voyages*, vol. 1, 230.   [34] Figueiredo, "Ayurvedic Medicine," 228.

[35] Teixera, *Relaciones*, 172.

[36] On theatre and Jesuit conversion as a pattern across Portugal's empire see César Braga-Pinto, *As Promessas da História: Discursos Proféticos e Assimilação no Brasil Colonial (1500–1700)* (São Paulo: Editorial da Universidade de São Paulo, 2002), 67–121.

these public performances and refused either to abandon their faith or to explain their medicine.[37]

Many of these exchanges unfolded behind closed doors, in the Jesuit Colegio de São Paulo, where members of the Order asked vaidyas – in all likelihood out of necessity – to work and to converse more privately on matters of faith and medicine. The superior of the Jesuit college, one Father Lancillotto, together with the director of Hospital dos Pobres, a certain Padre Paulo, wrote to their colleagues in Lisbon in 1548 that

> We have a doctor (*medico*) that cures here in our house, a Brahman ... and when the Fathers dispute with him for an hour or more he is so pertinacious (*emperado*) that he refuses to believe anything. Many times I have wished that Father António Gomez were here to see him and question him for he [the Brahman] is so terrible that, when the Fathers begin to have the upper hand, he becomes malicious, very malicious, and there is nothing in him but the worst poison.[38]

António Gomez, the man that Lancilloto wished were on hand to observe these exchanges, was himself a zealous defender of the Catholic faith. Gomez held an advanced degree in theology and was named by Xavier as rector of the Jesuit college in Goa, where his curricular reforms included the expulsion of native seminarians and the institution's eventual transformation into a school exclusively for students of Portuguese parentage. He was removed from his post in 1552, after barely four years in Goa, amid a reprimand from the city's bishop, and in the face of a popular backlash.[39] The contest for medical primacy that would find expression later in both Church policy and a series of ambiguous secular measures was part of the curative landscape from at least the 1540s.

For the Jesuits, these policies were not merely an effort to compel conversion but part of a campaign of medical reconnaissance. And it took on particular significance in Portugal's colonies, where medicine was at the heart of their work.[40] After mid-century, they assumed responsibility for Goa's Hospital Real do Espírito Santo – then the largest and best financed medical facility in the city. Its patients were wealthy casados, influential travelers, and soldiers in the service of the king. In addition to

---

[37] Sousa, *Oriente Conquistado*, 148–151; Županov, *Disputed Missions*, ch. 3.

[38] *DI* vol. 1, 254.   [39] Gonçalves, *História*, vol. 3, 446.

[40] On Mozambique Island, in Bahia, and in the Brazilian Amazon, the Company focused heavily on the treatment of illness. On Brazil, see Chapter 6. For Mozambique, letters between the Portuguese king and Jesuit leaders in Goa reveal lengthy seventeenth-century exchange over when, after much hesitation, the Company might finally fulfill its promise to finance repairs to the hospital and begin to staff it. See Souza, *Oriente Conquistado*, 34, 55, 317, 319.

the royal hospital, the Jesuits also ran two other hospitals in the area, which placed them among the single largest providers of medical care in and around Goa.[41] And yet, at the same time, periodic outbreaks of disease forced them to abandon even their own college. So when in 1567 they left what was at the time a newly renovated Colegio de São Paulo, they absconded under the cover of night to disguise their departure and hide the fact that the edifice lay vacant, essentially (if only temporarily) condemned.[42] If medicine was a cornerstone of their activities, then the prevalence of disease posed a major threat to the viability of the project and to the prestige of the order. The success of the Jesuit enterprise in Goa hinged in part on their success as healers not just of the soul but of the body.[43]

Once the Company took over the administration of the royal hospital in 1579, the same concern for the credibility of its medical practice drove its policies toward the acquisition of *materia medica*. They began to establish their own network for securing and circulating Asian therapeutics – one that was independent of the commercial networks that, as I have already argued, plagued Garcia de Orta's work. A standard list of medicines and their market prices had been compiled for the hospital decades earlier in 1552 but the Jesuits revoked it, arguing that it had become too convoluted and confusing. They preferred one that emphasized instead only medicinal plants in their unprepared state (medicinal simples) so that anyone in the hospital might readily combine them as needed.[44] Since the royal hospital served as a purveyor of drugs to Goa's other hospitals and to Portuguese colonial apothecaries,[45] the move was also a tactic in part of the Jesuits' larger strategy of curative exclusion.[46]

As it would in Brazil, the growth of Jesuit wealth and influence earned the Company powerful adversaries in Goa. The missionaries had become

---

[41] Sá, *Quando o rico se faz pobre*, 160. On medical care in neighboring Bijapur and elsewhere, see S. H. Askari, "Medicine and Hospitals in Muslim India," *Journal of the Bihar Research Society* 43 (1957): 7–21.

[42] Sousa, *Oriente Conquistado*, 216–217.

[43] Here I have to disagree with Ines G. Županov, "Drugs, Health, Bodies and Souls in the Tropics: Medical Experiments in Sixteenth-Century Portuguese India," *Indian Economic and Social History Review* 39 (2002): 1–43, in which the author has drawn a dichotomy between Orta, who wanted to heal the body, and the Jesuits, who focused on the health of the soul.

[44] José F. Ferreira Martins, ed., *Historia da Misericordia de Goa (1520–1620)*, 2 vols. (Nova Goa: Imprensa Nacional, 1910), vol. 2, 301–311.

[45] Walker, "Stocking Colonial Pharmacies."

[46] See the discussion in Xavier and Županov, *Catholic Orientalism*, 103–107.

embroiled in what was by 1618 a protracted and bitter struggle with the Santa Casa da Misericôrdia – that elite confraternity of prosperous casados that had once run the royal hospital and continued to perform its traditional role as a charitable institution charged with the care of Goa's infirm and incarcerated. The Jesuits, so claimed the brothers of the Misericôrdia (and echoing charges that would be common in Brazil too) commanded undue wealth and property, especially given their vows of poverty and missionary orientation. The order was at that time seeking to extend its own charitable work and its land holdings, both of which worked to the detriment of the Misericôrdia. The two bodies had earlier written to João III, who initially favored the secular confraternity but finally decided to allow Jesuit plans to go ahead. Members of the Misericôrdia, however often sat on Goa's municipal council or, if not, had friends and family who did.[47] As a result, the contest between charitable organizations – for land, patronage, and influence over city's poor – quickly manifested itself as a municipal ordinance on medical practice.

In the fall of 1618 the municipal council approved a comprehensive set of new measures aimed at regulating the practice of medicine in Goa. The new "policies pertaining to physicians, surgeons, blood-letters, and apothecaries," made six basic stipulations. "No one," it established, "regardless of Law [*sic*], quality, or nation" would be allowed to practice medicine without joint approval of the físico-mor of Goa and the city's municipal council. The total number of vaidyas and other non-Christian physicians ("físicos gentios" – literally "gentile physicians") would be limited to thirty, apparently following a measure taken by Goa's clergy some years earlier. The new policy added that when these physicians were making rounds, they would no longer be permitted to travel outside of Goa personally in order to procure medicines but must instead send their apprentices to do so. The council also required blood-letters to post above their doors a notice visible to all passers-by testifying to their medical certification. Apothecaries now had to submit to periodic examinations of their shops and storehouses so that the councilors could verify that the drugs in which they trafficked were not "rotten, old, or falsified." If some *materia medica* were found to have lost the "virtue and efficacy to do their work" they were to be destroyed – burned under the supervision of

---

47 Sá, *Quando o rico se faz pobre*, 160–168; Charles J. Borges, "Foreign Jesuits and Native Resistance in Goa, 1542–1759," in *Essays in Goan History*, ed. Teotonio R. de Souza, (New Delhi: Concept Publishing Company, 1989), 69–80; Martins, *Historia da Misericordia de Goa*, vol. 1, 385–389, and vol. 2, 294–298.

the councilors and the offending apothecary. Apothecaries would be required to sell their medicines in smaller quantities so that patients in need of only small doses could afford to buy them. And finally, apothecaries were prohibited from vending their medicines (simples or otherwise) to non-Christians or slaves of any faith.[48]

By the end of the sixteenth century, two patterns had taken shape. Various Portuguese factions had come to share a mutual distrust of native physicians. Despite what were at times pronounced differences among councilors, governors, Jesuits, and Inquisitors, the contest for control over medical practice amounted to a joint attempt to restrict and control the work of non-Portuguese, non-Christian physicians. Because what was at issue was not the validity of their medicine but rather the authority and influence of the native physicians who practiced it, Portuguese efforts on all sides increasingly sought to acquire – forcibly if necessary – the skill and learning of Goa's vaidyas. At the same time, native physicians remained inextricable members of Goa's medical community and often found employment even with many prominent officials. Attempts to reign in their influence and thereby circumscribe their presence, focused as they were on the appropriation of their knowledge, was but a tacit recognition that native physicians continued not only to wield medical authority but that their medicine remained credible even as that of Portuguese practitioners and the medicine they proffered did not.[49]

RUMOR HAS IT

It was one of the countless contradictions of colonization that the expulsion of Konkani villagers and the removal of their Hindu temples meant, first, that a great many young men and women were kidnapped and brought not only into missionary communities but into Portuguese households throughout the city and, second, that Goa – that bastion of Portuguese Catholicism in Asia, became evermore surrounded by concentric rings of Hindu sites of worship set up just beyond the pale of Portuguese settlement. The density of Hindu communities thickened around Goa while Hindu servants and slaves populated the anterooms, corridors,

---

[48] "Postura dos Fizicos, Cirurgiões, Sangradores e Boticários," dated 3 November 1618, in *O Senado de Goa: Memória Histórico-Arqueológico*, ed. Viriato A. C. R. de Albuquerque, (Nova Goa: Imprensa Nacional, 1909), doc. 211, 423–425.

[49] This was true even as the authority of their legal testimony was formally curtailed. See HAG, PAR, "Provisões a favor da Cristandade," 75–77v.

and kitchens of its most intimate spaces. Over the course of a day, Konkani servants – men, women, and children – moved back and forth across the domestic, geographic, and religious frontiers of Portuguese Goa in an ebb and flow of traffic that paralleled the coming and going of boats in Goa's port.[50]

In tandem with their displacement from Goa's center and simultaneous incorporation into Portuguese households, a number of rumors about young Indian women in particular had begun to circulate among the Portuguese. One account told of a man whose long-standing bout with dysentery drove his exasperated wife to murder. Finding her husband's illness utterly abhorrent, she resolved to poison him, for which task she secretly acquired a small quantity of finely crushed diamonds. Her hope was that that, by mixing them with his food, their toxic virtue would slowly drain him of life and put an end to their shared misery.[51] Another tale related the thievery exacted upon one unwed but wealthy Paula de Andrade. Her servant had conspired with a lover to poison Andrade and then to steal as many of the woman's jewels as the two could carry in their escape to neighboring Bijapur.[52]

Similar rumors of the use of poison in high diplomacy and low politics were pervasive in Goa. Jesuits corresponding from the Mughal court in Delhi plotted strategies for mass conversion based on reports that emperor Akbar had been poisoned by one of his sons and would soon die.[53] In Goa, a falling out between Archbishop João de Albuquerque and Vicar General Miguel Vaz was likewise rumored to have been settled by poison.[54] But the associations between women and poison that were rife in Goa during the middle and late sixteenth century had more immediate sources. Fears that Portuguese men might easily fall prey to their prowess reflected the profoundly ambiguous position of women in the domestic life of Goa – one enabled by a contradiction between the idealized gender norms of metropolitan Portugal and the exigencies of Portuguese settlement in Asia.

---

[50] Paul Axelrod and Michelle A. Fuerch, "Flight of the Deities: Hindu Resistance in Portuguese Goa," *Modern Asian Studies* 30 (1996): 387–421, reconstruct this history.

[51] Orta, *Colóquios*, vol. 2, 197. The diamonds failed to do the trick and the ailing man succumbed to death only a long time later.

[52] Orta, *Colóquios*, vol. 1 295–296.

[53] Sanjay Subrahmanyam, *Mughals and Franks: Explorations in Connected History* (New Delhi: Oxford University Press, 2005), 3–7; Sousa, *Oriente Conquistado*, 53–54; Correia *Lendas*, vol. 1, 59.

[54] Correia, *Lendas*, vol. 2, 188.

Women in Goa were by all accounts skilled herbalists. In the *Colóquios*, Orta took it as common knowledge that Goan and mestiço women used hashish (*bangue*) to seduce Portuguese men.[55] The plant datura was more dangerous, still – both as an aphrodisiac but also as a poison. It was datura that rendered Paula de Andrade helpless before her ill-intentioned servants. At home and in bed, women's possession of herbal knowledge seemed to threaten not only men but the wealth and integrity of the broader Portuguese community in Goa. The Dutch traveler Linschoten recorded similar stories of datura's use. "Indian and Portuguese women," he wrote,

> use much to give unto their husbands [i.e. as an aphrodisiac] and often times when they are disposed to be merry with their secret lovers, they give it him, and go in his presence and perform their lechery together, and taking their husband by the beard they will call him *cornudo* [cuckold], with other such like jests, the man not knowing anything thereof, but sit with his eyes open, not doing or saying anything, but laugh and grin like a fool, or a man out of his wits.[56]

Linschoten also confirmed the moral of the story of thievery in the Andrade household: "the herb [datura] the slaves use likewise to give [to] their masters and mistresses, [and] thereby ... rob them." It was a measure of their skill that wives, lovers, servants, and slaves could not only render men helpless with datura but that they could do so without killing them; both Orta and Linschoten noted that datura was a potent drug and had to be administered with great care lest, in Linschoten's words, it "bring a man to his end."[57] When it came to identifying the threat that such knowledge posed to the gendered colonial order, Orta was more pointed still: "a dead man," he wrote, "is no man at all."[58]

Rumors that percolated into the city from the vast and inaccessible South Asian interior seemed to confirm this image of women – and particularly Hindu women – as crafty and duplicitous temptresses. Duarte Barbosa reported that women at the court of Vijayanagar – the Hindu kingdom that controlled the southern reaches of the Deccan – poisoned one another out of jealousy and competition for royal favor – reports that resonated with the account of the missionary Gonçalo Fernandes Trancoso who journeyed there.[59] And Linschoten balked at what he described as "the boldness and inclination of the Indian women," for

---

[55] Orta, *Colóquios*, vol. 1, 95–98.   [56] Linschoten, *Voyages*, vol. 2, 69.
[57] Linschoten, *Voyages*, vol. 2, 69.   [58] Orta, *Colóquios*, vol. 1, 209.
[59] Barbosa, *Livro*, 59–91; Correia, *Lendas*, vol. 3, 243; Gonçalo Fernandes Trancoso, *Tratado do Padre Gonçalo Fernandes Trancoso sobre o Hinduísmo*, ed. José Wicki (Lisbon: Centro de Estudos Históricos Ultramarinos, 1973 [Maduré, 1616]), 224.

not a year went by, he insisted, without "twenty or thirty men poisoned, and murdered by their wives."[60]

Such accounts had a powerful influence on perceptions of women in Goa. Few Portuguese, including Orta (who had diplomatic connections and personal relationship with physicians at the courts of Gujarat and Ahmadnagar) knew much beyond unconfirmed reports of the interior.[61] That very uncertainty gave tales of domestic treachery some of their purchase on colonial imaginations. For the power of these rumors lay precisely in the fact that they could be neither confirmed nor falsified. The worries they evinced, however, were real enough.

From the beginning, Konkani women had been integral to the production and reproduction of Portuguese Goan society. No sooner had Afonso de Albuquerque taken the city than he encouraged his men to wed Goan women. Historians have long argued over the reasons for that decision and explanations range from the Luso-tropicalist myth of a uniquely syncretic Portuguese character to others rooted in more prosaic concerns for inheritance and commercial contacts.[62] But the policy did lead to widespread intermarriage, forging commercial bonds grounded in those of the family. Frequently enough – and paradoxically – intermarriage would draw many would-be settlers away from Goa and beyond the sphere of Portuguese rule altogether, forging the very Indo-Portuguese families who would later compete with those of Goa's casados and of the Portuguese Crown itself, most notably in the Bay of Bengal.[63] Here was one ineluctable tension that came with intermarriage: it could both facilitate and dissolve the creation of a stable colony in Goa.

The rhythms of daily life for what were at midcentury the approximately four thousand Portuguese householders in Goa depended upon women drawn from Goa's indigenous, Hindu communities – and not only as wives, servants, and slaves. Konkani and increasingly mestiço women, as well as others from as far afield as Java,[64] became nurses,

---

[60] Linschoten, *Voyages*, vol. 2, 215.
[61] For the unfolding of cross-cultural encounters in the Deccan between the Portuguese and the peoples of the Vijayanagar kingdom, see Rubiés, *Travel and Ethnology*, especially 164–200.
[62] See the discussion of Pearson, *Portuguese in India*, ch. 4, and especially 105–106.
[63] Subrahmanyam, *Improvising Empire*.
[64] According to Agostinho de Santa Maria, *História da fundação do Real Convento de Santa Monica* (Lisbon: Antonio Pedrozo Galram, 1699), bk. 2, ch. 1, Javanese *daias* (specialists in a form of midwifery in Santa Maria's presentation) had long been employed in this Carmelite convent in the heart of Goa.

midwives, wet-nurses, and healers of first resort (Figure 5.1). Their skill in wielding the medicinal power of Asian flora – and, to be clear, that was what underwrote rumors of poison and seduction alike – was common knowledge. That, at least, was the impression left on Jean-Baptiste Tavernier, who traveled extensively not only along the Malabar Coast but across much of the Deccan in the 1640s. "As for the commonalty [*sic*]," he later wrote:

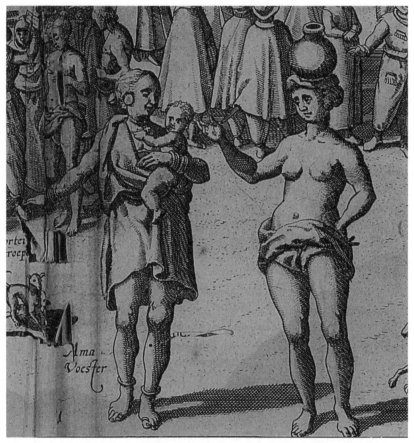

FIGURE 5.1 Intimacy and Expertise. Konkani-speaking servant (right) and wetnurse (left) as depicted in Jan Huygen van Linschoten, *Histoire de la navigatione de Jan Huygen van* Linschoten aux Indes Orientales (Amsterdam: Jan Evertz Cloppenburgh, 1619). I thank Jessen Kelly for assistance with this and other translations from Dutch.
Courtesy of the Biblioteca Nacional de Portugal.

When the rains have fallen and it is the season for collecting plants, mothers of families may be seen going in the mornings from the towns and villages to collect the simples[,] which they know to be specifics for domestic diseases.[65]

Such knowledge of nature gave women access to many of Portuguese Goa's men, women, and children when they were ill, dying, or giving birth – when, in other words, they were at their weakest or most vulnerable.[66]

AGNOTOLOGY AND A SUBVERSIVE LEAF

Its tendency to strengthen Portuguese reliance on the medical work of women of Indian descent seemed to be one of a number of ways that intermarriage threatened to dissolve the ethnic ties that underwrote all that was Portuguese in Goa. A deep reliance on them and the consequent anxiety that percolated throughout Portuguese Goa was only the most intimate instantiation of the wider situation between native healers and Portuguese colonists. And as the strictures on movement, association, and patronage announced by the archbishop in 1578 suggest, the prominence of the unconverted in the domestic sphere and throughout Goa helped initiate a broader process of intercultural exchange and interaction that many religious and secular leaders were at pains to control.

It was in part for that reason that, among many Portuguese in Goa, Asian medicinal plants were often loaded with significance that went far beyond their curative value. One such item of nature was the diminutive betel leaf. By 1516, the widespread and pervasive use of betel leaves not only along the Konkan and Malabar coasts but throughout Southeast Asia as well had brought them to the attention of the apothecary Pires. So taken was he with their uses and the "subtlety" of their "virtue," that he included mention of them in his 1516 list to Manuel I – even though, judging by Pires's tone and language, the king not only did not inquire about it but had no idea what it was. Indeed, the entry on betel leaves was one of the longest in the letter and was one of the very few places where medical curiosity got the better of Pires (Figure 5.2).

---

[65] Jean Baptiste-Tavernier, *Travels in India of Jean Baptiste-Tavernier, Baron of Aubonne*, ed. William Crooke, trans. V. Ball., 2nd ed., 2 vols. (London: Oxford University Press, 1925 [facsimile of the 1676 edition]), vol. 1, 240.

[66] Santa Maria, *História da fundação*, bk. 2, ch. 1; and HAG, PAR, "Provisões a favor da Cristandade," fls. 181v–182.

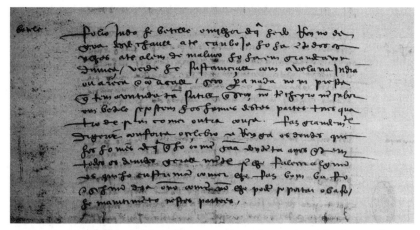

FIGURE 5.2 In Praise of Things Common. Entry from a letter by the apothecary Tomé Pires praising the uses of betel leaves. Detail from "Carta de Tomé Pires para o rei, dizendo que as coisas que o senhor lhe mandara pedir, as mandaria para o ano," dated January 27, 1516.
Courtesy of the Arquivo Nacional da Torre do Tombo.

Almost the entire section related to the medicinal – as opposed to commercial – value of betel leaves. "The men of these parts," Pires wrote,

can go for three or four days [at a time] without eating anything else. It is a great medicine ... [as it] clears the mind and fortifies the teeth such that the men here who eat it ... [still] have all of their teeth without missing any even at eighty years of age. Those who are used to eating it have good breath [but] those who do not take it have breath that is insufferable. [This drug] is a form of nourishment in these parts.[67]

These invaluable leaves, Pires noted, grew "in great abundance" from "Chaul to Cambodia, and in all the islands, even beyond the Moluccas."[68] For this apothecary, betel was a readily available and highly valued commodity with a number of promising medicinal virtues. It deserved attention.

But by midcentury, the humble, ubiquitous betel leaf had become one of the multiplying sites in which the ethnic, religious, and gender tensions that accompanied colonization had begun to converge. Social and cultural anxieties set the parameters for what, if anything, could be said about it. When Álvares took up the pen in 1548 to respond to the inquiry from

[67] ANTT, CC, pt. 1, mç.19, n. 102, f. 3v.   [68] ANTT, CC, pt. 1, mç.19, n. 102, f. 3v.

João III, the use of betel leaves had become heavily coded with subversive associations. What was for many peoples throughout the region not only a commonplace accompaniment to casual conversation but an indispensable accessory in the celebration of such life-defining moments as marriage and the birth of children[69] was, for the Portuguese, increasingly taken as a marker of all that was unbecoming to a devout and properly ordered life.

When Álvares wrote to João III he did not so much as mention the plant. In the *Colóquios*, Orta certainly did. He made explicit what Álvares's omission only insinuated. Orta knew the chewing of betel leaves to be a common habit and reported that women in particular enjoyed it. But he said he found it "odious," and that he had "no appetite for it." His own "stubborn persistence," he confessed, was no more than an expression of his wish to "remain only in the faith of a Portuguese."[70] Clearly, to some among Orta's readers, betel had come to seem incompatible with orthodox Catholicism. Such pointed commentary notwithstanding, Orta never actually devoted a chapter to the betel leaf but instead lodged his impressions of it, together with broken pieces of information about it, in four other chapters – in one on the areca nut (with which it was – and still is – often chewed), in another on a similar leaf, the "folio indo," and in the book's last two chapters which, taken together, amounted to a collection of things Orta claimed to have inadvertently "left out" due to his own "forgetfulness."[71] Colonial cultural preoccupations had led to a carefully cultivated ignorance.

The tensions to which colonization gave rise did not simply influence natural knowledge; they had begun to substantively determine it. Some years later, when Costa produced his *Tractado*, in which he tried to "verify much of what the doctor Garcia de Orta had written," the betel leaf was not to be found at all.[72] What was known and what was not about South Asian nature were artifacts of the culture of inquiry that obtained in colonial Goa.

---

[69] Anthony Reid, "From Betel-Chewing to Tobacco Smoking in Indonesia," *The Journal of Asian Studies* 44 (1985): 529–532.

[70] Orta, *Colóquios*, vol. 2, 389–392.

[71] The strategic nature of the placement appears to have been lost on the Conde de Ficalho who, in editing the work, considered taking all of the bits and pieces lodged in this last chapter and inserting them back into the chapters for which they seemed – to him at least – best suited. Orta, *Colóquios*, vol. 2, 389, and the unnumbered note at the bottom of the page.

[72] Costa, *Tractado*.

The imperative to eradicate the ties that helped bond together members of an alternative community – to eliminate as much as possible the markers of an alternate ethnicity – would wax and wane with time. It was not until the early eighteenth century that Inquisition officials were compelled to issue an injunction against betel leaves. When they did so, the new law stipulated in extensive detail every occasion in which they were *not* to be used.[73] That Orta was so evasive in his coverage of the leaf suggests that the production and presentation of natural knowledge had begun to bend under the strain of social and cultural pressures much earlier. Colonial settlement propelled curiosity and the production of natural knowledge but it produced ignorance as well.[74] In this and other ways, elision and obfuscation would prove important for Orta in the production and circulation of natural knowledge.

INDIA HOUSE

Place mattered. When Orta took up more or less permanent residence in Goa in 1538, he was thrust into the epicenter of these conflicts. It was no small adjustment and the contrast between this new circumstance and his first four years in South Asia could not have been starker. Between 1534 and 1538, Orta was on the move. That put him in direct contact with medical specialists and experienced commercial agents up and down the Indian littoral. As others have argued and as I have explored in Chapter 4, Orta's technique for producing certain knowledge of nature depended upon his ability to compare reports on *naturalia* from widely varied personal and geographic sources. Trooping from port to port with Sousa and his men made that kind of collaboration a fairly uncontentious affair. Sousa himself was the senior Portuguese official. Orta was hardly at risk of persecution. And because many of his exchanges with Hindu and Muslim physicians took place in the course of diplomatic maneuvers that placed him in the company of Deccani rulers, peaceable intellectual discourse itself could be – indeed was – passed off as part of the work of diplomacy.[75] Orta, however, undertook most of his investigations not during those first years but after his settlement in Goa.

---

[73] *APO* vol. 4, pt. 2, 133.

[74] This is the dynamic variously explored in a series of essays in Robert N. Proctor and Londa Schiebinger, eds., *Agnotology: The Making and Unmaking of Ignorance* (Stanford, CA: Stanford University Press, 2008).

[75] As, for example, in Orta, *Colóquios*, vol. 2, 397–398.

To produce medical and more broadly natural knowledge, Orta needed
to affiliate himself with the precisely the sorts of people whom religious
authorities viewed with suspicion – and that in what was perhaps the most
violently invigilated place in Portugal's Asian empire. Goa's Inquisition was
notoriously predacious in its efforts to enforce Catholic orthodoxy.[76] The
specter of the Inquisition loomed hauntingly over Orta after its 1560 arrival.
His situation in Goa was a precarious one from the start. Orta was from a
New Christian family. In what turned out to be a harbinger of things to
come, religious officials in the late 1530s twice prosecuted physicians in Goa
on suspicion of their adherence to Judaism.[77] In life, Orta managed to escape
that fate, though a decade after his death he too was found guilty of the same
offense. His decayed body was exhumed and burned in the heart of Goa in
1580. The protection afforded to Orta by Sousa during his governorship was
not only instrumental in facilitating Orta's work; it probably also protected
him from the flames of the Inquisition. Yet the relationship between Sousa
and Orta was almost certainly neither as one-dimensional nor as purely
amicable as it is so often taken to be.[78] Sousa's power and the protection
afforded by his patronage created opportunity but entailed obligation too. It
is difficult to imagine a person of Sousa's position, ambition, and commercial inclination securing the protection of an authority on matters of medicine and natural philosophy and enabling so much investigative
collaboration without also hoping to reap some reward in return.[79] Patronage, then, was a compromise. It came at a cost and the recipient, including
those inclined to natural inquiry, could pay dearly.[80] The claim that Orta

---

[76] Priolkar, *Goa Inquisition*; Ana Cannas da Cunha, *A Inquisição no Estado da Índia:
   Origens (1539–1560),* (Lisbon: Arquivo Nacional Torre do Tombo, 1995); António José
   Saraiva, *The Marrano Factory: The Portuguese Inquisition and Its New Christians,
   1536–1765* (Boston, MA: Brill, 2001).

[77] Jon Arrizabalaga, "Garcia de Orta in the Context of the Sephardic Diaspora," in Costa,
   ed., *Medicine, Trade and Empire,* 11–32; Županov, "Drugs, Health, Bodies, and Souls";
   Cunha, *A Inquisição no Estado da Índia,* 252–253.

[78] Pearson, "Locating Garcia de Orta in the Port City of Goa and the Indian Ocean World,"
   in Costa, ed., *Medicine, Trade and Empire,* especially 42–43; Ficalho, *Garcia da Orta,*
   151–166, 313; Carvalho, *Garcia d'Orta,* 20–23. But see also Arrizabalaga, "Garcia de
   Orta in the Context of the Sephardic Diaspora," 16.

[79] See Chapter 3. Sousa and Orta shared an interest in the investigation of nature. Sousa was
   from the lower nobility, which itself, according to Subrahmanyam, *Portuguese Empire,*
   89–90, tended toward commercial pursuits. Hence the relations of patronage to which
   I refer need not be only those between an official and his subaltern but also a form of
   mutual exchange between two members of the maritime commercial diaspora as outlined
   by Studnicki-Gizbert, *Nation upon the Ocean Sea,* 57–58.

[80] See also the discussion in Biagiolli, *Galileo Courtier,* 313–352.

had once worked in the royal household has become an unsubstantiated commonplace in studies of the *Colóquios*.[81] But if it is indeed true, then Orta was probably already aware of the price Tomé Pires had paid in the service of D. Manuel. If not, then he certainly would have heard the stories that circulated in Goa, where he also saw the misery and isolation that the webs of princely patronage had exacted from Álvares.[82]

With Sousa's final departure from Goa in 1545 and the arrival of the Inquisition, Orta, like Álvares, was vulnerable to suspicion and intrigue – a position in which his New Christian background was a severe liability. Here was the problem: Garcia de Orta needed to interact with vaidyas and other knowers of nature with backgrounds and geographical exposures that were wider and still more diverse and extended than his own. In that way he could replicate the dynamic of travel even when he could not personally leave Goa. He had to do so in a way that would provoke as little suspicion as possible from his countrymen. That was not all. As I argued in the last chapter, Orta's epistemology was one that encompassed the accounts of his own contemporaries in Goa and correspondents from throughout Indian Ocean Asia, as well as an array of classical texts, and combined all of that with impressions derived from his own somatic encounters with the things of nature. People, books, and things all had to be collected. The variety of evidence they offered had to be compared. Orta needed a space in which he could both engage with native specialists and to collect, examine, sort, and store both specimens of nature and books about them.

Orta's solution was to move science into the household. For Orta in Goa no less than for naturalists in Europe at the same time sites of knowledge production had begun to proliferate.[83] And yet, similar outcomes notwithstanding, the particular circumstances were different. The household lay at the very heart of Iberian notions of colonial Catholic propriety. As an ideal, the colonial household was a profoundly private and even cloistered space. Its theoretical inviolability underwrote notions of male honor and female virtue in Portuguese colonies in both the

---

[81] Arrizabalaga, "Garcia de Orta in the Context of the Sephardic Diaspora," 16, notes that it was a powerful relative, Thomaz de Orta, who was in fact a physician of the royal household.

[82] On patronage and the fates of Pires and Álvares, see Chapter 3.

[83] Ogilvie, *Science of Describing*, 141–174; Findlen, *Possessing Nature*, 97–150; Steven Shapin, "The House of Experiment in Seventeenth Century England," *Isis* 79 (1988): 373–404; Deborah E. Harkness, "Managing an Experimental Household: The Dees of Mortlake and the Practice of Natural Philosophy," *Isis* 88 (1997): 247–262.

Atlantic and Indian Ocean worlds.[84] Cristovão da Costa, another Portuguese naturalist and one of Orta's near contemporaries in Goa (his Spanish version of the *Colóquios* appeared in Burgos in 1628), penned a treatise "in praise of women" in 1592 and singled out their "chastity, honesty, fidelity, [and] silence."[85] In Portugal's colonies, a secure and well-ordered household served, among other things, as the guarantor of precisely those qualities.[86] Orta's decision was informed by the deepening religious trouble in Goa and the ideological significance of the household – the inviolable space offered a place for the investigative exchange of specimens and knowledge about them that was removed from the prying eyes of officials – as well as by the practical imperatives of natural inquiry in Goa, which demanded a physical workspace in which to accumulate, compare, and keep to hand the tools (books) and materials (plant and mineral matter) that he needed to carry out his work.

The Orta household stood one block west of Rua Direita (to the right in the Linschoten illustration), on Rua dos Namorados.[87] It was just about three blocks from the city's cathedral and two blocks from the seat of the Inquisition. It sat atop a slight hill that looked down over Goa's *ribeira*. From his veranda Orta could see ships coming to port and could watch his own visitors climbing up the long steady slope toward him. Behind the house was a garden in which grew *negundo* and *jambo*, and perhaps many of the other plants Orta discussed in his book. From the street, the garden was probably not visible.[88] Linschoten's map, which is roughly contemporary, shows that façades enclosed the whole of the block, which meant Orta's

---

[84] The analytical framework here has been worked out with particular reference to Brazil. See Roberto da Matta, *A casa e a rua: Espaço, cidadania, mulher, e morte no Brasil* (São Paulo: Brasiliense, 1985); Sueann Caulfield, *In Defense of Honor: Sexual Morality, Modernity, and Nation in Early Twentieth-Century Brazil* (Durham, NC: Duke University Press, 2000), 5–9, which surveys the intertwined concepts of honor and virtue as they pertained to Portuguese America from 1492 to 1900; Ronaldo Vainfas, *Trópico dos pecados: moral, sexualidade, e Inquisição no Brasil* (Rio de Janeiro: Editora Campus, 1997), explores at length Inquisitorial influences on quotidian behavior in the colony; and Coates, *Convicts and Orphans*, 120–177 examines the way these concepts fostered empire-wide institutions and colonization schemes involving the *órfãs del rei* ("king's orphans").

[85] Cristovão da Costa [Cristobal Acosta], *Tratado en loor de las mvgeres. Y dela Castidad, Onestidad, Constancia, Silencio, y Iusticia. Con otras muchas particularidades, y varias Historias* (Venice: Giacomo Cornetti, 1592), 79v–86; Cagle, "Botany of Colonial Medicine."

[86] Studnicki-Gizbert, *A Nation upon the Ocean Sea*, 76–89.

[87] This the location according to Carvalho, *Garcia d'Orta*, 31.

[88] Orta, *Colóquios*, vol. 2, 99–108 and 163–164; Carvalho, *Garcia d'Orta*, 29–31.

garden abutted those of his neighbors. Whether neighbors could view one another from these interior spaces is uncertain. But in the *Colóquios* Orta made it abundantly clear that he was not directly accessible.

The interior space of the house was, in short, impenetrable to the gaze. It was within these walls that he collected news and information from correspondents he deemed "worthy of credit" spread from Tunis to Malacca. Orta rarely named his sources but – in a tacit recognition of the role of male honour in the making of credible witnesses – he often anchored claims to their reliability by referring to them as married men.[89] Orta's contacts ranged from a certain Jewish merchant in Cairo to Crown-appointed officials of the Estado. They included colorful characters like the Portuguese renegade Sancho Pirez – a Matosinhense artilleryman who had abandoned Nuno da Cunha in Diu in 1534 and whom Orta met at the court of Burhan Nizam Shah – and one Coje Çofar, "a native of Puglia who had become a Moor."[90] In the garden that spread out behind Orta's home, he discussed the negundo trees with Ruano, his principal interlocutor in the dialogues that comprise the *Colóquios*. In this garden too, his servant Antonia told Ruano the wonders of the negundo tree, which Orta explained was in common use in Goa and "for which one need not a physician … for you cannot enter a house to treat anything without there being someone insisting on the use of negundo, either cooked or fried in oil."[91] It was within the protected confines of Orta's home that the vaidya Malupa, who visited each morning to look after the health of Ortas maidservants, answered Orta's queries on the origins of turbith and the use that might be made of it when mixed with ginger.[92] Within Orta's walls, a Milanese lapidary named André visited briefly to arrange the sale of some of Orta's emeralds and, in the course of conversation, related what he had seen of a hunt for elephants and their ivory during a recent journey to Pegu.[93] And there, too, the Portuguese physician and Orta's younger colleague Dimas Bosque gathered with Ruano to share word of a vermilion stone said to be better than even a bezoar in staving off the effects of poison.[94]

---

[89] For example, see Orta, *Colóquios*, vol. 1, 260; and vol. 2, 184, 202, 378.

[90] Expressions like "worthy of faith" (*dino/digno de fé*) or "worthy of faith and credit" (*dino/digno de fé e credito*) are repeated when Orta introduces information from unnamed sources. See, for example, Orta, *Colóquios*, vol. 1, 19, 25, 48, 120, 154, 155, 157, 195, 308, 314; and vol. 2, 26, 33, 76, 182, 184, 234, 246, 250, 322, 354.

[91] Orta, *Colóquios*, vol. 2, 163.   [92] Orta, *Colóquios*, vol. 2, 327–343.

[93] Orta, *Colóquios*, vol. 1, 303–314.

[94] Orta, *Colóquios*, vol. 2, 371–384. On Bosque, see Jaime Walter, "Dimas Bosque, físico-mor da Índia e as Sereias," *Studia* 12 (1963): 261–271.

WHERE THE TRUTH LIES

The contradiction of course was that, if Orta's work were to be of any use to anyone, it had to follow the cast of characters who had helped produce it as they ventured back across the threshold of Orta's household and back into the streets of Goa. Knowledge might be produced and certified within the household, but it would only be taken as an authoritative account of nature if it secured the assent of the wider Portuguese-speaking community. Enacting that translation was the most elemental function of the *Colóquios*: to take knowledge produced within the more or less private and exclusive confines of the household and transfer it as an intact, credible, authoritative, and actionable statement of certain natural knowledge into the bustling, uncertain hubbub of Portuguese Goa.[95] The question for Orta was how to craft a text that did just that – present natural knowledge that was credible and authoritative. It was not a simple task. Why a book by a Portuguese physician should be taken as credible, let alone authoritative, when there was widespread recognition that vaidyas, hakims, daias, and domestic servants of varied extraction wielded so formidable a knowledge of nature was an open question.

If local healers were taken as authorities on matters of natural fact, then some indication of Orta's affiliation with them would buttress his own credibility and lend weight to his claims to truth. Yet an open acknowledgement that he had been clandestinely collaborating with Hindu and Muslim physicians, together with women of various backgrounds, in the production of natural knowledge meant rendering visible the very interactions he sought to occlude. In this, the dialogue turned out to be the perfect representational instrument. By carefully scripting his interactions with Antonia, Malupa, and the many other figures who appear in the *Colóquios*, Orta could mingle fact and fiction with considerable impunity. He could strategically signify affiliation for the sake of establishing his own credibility, while at the same time fashioning an investigative persona for himself that subscribed to conventional notions of honor and propriety in the colony, thus allaying the suspicion of Jesuits, Inquisitors, and other skeptics. Since permission to print the *Colóquios* had ultimately to come from Aleixo Dias Falcão, a Jesuit and

---

[95] Pace Shapin, "The career of experimental knowledge is the circulation between private and public spaces," in "House of Experiment," 400. I am not concerned with *experimental* knowledge *per se*, but I believe the observation holds equally true for Orta give the parameters within which he worked in Goa.

Inquisitor in Goa, the book's very existence is a testament to the skill with which Orta managed the contradictory demands of credibility, religious orthodoxy, and colonial cultural propriety.

How did he do it? The *Colóquios* entailed at least one substantial omission: Orta was a married man. Yet the *Colóquios* said nothing of either his wife or his children. Orta's family and friends had already appeared before the Inquisition in a string of trials in which they were called not to stand for judgment but to testify about those who did. Advertising those encounters with authority could undermine his credibility and, indeed, endanger not only his own life but those of his kinsmen as well. Given the perception of domestic relations as a measure of honor and integrity, a second reason for the omission must surely have been Orta's own turbulent married life. Orta and his wife no longer lived together; she had taken up residence on the family estate on the island of Bombay.[96] Orta remained in Goa.

Just as Orta expunged certain details that might prove injurious to his image as a capable patriarch, he also subtly insinuated suggestions of his own devout Catholicism.[97] He referred to himself as a stubbornly faithful Portuguese.[98] And on the matter of a New Christian in Tunis, upon whom he relied at several points in the text, Orta noted accusingly that he was "Spanish by his language" but a "Jew by his false religion."[99] Orta also portrayed himself as a wise and compassionate but disciplined physician. In the treatment of D. Geronimo's brother, Orta advised that the illness, colerica passio, "would brook no delay" and asked to be kept informed of its course. He promptly issued a list of medicaments to be variously combined by an apothecary (barley, cumin, sugar, castor oil, honey, quinces, white wine, cinnamon, and rosewater) and taken intermittently by the ailing man. Orta and Ruano then left the scene. As they did so, Orta bid everyone farewell, suggestively adding, "may God bestow health upon this house."[100]

He dispensed orders to procure certain medicines from Goa's native apothecaries but there was not so much as the intimation that he might

[96] Carvalho, *Garcia d'Orta*, 16–23.

[97] On the question of Orta's New Christian background and Jewish ancestry, see Jon Arrizabalaga, "Garcia de Orta in the context of the Sephardic diaspora."

[98] Orta, *Colóquios*, vol. 2, 389.   [99] Orta, *Colóquios*, vol. 1, 60; vol. 2, 108.

[100] This and similar expressions are used repeatedly: Orta, *Colóquios*, vol. 1, 263. See also vol. 1, 49, 107, 183, 243, 262, 356, 362; vol. 2, 37, 107, 234, 260, 401.

retrieve them himself. Despite the opportunity to highlight his discrimin-
ating eye for the choicest *materia medica*, rarely in the *Colóquios* did Orta
mention venturing into Goa's apothecary quarter. That was the servant
Antonia's charge. The issue was not simply one of the division of investigative or curative labor. Goa's geography was saturated with moral
significance. It abounded with places of profligacy and debauchery,
houses of pagan worship, and of Catholic propriety, and markets where
the medical and commercial worlds mingled. Goa's *boticas* (apothecaries)
were gathered together in a quarter of the city still dominated by native
Goans. The street they lined ran parallel to one dominated by the vanias
who financed much of the drugs trade in Goa. None too subtly separating
this quarter from that of Goa's casados was the city's pillory (Figure 5.3).

Omission and aversion were two key elements of Orta's literary self-
fashioning. That refusal to venture past the *pilourinho velho (sic)* – the old

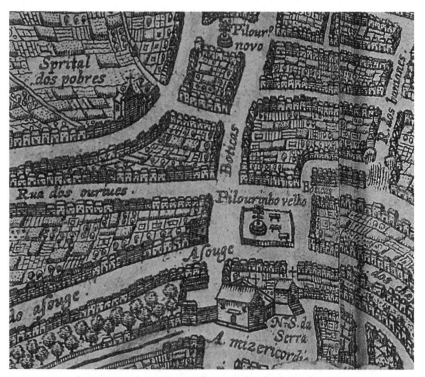

FIGURE 5.3 Separation Anxiety. A pillory marks the boundary between
Portuguese Goa and the apothecary and merchants' quarters. From Jan Huygen
van Linschoten, *Tertia pars Indiae Orientalis* (Frankfurt: Matthias Becker, 1601).
Courtesy of the Beinecke Rare Book and Manuscript Library, Yale University.

pillory – was part of a third. Since too close a tie with Goa's Hindu community might stir suspicion, Orta took care not to conjure that affiliation in any way – even when talking about things he had learned from them. One way to do this was simply to diminish the significance of various elements of local *materia medica*, which is precisely what Orta did when he addressed substances in the *Colóquios* that had come to be associated with the most subversive aspects of local social life. Betel leaves provoked disgust. Opium was dismissed as morally and physically harmful. The drug provoked "indecency" – it led all too quickly to the "act of Venus" – but as a medicine was at best useless and at worst likely to kill a person; Orta was always suspicious when a compound medicine had "the scent of opium."[101] And hashish (*bangue*), Orta pointedly noted, was "not one of our medicines" and made a fool of those who took it.[102] The problem was not simply that these were either rare or unfamiliar substances among the Portuguese. Orta handled those in quite another way (Chapter 3). Rather, as with the betel leaf, the consumption of these seemed to either threaten or actually invert an idealized colonial order.

Some of the once unfamiliar but most commonly used *materia medica* were simply too efficacious to be ignored. *Raiz da China* was an invaluable treatment for intermittent fevers.[103] Another novel drug had proven an indispensable treatment for "chronic dysentery," though Orta "could not but confess" that it was "not so prized nor so certain as the herb which the people of Malabar give."[104] The reason for such candor was twofold. First, the medicine was already widely used among the Portuguese in the royal hospital and, second, Orta was known for prescribing this and a few other related medicines used by healers he met along the Konkan and Malaber coasts.[105] The day-to-day business of healing required a pragmatism that the printed word could not easily extinguish from memory. If Orta was known to use local remedies, he could hardly deny it in print. It was better to "confess" the transgression – to attenuate the corrosive influence of rumor – in an account of the several available treatments for a common illness.[106]

---

[101] Orta, *Colóquios*, vol. 2, 172–173.

[102] Orta, *Colóquios*, vol. 1, 98. An unnamed Portuguese who had allegedly fallen victim to its intoxicating virtue ended up a jester at the court of Vijayanagar. See Orta, *Colóquios*, vol. 1, 97.

[103] Orta, *Colóquios*, vol. 2, 259–270.   [104] Orta, *Colóquios*, vol. 2, 15.

[105] He had done so in the case of the treatment in question, a compound of cumin seeds and sour milk, for one *liçenciado* Alvaro Fernandes. Orta, *Colóquios*, vol. 2, 14.

[106] Orta, *Colóquios*, vol. 2, 140, tendered a similar "confession" in his account of his treatment of Martim Afonso de Sousa during their trek toward Ahmedabad.

And in any case, when such wholesale adoption of treatments were unavoidable, Orta argued for the application of a certain protocol: local remedies ought to be integrated into a Portuguese colonial pharmacopoeia used to treat any illness but only after treatment with what Orta referred to as the "medicines of my [Western] doctors" had failed to do the trick.[107]

This is not to dismiss Orta's regard for accounts offered by South Asian specialists. All too frequently he claimed to have gotten key pieces of information from them. But he portrayed such instances of reliance as matters of practical necessity,[108] and the relationships by which they were ascertained as impersonal and even strictly transactional.[109] So for example: lest his connection to Burhan Nizam Shah, the ruler of Ahmadnagar, raise Inquisitorial eyebrows, Orta took care to tell his readers that he had been "well paid" for the work.[110] Their relationship was strictly medical and all debts had been satisfied.[111] Accounts of his reliance on Indian specialists, moreover, did not mean that Orta took them on their word. Rather, he portrayed Indian healers as both ignorant of anatomy and beset with a lack of curiosity,[112] and he portrayed Indian merchants as cunning and backhanded.[113] For example, Orta related that since he and most other Portuguese were "very little conversant with the things of the Kingdom of Delhi," errant yogis were necessarily taken as informants on a prized cure for poison (Orta called it *baçaraga*) thought to come from there. But what they said about it, so Orta claimed, "was contrary to all good philosophy," and at any rate, he insisted, "what they say one day they deny the next."[114]

In carefully staging these exchanges through the use of the dialogue, Orta could dramatize his engagement with potentially suspect figures – touting his own manipulation of their confidence in order to ferret out their deceptions. So, for example, when a vania revealed how he adulterated the camphor that came from Borneo with a Chinese variety that was cheaper and of poor quality, Orta turned that knowledge over to his readers: "all such things must be prepared for by those who wish to speculate in camphor," he warned.[115] It was a caveat that, as Orta and his readers well knew, extended to countless other drugs as well.

---

[107] Orta, *Colóquios*, vol. 2, 139.   [108] Orta, *Colóquios*, vol. 1, 142–143.
[109] See for example Orta, *Colóquios*, vol. 2, 69, 121–122, 389–402.
[110] Orta, *Colóquios*, vol. 1, 64–65, 144–145.
[111] Studnicki-Gizbert, *Nation upon the Ocean Sea*, 57–58.
[112] Orta, *Colóquios*, vol. 2, 137, 328–329, 332.
[113] In addition to the following examples and my discussion of these concerns in the previous chapter, see Orta, *Colóquios*, vol. 2, 134–138.
[114] Orta, *Colóquios*, vol. 2, 400.   [115] Orta, *Colóquios*, vol. 1, 154–155.

If the dialogue was a conventional and increasingly outdated genre of scientific exposition among many naturalists at work within Europe,[116] Orta's embrace of it in Goa should not be taken as a mark of intellectual backwardness any more than his emphasis on firsthand experience should be taken as evidence of singular foresight and innovation.[117] The dialogue form of presentation enabled Orta to script potentially incriminating interaction in ways that that the expository form so fashionable in the West could not. Instead of making a claim outright, Orta was able to make visible the process by which he reasoned his way through an array of evidence toward a conclusion with collaborators, themselves widely held to be authoritative. He advertised his own personal affiliations in a way that enhanced his intellectual credibility in Goa and buttressed the authority of the *Colóquios*. But rather than leave his exchanges to the Inquisitorial imagination, he offered a portrait of his domestic life and work that might mitigate suspicion, intrigue, and accusation. Hence the dialogue provided a way for Orta to manage the risks attendant upon the production of knowledge and the practice of medicine in Goa.

In effect, Orta was able to display a command of natural knowledge without personally claiming ownership of it and without tying himself too closely to the mestiço and native women and other indigenous specialists who did. Here was a situation analogous to the one facing the apothecary Pires and the pilot Rodrigues a half-century earlier. A credible and authoritative account of the natural world demanded not the appropriation and occlusion of peoples and their knowledges but their visible embrace. And yet colonizing ambitions had engendered tensions that made the easy and open embrace of native physicians and alternate knowledges much more problematic. In Goa, Orta's insinuation within colonial networks of patronage, protection, and investigation made his position considerably more precarious and the politics of visibility and occlusion – fact and fiction – more fraught.

---

[116] On which see Virginia Cox, *The Renaissance Dialogue: Literary Dialogue in its Social and Political Contexts, Castiglione to Galileo* (New York: Cambridge University Press, 2008); and Roger Friedlein, "El diálogo renacentista en la Península Ibérica," in Klaus W. Hempfer, Gerhard Regn, and Sunita Scheffel, eds., *Text und Kontext. Romanische Literaturen und Allgemeine* (Stuttgart: Franz Steiner Verlag, 2005), 141–146.

[117] Stefan Halikowski Smith, "Perceptions of Nature."

PART III

THE PORTUGUESE ATLANTIC, 1550–1700

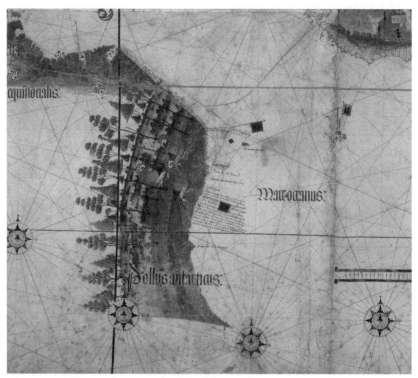

FIGURE 6.1 The Dubious Allure of an Atlantic Island. Detail of Brazil, the "Island of Santa Cruz" (*Ilha de Sancta Cruz*), from the Cantino Atlas. © Getty Images.

6

Moral Hazards

> For those with little faith, the world turned inside out.
>
> Francisco Pires (Bahia, 7 August 1552)[1]

THE AMBIVALENCE OF WONDER

Pero Vaz de Caminha might have been right. That unfamiliar coast in the southwestern corner of the Atlantic may indeed have been marked by prodigious fecundity. Its peoples might well have been as comely and as fit for political and religious submission as Caminha had claimed. His letter to Manuel I in late April 1500 was certainly not the last account filled with assertions like those. By midcentury, material in print and manuscript detailing the flora, fauna, and native peoples of a place Caminha had called the "Island of the True Cross" (*Ilha de Vera Cruz*) – soon to be known simply as Brazil – had begun to multiply in Lisbon, Paris, Antwerp, and Venice.[2] Among the most widely circulated accounts were those of André Thevet, Anthony Knivet, Jean de Léry, and Hans Staden. Thevet gathered his notes while in the French settlement at Guanabara Bay – the auspiciously named colony of "France Antarctique" at modern

---

[1] *MB* vol. 1, 397.
[2] On the persistence of manuscript culture in Portugal see Diogo Ramada Curto, "A história do livro em Portugal: Uma agenda em aberto," in *O livro antigo em Portugal e Espanha, séculos XVI–XVIII*, a special edition of *Leituras: Revista da Biblioteca Nacional* 9/10 (2002): 13–62; and the discussion in Anson C. Piper, "Jorge Ferreira de Vasconcelos: Defender of the Portuguese Vernacular," *Hispania* 37 (1954): 400–425. See also Chapter 8.

Rio de Janeiro. Extracts from Thevet's published account, including one of its woodcuts, found their way into Clusius's *Aromatum et simplicium*, where it sat alongside of the material on India that Clusius had culled from Orta's *Colóquios*.[3] Accounts like these piqued the interest of European rulers and fired the imaginations of merchants and missionaries. They would help transform the South Atlantic into a principal theatre of imperial rivalry, commercial competition, religious proselytization, and plantation slavery.

Yet back in Lisbon, late in the spring of 1500, D. Manuel's reaction to Caminha's news was most notable for its restraint, and for what the Portuguese monarch did not – indeed could not – do. Having read Caminha's letter and listened to reports of captain Gaspar de Lemos and his crew (their supply ship was originally to follow Cabral to Cochin but returned straightaway to Lisbon with news of the landfall), Dom Manuel had good cause to ask that most intractable of questions: So what? The answer was anything but clear. By 1500, sugar from Portugal's Madeira colony poured into European pantries; the São Jorge da Mina Castle was now one of a number of ports in West Africa where royal factors busily accumulated gold, ivory, and slaves; and over a half-century of lucrative trade and intermittent exploration along the western littoral of Africa had only two years earlier left Portugal with direct and (for the moment) unrivalled access to the spices, drugs, and other riches of Asia.[4] Cabral's South American landfall took place in the wake of all that. So Caminha's exuberant description of Edenic verdure, supreme health, and prelapsarian innocence at the western edge of the Atlantic must have seemed a lackluster footnote to da Gama's tales of ivory, silver, spices, textiles, and a kind of exotic Christianity that was all the more remarkable for its very strangeness. And even after some of those South Asian Christians turned out to be Hindu pagans (da Gama famously mistook a Hindu shrine for a Christian chapel), the vegetable and material richness of the Indian Ocean world seemed not to disappoint. What, by comparison, was this uncharted "island" to offer?[5]

---

[3] This, as I have discussed in Chapter 4, was a metropolitan juxtaposition that made manifest a region the Flemish naturalist referred to as "the Indies."

[4] Although Spanish and Portuguese ships clashed in the Moluccas in the early 1520s as discussed in Meilink-Roelofsz, *Asian Trade and European Influence*.

[5] Here my interpretation of what Pagden, *Fall of Natural Man*, has termed the "problem of recognition" differs from that of J. H. Elliott, *The Old World and the New, 1492–1650* (New York: Cambridge University Press, 1970), who was concerned with a developing appreciation for the novelty of the Americas.

It was in part to answer that question that in May 1501 D. Manuel sent an exploratory voyage back across the Atlantic. Under the command of one Gonçalo Coelho and including the Florentine financier-cum-chronicler Amerigo Vespucci, the expedition was to establish a fixed route, chart the coast, and determine what, if any, commercial value the region might promise. Vespucci confirmed Caminha's account of health and verdure but he was decidedly unimpressed with the region's commercial potential. Its dyewood was marketable and such creatures as macaws and monkeys became part of a metropolitan gift economy. But otherwise, Brazil did not fail to disappoint. As Vespucci noted, "One can say we found nothing of profit there except an infinity of dyewood trees, canafistula ... and other natural marvels that would be tedious to describe."[6] Outspoken observers agreed. Julius Caesar Scaliger, for one, did not mince words. The spices of Brazil, he wrote, were "scarce, ignoble, and bad."[7]

Wonder had its limits. Marvel need not have compelled possession and did little to underwrite the conquest and subordination of Brazil.[8] That ambivalence was all too evident on the Cantino atlas. If Caminha's letter of 1500 had lodged Brazil into the imperial imagination, the 1502 expedition put it firmly on the imperial map: the last round of corrections to the atlas (just before it was smuggled to Ferrara) included such details from the Coelho-Vespucci voyage as names and landmarks (Monte Pascual, the inland mountain whose summit was the first evidence of dry land spotted by Cabral's crew two years earlier, was now made into an orienting point for Portuguese sailors). On the atlas, a profuse and colorful interior was populated only by tall trees and the kinds of colorful birds whose plumage, according to Alessandra Russo, increasingly denoted an exotic and remote New World.[9] Yet unlike Africa, which on the Cantino atlas was depicted in its continental entirety, or Sumatra, which was already clearly distinguished from the long arch of the Malay peninsula, Brazil was neither firmly attached to other lands nor were its limits demarcated – not even speculatively. It was a land inhabited but unbound. The only feature that lent it any location at all was the verdant,

---

[6] Quoted in H. B. Johnson, "The settlement of Brazil, 1500–1580," in *Colonial Brazil*, ed. Leslie Bethell (New York: Cambridge University Press, 1987), 6. I have added italics for emphasis.

[7] Quoted in Cañizares-Esguerra, *Nature, Empire, and Nation*, 73.

[8] The case for wonder is made by Stephen Greenblatt, *Marvelous Possessions: The Wonder of the New World* (Chicago: Chicago University Press, 1991).

[9] Russo, "Cortés's Objects," 236.

sinuous edge where the sea met the shore. And indeed, for the first half-century after Caminha's report many Portuguese were concerned only with transactions across that line. If maps were instruments for and indices of the extension of colonial power,[10] the Cantino atlas accurately reflected Portugal's limited interest in, knowledge of, and influence over the South American littoral.

That same ambivalence – Brazil was lush and healthy yet largely ignored – would characterize the earliest approaches to disease and the study of nature in Portuguese America. As with Garcia de Orta in Goa, situating Brazil within the history of natural inquiry in Portugal's empire in the sixteenth and seventeenth centuries, and in the history of the tropics more broadly, affords an opportunity to critique a set of dominant narratives in the history of science – now from an Atlantic rather than Indian Ocean perspective. To recapitulate briefly: overseas encounters in general and New World discoveries in particular were supposed to have helped fuel the widespread obsession with collection and display – an activity that, as it grew over the century, encompassed an expanding number of people, institutions, and social groups. Curiosity, once viewed as vain and dangerous – for how could the human mind comprehend divine creation?[11] – became a prestigious intellectual posture. Knowledge of the wider world opened pathways for social mobility and professional legitimation. An obsession with collecting helped to strengthen attention to the physical and material characteristics of plants, animals, and humans, and all things that could be either gifted or bought and sold. In short: discovery fueled inquiry, invited curiosity, and begot empiricism.[12]

The example of Brazil calls into question that account in two important ways. Despite the widespread fascination with the new and the exotic – and in contrast to events unfolding in Goa, where apothecaries had begun to catalogue the natural world from the inception of the Estado da Índia (see especially Chapter 3) – the natural abundance of

---

[10] The classic statement is that of Denis Wood, "How Maps Work," *Cartographica* 29 (1992): 66–74. His assertion that "*maps are weapons*" (italics in the original) was argued in the case of colonial Latin America by Walter Mignolo, *The Darker Side of the Renaissance: Literacy, Territoriality, and Colonization*, 2nd edn. (Ann Arbor, MI: University of Michigan Press, 2003). But if maps are instruments of empire, they can often be dull and their purposes deflected. On the ambiguities of maps and mapping in colonial Latin America see Mundy, *Mapping*; Padrón, *Spacious Word*; and Safier, *Measuring the New*.

[11] Daston, "Curiosity in Early Modern Science."

[12] Daston and Park, *Wonders*, 148–159.

Brazil so praised by Caminha was all but ignored. Nearly a century passed before a generation of observers took to cataloging Brazilian nature and even then reports were cursory and often discounted.[13] Pero de Magalhães Gândavo's *História da próvincia de Santa Cruz* was published in Lisbon in 1576.[14] Gabriel Soares de Sousa authored a *Tratado descritivo* in 1587.[15] And it was over the same decade of the 1580s that the Jesuit Fernão Cardim wrote three descriptive treatises now collectively known by the title *Tratados da terra e da gente do Brasil*.[16] Those several accounts each canvassed a nearly identical list of some four dozen plants and animals. They installed a relatively small and frequently reiterated catalog of Brazilian nature in metropolitan imaginations, collections, and apothecary shops.[17] Despite the intensification of colonial settlement in Brazil, even as the number of apothecaries swelled in Portugal (and especially in Lisbon) in the sixteenth and seventeenth centuries, the presence of Brazilian *materia medica* did not.[18] The earliest published treatment of disease in the Atlantic – Aleixo de Abreu's *Tratado de las siete enfermedades*, published in Lisbon in 1623 – stressed the use of South Asian medicines almost to the complete exclusion of those from South America.[19] In 1709, a personal physician to the Portuguese king João

---

[13] Readers may find it useful to recall events in Asia, where a stream of apothecaries, most famously Tomé de Sousa and Simão Alvares arrived at India's Malabar and Konkan Coasts with Afonso de Albuquerque's conquests beginning in 1510. Physicians came too, most famously (but by no means exclusively) Garcia de Orta, who arrived in 1534.

[14] Pero de Magalhães Gândavo, *História da provincial de Santa Cruz a que vulgarmente chamamos Brasil* (Lisbon: António Gonçalves, 1576),

[15] Gabriel Soares de Sousa, *Tratado Descriptivo do Brazil*, ed. Francisco Adolpho de Varnhagen (Rio de Janeiro: Typographia Universal de Laemmert, 1851 [1587]).

[16] John Monteiro provides a brief discussion of these texts and their authors at the beginning of "The Heathen Castes of Sixteenth-Century Portuguese America: Unity, Diversity, and the Invention of the Brazilian Indians," *Hispanic American Historical Review* 80 (2000): 697–719.

[17] Fernão Cardim, *Tratados da terra e da gente do Brasil*, eds. Baptista Caetano, Capistrano de Abreu, and Rodolpho Garcia (Rio de Janeiro: Editores J. Leite, 1925), 61–67, for example, identified sixteen medicinal plants in Brazil. James Nelson Novoa has detailed the accumulation of exotica from the Portuguese colonies in "Unicorns and Bezoars in a Portuguese house in Rome: António da Fonseca's Portuguese Inventories," *Ágora: Estudos Clássicos em Debate* 14 (2012): 91–111.

[18] Braga, *Assistência, saúde pública e prática médica em Portugal*; José Pedro Sousa Dias, *Droguistas, boticários e segredistas: Ciência e Sociedade na Produção de Medicamentos na Lisboa de Setecentos* (Lisbon: Fundação Calouste Gulbenkian and the Fundação para a Ciência e Tecnologia, 2007).

[19] I explore the author and his work at length in Chapter 7. Aleixo de Abreu, *Tratado de las siete enfermedades: de la inflammacion universal del higado, zirbo, pyloron, y riñones, y de la obstrucion de la satiriasi, de la terciana y febre maligna, y passion hipocondriaca:*

V authored a dietary guide (*regimen sanitatis*) that left out New World comestibles altogether – with, that is, the exception of the tomato, which he discounted out of hand as poisonous.[20]

Meanwhile, as missionaries fanned out among the native peoples of Portuguese America, as quotidian microbial exchanges led to pervasive and devastating epidemics, and as lurid and pained accounts of human suffering – native and European alike – were printed and circulated, the image of Brazil inaugurated by Caminha would persist for almost two centuries. Despite epidemic disease, Brazil remained a paradise.

That assessment distinguished Brazil from every other theatre of Portuguese empire. West Africa, once an earthly paradise, became seen as a place of debilitating illness. In India, concern for disease mounted and uncertainty ran high almost from the outset of Portuguese settlement. But instead of the kinds of blanket assertions of ill-health that became common in reports of West Africa, writers in Portuguese Asia drew finer distinctions. By the 1530s, the Malabar port of Cannanore had earned a favorable reputation among the Portuguese; its drugs and spices, airs and waters were favorably compared even to those of Goa, and it became a favored place to convalesce.[21] Accounts of Brazil were different. Of the Tupí-speaking peoples the Portuguese met along the east coast of Brazil, Gândavo found them "too numerous to comprehend."[22] As epidemic disease – fevers, cough, dysentery, and pox – spread among them, unknown thousands perished.[23] In just the decade and a half after

---

Lleva otros tres tratados, del mal de Loanda, del guzano, y de las fuentes y sedales (Lisbon: Pedro Craesbeeck, 1623).

[20] BNP Res. Cod. 5073: "Variologia medicinal Galenica e Kymica. Repartida em varios tractados por Manoel Lopes Pereyra, medico da camara de sua magistade," [1709]. The most detailed study of the reception of this New World food is probably David Gentlecore, *Pomodoro!: A History of the Tomato in Italy* (New York: Columbia University Press, 2010), ch. 1.

[21] Correia, for example, repeatedly addresses this in *Lendas*, vol. 1, 729, 961; vol. 2, 26, 118, 537, 969–970; and vol. 3, 17.

[22] Gândavo, *Tratado*, 52.

[23] John M. Monteiro surveys the cultural landscape of sixteenth-century Brazil in "The Crises and Transformations of Invaded Societies: Coastal Brazil in the Sixteenth Century," in *The Cambridge History of the Native Peoples of the Americas*, 3 vols., eds. Frank Salomon and Stuart B. Schwartz (New York: Cambridge University Press, 1996), vol. 3, pt. 1, 973–1023. For a survey of shifting ecology and epidemiology of sixteenth-century Brazil, see Alida Metcalf, *Go-Betweens and the Colonization of Brazil, 1500–1600* (Austin, TX: University of Texas Press, 2005); and David Noble Cook, *Born to Die: Disease and New World Conquest, 1492–1650* (New York: Cambridge University Press, 1998), 149. Exactly how many people inhabited lowland South America remains an open question.

renewed colonization got underway in 1549, there were at least a half-dozen separate epidemics.[24] And yet, for the better part of two centuries, observes accounted Brazil a healthy place. In prose, poetry, and polychrome atlases, they asserted and reiterated the health of its airs and waters and the exuberance of its nature. Until that changed, it would be impossible to imagine the intertropical zone as an epidemiologically coherent region.

If, as so many studies contend, early modern empires helped redefine metropolitan sensibilities and authorized alternative epistemologies, they could also deflect the study the nature, deprioritize empirical inquiry, render some bodies less evidentiary than others, and make widespread epidemics invisible, effectively coding whole regions as healthy where there was every evidence to the contrary. Brazil was a historical exception and it remains a historiographical conundrum. What can explain such a situation? When and why did attitudes toward nature and disease in Brazil finally change?

Imperial comparisons and distinct colonial histories provide partial explanations. If the attraction of Asia lay primarily in the multitudinous and lucrative spice trade, in Brazil it lay of course in the cultivation of sugarcane – a single plant of Old World provenance (originally domesticated in southeast Asia[25]), that was well known and could be profitably sold. If Asian drugs and spices were in high demand, those from the Americas were not,[26] and on both sides of the Atlantic, fears ran high in many quarters over what might happen were one to regularly consume them. [27] And if the accumulated accounts of disease and death transformed impressions of West Africa and suffused those of India, differential susceptibility to disease and the consequently disproportionate impact of epidemics on Brazil's native peoples surely seemed to support claims that, at least for metropolitan migrants, Brazil was indeed a healthy destination.

---

[24] Cook, *Born to Die*, 149.

[25] Andrew F. Smith, *Sugar: A Global History* (London: Reaktion, 2015), ch. 1.

[26] Hence the vigorous efforts by some Spaniards to liken American spices to Asian ones. See, for example, Paula de Vos, "The Science of Spice: Empiricism and Economic Botany in the Early Spanish Empire," *Journal of World History* 17 (2006): 399–427; Barrera-Osorio, *Experiencing Nature*; Daniela Bleichmar, "Atlantic Competitions: Botany in the Eighteenth-Century Spanish Empire," in Delbourgo and Dew, eds., *Science and Empire*, 225–252.

[27] Earle, *The Body of the Conquistador*.

At the center of both of these patterns was the Company of Jesus. Jesuits did not inaugurate metropolitan ambivalence. After all, they did not arrive to Portuguese America until 1549 and their letters from the 1550s are the earliest, (albeit limited) inventories of the flora and fauna of Brazil. Nor did Jesuits deny the pervasiveness of disease in the colony. From their arrival onward, missionaries stationed in coastal villages and outlying towns tended to the ill and dying, and their urban colleges housed the apothecary shops that supplied medicines to the residents of colonial cities like Salvador and Olinda[28]. But more than any other single colonial organization, due to the volume of material its members produced and the ease with which that material found its way into print,[29] the Company reinforced and ultimately perpetuated particular attitudes toward nature and disease in Brazil. The first generation of Jesuits in Portuguese America encouraged both a learned ignorance of Brazilian nature, as well as a tendency among colonial contemporaries to dismiss the bodily manifestations of epidemic disease.

A great deal of scholarship on the intellectual endeavors of the Company of Jesus portrays them as champions of the disciplined, empirical study of natural phenomena – and for good reason: over the more than two hundred years in which they operated in Portuguese America, Jesuit missions along the Brazilian coast and well into the Amazonian interior came to constitute a *de facto* bioprospecting network. Through their missions, Jesuits canvassed much of the Brazilian interior for what they believed to be the most useful medicinal plants.[30] By the time of their expulsion from Portugal's empire in 1759, their Brazilian colleges had not

---

[28] Serafim Leite, *Artes e ofícios dos Jesuítas no Brasil (1549–1760)* (Rio de Janeiro: Livros de Portugal, 1953), 295–300; and more recently Timothy D. Walker, "Medicines Trade in the Portuguese Atlantic World: Acquisition and Dissemination of Healing Knowledge from Brazil (c. 1580–1800)," *Social History of Medicine* (2013): 403–431.

[29] Laura de Mello e Souza, *Inferno Atlântico: Demonologia e colonização, séculos XVI-XVIII* (São Paulo: Companhia das Letras, 1993), particularly chapter 3, makes the case for the Portuguese Atlantic. Clossey, *Salvation and Globalization*, especially ch. 9, surveys the wider pattern.

[30] Whereas Harris, for example, in "Long-Distance Corporations"; and "Jesuit Scientific Activity," has helped develop a conceptual framework for such a study, to my knowledge there is no in-depth examination of the Company's bioprospecting networks for Brazil in this period. A useful starting point would be Leite, *Artes e ofícios*, especially 89, n. 1. Walker, "Medicines Trade," provides a brief discussion; and Russell-Wood, *Portuguese Empire*, 154–156, surveys Jesuit bioprospecting efforts and attempts at acclimatization. For the nearby Platine region of Spanish America in roughly the same period, see Eliane Cristina Deckmann Fleck, *Entre a caridade e a ciência: a prática missionária e científica da Companhia de Jesus (XVII e XVIII)* (São Leopoldo: Editora Unisinos, 2014).

only carried a lucrative trade in medicinal simples but Jesuits had used their unparalleled networks, extensive contact with native peoples, and unrivalled access to Brazilian flora to create a therapeutic panacea. Brazilian theriac (*triaga Brasilica*) was so prized that a when a copy of the recipe was rummaged from their hastily abandoned college in Bahia sometime around the beginning of June 1760, one of the sequestration judges (*desembargadores do sequestro*) guessed it could be auctioned off for a small fortune.[31]

Histories of colonial Brazil that examine the epidemiological catastrophe that unfolded in Jesuit missions have produced divergent portraits of the Company's clinical labor. These have stressed either the Jesuits' tireless and devoted medical work, intended to ease the suffering of would-be Amerindian converts,[32] or they have argued that Jesuit policies were singularly self-serving, and that Company members crowded natives together into missionary encampments even as they knew it would lead to medical catastrophe.[33] Elements of both seem true enough: based on their letters and contemporary accounts, Jesuits often did work tirelessly to mitigate the impact of disease, and their tactics were calculated and self-serving. But the interpretation of cross-cultural medical interactions in the face of epidemic disease defies both historical apologetics and postcolonial indictments. And the story of an emergent missionary empiricism is far more complex.

For the first generation of Jesuit missionaries and for the indigenous communities who were the targets of their evangelical efforts, the experience of epidemic disease could be culturally fraught and emotionally and spiritually disorienting. In the inimitable phrasing of Serge Gruzinski, among participants on all sides of the colonial encounter (for Portuguese settlers and Jesuit missionaries, for Tupí-speaking peoples, and for the growing number of colonial inhabitants whose descent such neat distinctions failed to accommodate), "the initial decades were a time of rapid choices and instant decisions – individual and collective, conscious and unconscious – on countless issues."[34] Interests, perspectives, and

---

[31] Leite, *Artes e ofícios*, 88.

[32] Serafim Leite, "Serviços de Saúde" in his *Artes e ofícios*; and Daniela Buono Calainho, "Jesuítas e medicina no Brasil colonial," *Tempo* 10, no. 19 (2005): 1–9.

[33] John Hemming, *Red Gold: The Conquest of the Brazilian Indians* (Cambridge, MA: Harvard University Press, 1978), especially 144–145. But see Metcalf, *Go-Betweens*, ch. 5; and for contemporary Jesuit activities in the neighboring parts of Spanish America see Fleck, *Entre a caridade e a ciência*.

[34] Gruzinski, *Mestizo Mind*, 51.

approaches could change suddenly and dramatically as part of the vertiginous processes of encounter and colonization.

Jesuit accounts of disease reveal disparate interpretations, dissonant views, dissenting opinions, and the emergence of doubts even within the Company over the cause and ultimate meaning of epidemic disease. In larger scale studies of the Company concerned with longer time lines, it is precisely the destabilizing impact of disease in these first years that has been lost. The precise chronologies of disease and interaction are crucial. They highlight the emergence of multiple and at times competing understandings of health, medicine, and disease among members of the Company. If, as so many modern historians suggest, the Jesuits became advocates of the careful, disciplined study of natural phenomena, I argue that for the mid-sixteenth century such a view is anachronistic. Members of the Company of Jesus came to Brazil at a time when the order itself was still quite new, its internal organization unsettled, and its position in Portugal's empire and beyond still uncertain. I argue that the first Jesuit accounts of both nature and disease in Brazil grew out of debates within the Company over the allocation of personnel and expertise. How epidemic disease was produced – how the terms in which it became an object of colonial management and a subject cross-cultural competition were established – and how that, in turn, helped pattern the study of nature more broadly are the subjects of this chapter. This story requires traipsing along the South American coast with the first Jesuit missionaries there, following a stream of letters that circulated not only across the Atlantic but between their earliest coastal encampments among the Tupí, Carijó, Ibiapirara, and others. It means shuttling back and forth between the colonial Brazilian capital of Salvador, the center of Catholicism in Rome, and the Portuguese imperial capital of Lisbon.

DISEASE AND DISSENT

Diogo Jácome came to the captaincy of Espírito Santo early in 1564 as one of four Jesuits charged with proselytizing the Tupínikin in the hinterland of the small Portuguese settlement of Espírito Santo. His was a short and troubled stay. The epidemic that would lead to his death broke out in the missions there only months after Jácome arrived. Its epicenter was the *aldeia* (mission village) of Nossa Senhora da Conçeição, the mission under Jácome's supervision. By September of that year, a community that according to one account was "large and full of people" – the author put the number at over four hundred – had been reduced "by the force of illness" to a contingent of scattered villagers whose number was evidently too small to record. The disease had spread quickly. According to one of Jácome's colleagues it "filled every house with the ill and the dying." "Homes," this missionary recalled, "became hospitals." Jácome and another Jesuit, Pero Gonçalves, tended to the sick and tried to confess and baptize the dying. But the pace of death – three and four a day – overwhelmed their efforts. The two spent much of their time digging graves and burying the dead.[35]

Toward the end of September, when the epidemic finally came to end, Nossa Senhora da Conceição was left with little more than the fetid odor of human decay to remind villagers of what had happened. And it was for both of those reasons – the smell and the memory – that Jácome and Gonçalves relocated the entire aldeia. In the process, the two Jesuits themselves began to sicken. Gonçalves died first, in early November. Days later, Jácome developed the fever that would end his life the following April, barely a year after he had come.[36]

For Pedro da Costa, the Jesuit who recorded all of these events, the story of Nossa Senhora da Conceição was a difficult one to tell. Precise details, Costa had to admit, escaped his recollection. Part of the issue was the loss of his first letter detailing the events. It had sunk with the ship that was to carry it across the Atlantic – a reminder of the fragility of these imperial networks. But with palpable sorrow Costa wrote that the real trouble was that the whole episode was simply hard to make sense of – or, as Costa himself put it, it was that "the acts of God" seemed utterly "incomprehensible."[37] By 1564, scarcely a decade and a half after they had come, that was precisely the issue facing Jesuits throughout Brazil. Placing disease within the broader project of conversion – identifying its causes, explaining its occurrence, and properly caring for the afflicted – had proven far more challenging than the first generation of Jesuits in Brazil had believed it would.

There was no mistaking the presence of epidemic disease and, in the disruptions it produced, a lot was at stake. Not only were the Jesuits central to the Crown strategy for easing tensions between Brazil's native peoples and Portuguese colonists (enslavement, although illegal, was rampant and the Crown would not enact a formal policy for decades) but Portuguese claims to sovereignty in the Americas were, like those of

---

[35] *MB* vol. 4, 270.   [36] *MB* vol. 4, 267–272.   [37] *MB* vol. 4, 265–266.

the Spanish, rooted in papal authority and predicated on the evangelization and conversion of native peoples to Catholicism.[38] The Company of
Jesus was charged with carrying that out. Virtually everywhere Jesuits
went, disease seemed to follow. It became an inevitable aspect of life for
native peoples all along the coast. The missionaries soon realized that the
reach, frequency, and severity of disease meant that credible explanations
for it and effective attempts to manage it were inseparable from the work
of conversion itself.

The Jesuits' peregrinations took them far beyond the colonial capital.
Five years after having disembarked in Salvador, the Jesuits had established three principal fields of missionary activity: one in Bahia (the
captaincy that was home to the colonial capital), another in Espírito
Santo to the south (where the tragedy of Nossa Senhora da Conçeição
would unfold), and a third still further south in São Vicente (where
Martim Afonso de Sousa, the would-be Governor of the Estado da Índia,
had earlier established some of Brazil's earliest sugar plantations).[39]

As disease moved unrelentingly through Portuguese America, the
Jesuits felt compelled to account for it and to demonstrate that they could
manage it. The results were dubious at best – even by the Jesuits' own
standards. Ultimately, epidemic diseases would not simply defy the ready-
made explanations that the Jesuits brought with them to Brazil. They
would also foster internal division, lead to competing accounts of their
causes, and sustain competing claims not only about how diseases should
be treated but about who should be called upon to treat them.

The earliest Jesuit letters were marked by a deeply held certainty about
the causes and ultimate purpose of these diseases, and by the Jesuits'
abiding confidence in their own ability to manage them. Diseases were,
to use Costa's words, "acts of God." Jesuits saw them as powerful forces
of good meant to facilitate the Jesuits' own missionary efforts. Diseases
abetted that work in various ways. They were divine punishment – as the
first Jesuit Superior in Brazil, Manuel da Nóbrega, frequently put it, "the
castigation of God"[40] – for the recalcitrant behavior of those who refused
conversion, for those who submitted to it only to abandon the spiritual
community of the missions later, and for those who remained in the

---

[38] A concise survey of these issues can be found in Johnson, "Settlement," 19–29.
[39] These were early foci but an overview of Jesuit mission development can be found in
Dauril Alden, *The Making of an Enterprise: The Society of Jesus in Portugal, Its Empire,
and Beyond, 1540–1750* (Stanford, CA: Stanford University Press, 1995). On Sousa and
his relationship with the Portuguese physician Garcia de Orta see especially ch. 3.
[40] *MB* vol. I, 310, 319.

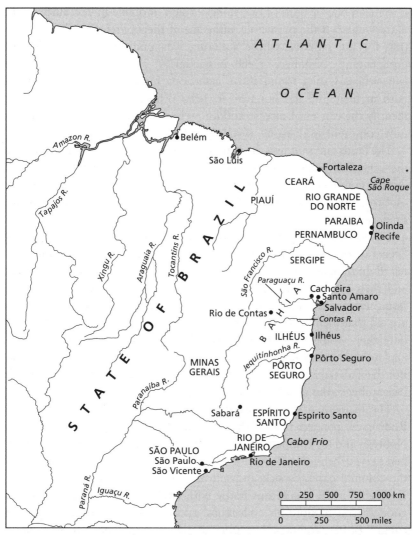

MAP 6.1 Portuguese Settlements and Principal Ports of Trade in Brazil. Adapted by David Cox from Bethencourt and Curto, eds., *Portuguese Oceanic Expansion*, xviii.

missions but who secretly persisted with diabolical rituals (cannibalism of course was a favored accusation[41]). For the faithful, death was understood as a reprieve. When children died – converted or not – Jesuits took

---

[41] *MB* vol. 1, 303–304, 316–319; *MB* vol. 2, 113; *MB* vol. 3, 386–387; and *MB* vol. 4, 77–78 and 120–181.

it to mean one or both of two things: a sign of divine mercy, since young natives escaped the pernicious influence of their parents, and as castigation for the parents, whose suffering was punishment for their own unrepentant resistance to the missionaries' efforts.[42] With time and experience, Jesuits found those assertions increasingly unsatisfying. If faith in their god did not waiver, Jesuits' faith in their own ability to identify the causes of disease and know how to respond – their ability to fully comprehend disease – certainly did.

The lands surrounding the new colonial capital of Salvador constituted the very first Jesuit mission field in Brazil. In 1551 that field grew to include contacts among a number of Tobajara settlements in the interior of Pernambuco, the captaincy to Bahia's north. Manuel da Nóbrega, Francisco Pires, and a handful of Jesuit neophytes were there for barely a year. It was enough time to erect a series of crosses and to note that a "general cough" had spread among their Tobajara hosts. One young girl fell ill and lingered near death. The villagers argued that Nóbrega, Pires, and their companions were to blame. On the contrary, countered the Jesuit Pires, he and his companions "brought only life."[43] Nóbrega argued that members of the Tobajara community could escape disease if only they would submit to the rituals of Catholic conversion. If that explanation satisfied the Tobajara, neither Nóbrega nor Pires said so. But the Tobajara refused the missionaries' advances. Rather than stay in Pernambuco, the Jesuits returned south.[44]

The incident made its way into a letter that another Jesuit, Vicente Rodrigues, penned from Bahia in May of the following year. When Nóbrega and his companions first left for Pernambuco, Vicente Rodrigues had stayed behind in Salvador to run a small hospital and to care for the colonial capital's sick and infirm. While his colleagues were away, Rodrigues' own calamitous battle with epidemic disease had given him good reason to note his colleagues' account of the ill-defined "general cough" of Pernambuco. As Nóbrega and the others built crosses among the Tobajara to the north, a "terrible" and "deadly" sickness engulfed the

---

[42] In addition to passages cited later, see *MB* vol. 1, 19; *MB* vol. 3, 52–53, 360–362, 452–455; and *MB* vol. 4, 8–10.

[43] *MB* vol. 1, 379.

[44] *MB* vol. 1, 320–321. The account is given by Vicente Rodrigues at the behest of the governor, Tomé de Sousa. As with his earlier visit to Porto Seguro in 1550, Nóbrega did not establish lasting missions here at this time.

whole of Salvador.[45] It overwhelmed Rodrigues's hospital before spreading beyond the city, where Rodrigues worried that it threatened to overtake the villages dotting the Bahian hinterland. These *aldeias* of Tupinambá – some had converted some had not – were in the throes of an epidemiological assault. Rodrigues knew precisely how to interpret the deaths. A large contingent of Tupí villagers had been poised to enter the Catholic fold until, at the last minute, they recanted. The epidemic and particularly the death of countless young children was, as Rodrigues had it, only one of the "many tests put to them by our god."[46] Only time would tell whether they could continue to refuse the new religion under such an assault.

Yet the Tupí and other native communities were not the only ones being tested. Jesuits themselves, Rodrigues included, also found the epidemics ever harder to bear. Especially troubling were the deaths of native children. It seemed "such a strange thing," Rodrigues reflected, "particularly among boys and girls so small, [for they] seem to have done nothing wrong at all."[47] That note of distress was not shared by all of Rodrigues's colleagues. Back from Pernambuco, Francisco Pires also recorded the events of 1552. He was less circumspect. The children, he wrote, had been "baptized in innocence and had died in innocence." Their parents and elders deserved no such mercy: disease and death were brought about by their own pervasive lapse in devotion and was intended to instill fear and obedience in the newly converted who might survive.[48] But Pires, too, was moved by what he had seen, and even he conceded some surprise to fine that so many Tupí continued to seek out the Jesuits' care and leadership even as, in Pires' words, so "many of them do die and many others are always sick."[49]

Doubt about the reasons why disease struck and about whether the Jesuits themselves could really know such things – even as they assured would-be proselytes that they in fact did know those things – crept slowly and unevenly among the missionaries. With time, as their missions grew more numerous, their doubts grew more pronounced. By 1553 Nóbrega and two other priests, José de Anchieta and Brás Lourenço, had sailed for the more southerly captaincies. They stopped first in Espírito Santo, where Lourenço joined the Jesuit Afonso Brás in a mission among the Tupinkin. It was Lourenço who established the mission at Nossa Senhora

---

[45] *MB* vol. 1, 318.
[46] *MB* vol. 1, 317, from among the letters discussing the event on 302–321.
[47] *MB* vol. 1, 303. [48] *MB* vol. 1, 391–400. [49] *MB* vol. 1, 395.

da Conçeição (among several others) that Jácome and Costa would find a decade later in the spring of 1564. Nóbrega and Anchieta continued on to São Vicente, where a mission among the Carijó in the Priatininga region was already underway.[50] That mission seemed especially promising to Anchieta. Much like the Company's work among the Ibiapirara who, despite their tendency to collect and display the severed heads of newly-vanquished foes, the Carijó seemed receptive to Jesuit overtures.[51] Yet in just over a year, many of the converted Carijó had died. The entire aldeia of Maniçoba had been emptied.[52] A few of the deaths, such as that of an elder who, according to Anchieta, had "abandoned the faith,"[53] seemed to fit comfortably into the salvific explanatory framework the Jesuits brought with them from the north.

But that was not what explained most of the deaths that year. It was in "seeing that they had embraced the truth and practice of the faith," wrote Anchieta, that "the Lord took this life from them in exchange for an eternal one."[54] But this was a reversal of his earlier logic. The ambiguity was subtle but palpable, as he added that such an explanation was, at least, "how it seemed to us."[55] Disease, it now appeared, fell most forcefully upon those who joined – and remained faithfully within – the missions. The closer new converts got to God, the more likely they were to die. So strong was the connection, so inevitable seemed death once disease began to strike the mission faithful, that survival itself became the noteworthy outcome. In the middle of the epidemic, a young girl nearing death approached Anchieta seeking salvation. Anchieta complied and after the baptism even Anchieta was struck by the effect: "unexpectedly," he wrote, the young girl recovered.[56]

When Pero Correia wrote of the same São Vicente epidemic of 1554, he was more circumspect. Death, he recalled, "came suddenly." That was true for some of the most recalcitrant natives but still more so for the "men and women who were very good [Christians]." God, it seemed, was castigating everyone.[57] Precisely why these illnesses afflicted the missions so completely, what the Jesuits could to do mitigate their damage, and how the missionaries were to continue the work of conversion were all thrown into question. As uncertainty deepened, care for the sick gave way

---

[50] According to *MB* vol. 1, 355, Afonso Brás had been in Espírito Santo since 1551 and Leonardo Nunes and Diogo Jácome were in São Vicente by the middle of 1552.

[51] *MB* vol. 2, 117–118.   [52] *MB* vol. 2, 107–108, 158–160, and 209.

[53] *MB* vol. 2, 108.   [54] *MB* vol. 2, 107.   [55] *MB* vol. 2, 107.   [56] *MB* vol. 2, 110.

[57] *MB* vol. 3, 379–381.

to rituals of contrition. Correia and other missionaries gathered in the village center where they mounted a procession. Only after nine full circuits through the village did "our Father" finally "show us mercy," and bring the epidemic to an end.[58]

Relations in the Piratininga mission continued to deteriorate. The combination of disease and death led to the dissolution of trust between the Jesuits and the same Carijó who had once seemed such promising proselytes. The Carijó hatched a plot to exterminate the missionaries. But disease soon spread among the conspirators and, when the time came to act, they had neither the numbers nor the strength to carry through with their plan.[59]

The idea that punitive death might somehow encourage conversion or enforce discipline among new adherents was now difficult to sustain. The lesson for Anchieta was clear. It was not their god but the Jesuits themselves who would need to compel conversion and enforce mission discipline.[60] In the matter of conversion, wrote Anchieta pointedly, "there is nothing better than a sword or [even] a rod of iron."[61]

Back in Espírito Santo, Bras Lourenço read the news of the events in Piratininga in Correia's letter dated 18 July 1554.[62] It was perhaps for that reason that Lourenço had already begun to enforce strict discipline in the Espírito Santo missions – a feature that was particularly striking to the Jesuit Diogo Jacóme and others when they came four years later.[63] Once again, disease had accompanied them. Fevers and dysentery first struck the Espírito Santo missions in 1558, and it did so with all of the increasingly familiar indecipherability of divine intent. The illness took no more than six days to claim a life. It showed as little mercy to the women and children of the Tupí missions as for the men. And it had as little patience for the converted as for those who were not. With the help of an interpreter, Lourenço baptized as many victims as possible *in extremis*, though many others died unconverted from what one young Jesuit – António de Sá – described as their own "stubbornness."[64]

Like desperate rituals of contrition, baptism *in extremis* was by now a standard measure in the missions. In moments of epidemic calamity, Jesuit missionaries directed their efforts to that stopgap rite of initiation. Children taken ill were regularly converted that way. Lourenço and Sá resorted to the measure in Espírito Santo in 1558. And there as elsewhere, what was for the Jesuits a gesture of mercy was for many grieving

---

[58] *MB* vol. 2, 70–71.   [59] *MB* vol. 2, 108.   [60] *MB* vol. 2, 118.   [61] *MB* vol. 3, 554.
[62] *MB* vol. 2, 70–71.   [63] *MB* vol. 4, 265–275.   [64] *MB* vol. 3, 20.

Amerindian mothers an unwelcome advance. In many cases native women hid their children to keep them from the hands of men like Nóbrega, Anchieta, Correia, Lourenço, and Sá. Women taken ill feared that, if they were to die, the Jesuits would steal their children and raise them as their own.[65]

This end-of-life battle between mothers and missionaries over the lives of their children was familiar to both Bras Lourenço and António de Sá. Lourenço's experience with it was plain enough: he had been in Bahia with Vicente Rodrigues during the epidemic of 1552. Sá was there too, though he had arrived well after it had begun. When the disease in Bahia had first broken out, he had been in Pernambuco with Nóbrega and Pires. At the time of the Bahia epidemic, Sá was but a young orphan – one of a number of Portuguese boys sent to Salvador from Lisbon under the watchful eyes of Francisco Pires in 1550.[66] With Pires, he bore witness to the "general cough" that nearly led to the demise of the Tobajara girl in Pernambuco. And it was by the sides of Nóbrega and Pires that Sá made it back to Bahia where he helped with the sick and dying in the missions surrounding Salvador. Now in 1558, a veteran of missions and medical emergencies, he was in Espírito Santo. How his own peculiar history and the accumulation of eight years of experience with increasingly inexplicable contagion might have shaped Sá's outlook is impossible to know. But the 1558 epidemic left its mark on Sá, traces of which remain in the form of a letter he penned in February of the following year.

In the throes of death, a Tupí woman (Sá did not give her name) gave birth to a healthy baby boy. In agony but still clinging to her newborn son, the woman refused to let either Sá or Lourenço lay a hand on him. And in her final, fleeting moment of life the unnamed woman turned to her son and explained, "your mother is about to die and you will be here alone, with no one to nurse you and no one to care for you; you must come with me."[67] Then she died. But her arms were still locked around

---

[65] *MB* vol. 1, 387; and *MB* vol. 2, 134.

[66] Here and elsewhere the place of children in imperial expansion, conquest, and colonization looms large but remains largely unexplored – especially where the Jesuits are concerned. An exception is Metcalf, *Go-Betweens*, 93–96, 99–100. For other cases in Portugal's empire and beyond see Coates, *Convicts and Orphans*; and Ondina E. González and Bianca Premo, eds., *Raising an Empire: Children in Early Modern Iberia and Colonial Latin America* (Albuquerque, NM: University of New Mexico Press, 2007).

[67] *MB* vol. 3, 19. Quotation is somewhat unusual in the Company's letters from Brazil but they are more common in Sa's letters. See also, for example, MB III, 38.

her son. And just like that the two were buried, "the child alive and his mother dead, together in one coffin, buried and un-baptized."[68] Sá penned these lines in utter incomprehension of her calculus: "What animal is this?" he pleaded. That he took the unusual license of recalling and quoting the mother's very words made this only the most vivid moment in a letter detailing an entire epidemic. But it was not the only scene he recorded. Indeed, Sá's letter consisted almost entirely of episodic depictions of death and desperation.

Writing similar letters, most of the early Jesuits in Brazil tried to make sense of what they had seen – to interpret events from within a more or less shared religious idiom, much as they had done until now with disease.[69] The several pages that Sá managed to write were marked by his near total refusal to do just that: interpret. Almost nowhere did he insist on the purposefulness, however unintelligible, of his god. It seems that, for an instant – in that letter – Sá abandoned the search for meaning. And yet, bereft of explanation, the young Jesuit could not stop himself from writing down what he had seen, even if he failed to understand it. The impulse was so strong that he finally excused himself for his compulsive literary reenactment: "because Our Father must draw good [from evil], I have to tell you [these things] so that all He does shall be praised."[70]

Sá left the praising to others. Long on detail but short on interpretation, the entire missive resembled less a letter than a list. Where explanation failed, bare enumeration would have to suffice. As in faraway Malacca or on the Konkan coast of India (see Chapter 3), the list was once again a way to navigate the ill-defined boundary between what was known and what was not. That the salvation of humanity[71] should ever hinge on such unthinkable acts as the burial of a living, "innocent" newborn child at the whim of its "pertinacious" and ultimately dead mother was just one of the most troubling and yet quotidian experiences of life on the missions. Less than a decade after the Company first came to the South American colonies, the cause of disease and its treatment had

---

[68] *MB* vol. 3, 20.

[69] This was a characteristic epistolary habit of many Jesuits. See the discussions in Thomas M. Cohen, *Fire of Tongues: António Vieira and the Missioary Church in Brazil and Portugal* (Stanford, CA: Stanford University Press, 1998); and John W. O'Malley, *The First Jesuits* (Cambridge, MA: Harvard University Press, 1993), 91–133.

[70] *MB* vol. 3, 21.

[71] This is not hyperbole. It was the project as the Jesuits and some Portuguese rulers conceived of it. See Cohen, *Fire of Tongues*.

become (to cite Costa again) utterly "indecipherable."[72] Some months later, after the same plague had swept through the Bahian missions, António Blazquez asked his readers in Lisbon to "imagine how one's heart was torn with pity."[73]

COMPANY SCIENCE

Up and down the coast, Jesuits offered increasingly tentative and contradictory explanations for the ills that befell their mission quarry. Even so, one of the things they could generally agree on was that the bodily ills they observed were somehow the consequence of moral lapses and spiritual failings. Inner corruption led to outer deterioration and even death. Disease was not a medical problem but a spiritual one. Tending to the soul would heal the body. If disease was a form of divine wrath brought by moral failing, then preventing it demanded redoubling the missionary effort among the Tupí and Guaraní peoples of the colony. Stricter, more thorough Catholic instruction would forestall deviant behavior. And that, in turn, would keep so many bodily afflictions at bay.

Their approach surely reflected ongoing theological shifts that had come to emphasize the role of the devil in quotidian earthly affairs, and which led Jesuits and many other missionaries to view Amerindian religion in general as a massive diabolical hoax.[74] The approach was also consonant with the longstanding proscription of medical study and private clinical practice for priests.[75] Yet the story is more complex. The Jesuits' initial approach to epidemic disease was not merely a consequence of their religious vocation or theological disposition, reinforced by clerical regulation. These would not have prevented the recruitment of physicians, apothecaries, or surgeons who might serve as lay brothers or (in the case of physicians) provide ancillary services for the

---

[72] The letters of Sá in 1558 and Costa in 1564 were not the only ones to evince this uncertainty. But they were two of the most pointed. See also the letter of Anchieta in *MB* vol. 3, 367–382.

[73] Afrânio Peixoto and Alfredo do Vale Cabral, eds., *Cartas avulsas de Jesuítas (1550–1568)* (Rio de Janeiro: Officina Industrial Graphica, 1931), 312–313, as quoted in Hemming, *Red Gold*, 141.

[74] Souza, *Inferno Atlântico*; Fernando Cervantes, *The Devil in the New World: The Impact of Diabolism in New Spain* (New Haven, CT: Yale University Press, 1997).

[75] By the seventeenth century, these restrictions circulated in pamphlet form in Lisbon. See BL Add. Mss. 15194, ff. 41–42v. Michael R. McVaugh, *Medicine before the Plague: Practitioners and Their Patients in the Crown of Aragon, 1285–1345* (New York: Cambridge University Press), 72–78, provides useful Iberian background.

Company – as in fact they did, and almost from the outset of Jesuit evangelization in Brazil.[76]

Defining disease as a moral problem was instead a carefully considered way of reconciling competing demands on scarce Company resources – the response to a pervasive problem by leaders of a small organization whose members held competing points of view and who had (at times) divergent priorities. Although an *ad hoc* strategy rather than a premeditated plan of action, Nóbrega would nevertheless articulate a compelling defense of the approach in the 1550s and then vigorously champion it long after he was replaced in 1560 as the Company's Superior in Brazil.

The whole plan hinged on language. As Nóbrega put it, "the principal" and "most necessary" kind of "knowledge" required for the success of the Brazilian missions was "the language of the land."[77] Nóbrega thought that the Company should develop this linguistic expertise over the long run by recruiting children on both sides of the Atlantic. Inspiration for the idea may have come in 1550, when the Company first received in Bahia a contingent of orphans dispatched from the kingdom (the same contingent that included the impressionable young António de Sá).[78] Children sent regularly from Portugal would complement the growing number of native children that Nóbrega believed the Company could recruit in the colonies. By 1550, he and his Jesuit colleagues had found they were given ready access to Tupí children, who often came to live among the missionaries. Nóbrega thought the emerging arrangement – the receipt and schooling of young boys from the colony and orphans from Portugal – could be the foundation of a kind of student exchange system. Under Company supervision, young Portuguese boys could learn native languages and the best young native converts – once they were fluent in Portuguese and possessed of the rudiments of Latin, could travel to Portugal to learn letters and "virtue" and become "hombres de confiança" (trustworthy men). Simultaneously and on both sides of the Atlantic, this exchange would produce men who knew the language of Brazil, who could be trusted, and whose account of Catholic doctrine and its requirements were in line with those of the Company and its supporters. Indeed, Nóbrega could already

---

[76] Leite *Artes e ofícios*, 96–100; Bella Herson, *Cristãos-novos e seus desvendentes na medicina brasileira, 1500–1850* (São Paulo: Edusp, 1996), 62–68. Alden, *Enterprise*, also discusses lay brothers who served in a medical capacity without ordination.

[77] *MB* vol. 3, 363.

[78] *MB* vol. 1, 173. According to *MB* vol. 3, 315, n. 13. The first orphans left Lisbon for Brazil on January 7, 1550.

point to the promising example of one "Cipriano do Brasil."[79] Until the arrangement bore fruit, newly arrived Jesuit missionaries would continue to struggle to acquire indigenous languages as best they could.[80]

As an element in the cultural work of conversion, the Jesuits' handling of indigenous languages is well studied.[81] What is important here is the therapeutic orientation that their focus on language signaled. For it meant problems of health which might have demanded medical acumen became instead problems of personnel and linguistic expertise. My point is not that Jesuits ignored the bodily suffering of their proselytes (they generally did not[82]), much less that they thought that spiritual and bodily health could somehow be neatly disentangled from one another (I have no evidence that they did). But over the course of their first decade or so in Portuguese America, members of the Company of Jesus chose a therapeutic emphasis that differed markedly from their bioprospecting work of later years. The question, then, is not simply about therapeutic priorities (the body or the soul) but why it made sense to define disease as a moral problem requiring linguistic expertise rather than as a medical problem requiring curative expertise. What did Nóbrega understand about the Company that motivated such an approach?

When the Company of Jesus arrived in Brazil in 1549, it was not yet a decade old. It had undertaken an overseas mission even as its leaders spread between Lisbon, Rome, and beyond were still trying to answer basic but substantive questions about the Company's internal operations. Not least among them were its educational priorities and uncertainty over the function of its colleges. Before 1551, the Company that would quickly gain a reputation for education across early modern Europe and beyond had no schools of its own at all. Its residential colleges were mere boarding houses situated near universities so that Jesuit neophytes could live together during their course of university studies. In these years, Loyola and other leaders of the Company in Rome debated whether the order should focus exclusively on apostolic activities, take on the formal education of its members, or provide an education to promising young students more generally. And if either of the latter, it was not at all clear

---

[79] See *MB* vol. 3, 363, n. 25.   [80] *MB* vol. 3, 363–364.

[81] See, for example, Adone Agnolin, *Jesuítas e Selvagens: A Negociação da Fé no Encontro Catequético-Ritual Americano-Tupi (séc. XVI–XVII)* (São Paulo: Humanitas Editorial, 2007).

[82] Calainho, "Jesuítas e medicina."

what a Jesuit education should include.[83] The opportunities afforded by empire helped answer those questions.

The growth of Portugal's seaborne empire created possibilities that the Company – new, small, underfinanced, and marginal especially to affairs at the papal court – responded to for the sake of its own self-preservation. The necessary pursuit of patronage and influence, recruits and reputation from Lisbon to the Roman curia helped shape the institutional development of the Company and define its intellectual priorities. Loyola and other members of the leadership in Rome defended their ultimate decision to establish schools as an act of charity and an extension of their spiritual mission. They also saw it as a way to generate recognition of, and support for, the new Company, as well as a way to recruit the most promising young men into its ranks.[84] By the middle decades of the sixteenth century, perhaps nowhere had the Company's fortunes changed so soon, so rapidly, and with so much influence as a consequence of its educational pursuits as in metropolitan Portugal. There, over the course of the 1550s, as Nóbrega was plotting a missionary strategy in Brazil, the Company of Jesus – a missionary order vowed to poverty and apostolic duty – quickly became the keeper of higher education.

Loyola's strategy worked a little too well. Jesuit colleges multiplied. But the decision brought problems of its own. Within a couple of years, Jesuits like the Italian Giuseppe Cortesono began to worry that the Company was "being ruined by taking on so many schools." In the view of Cortesono and others, Jesuits now spent too much time teaching and too little time on their own education. Staffing schools not only exacerbated the already endemic shortage of personnel but also led the Company to take candidates it might not otherwise admit.[85] That particular problem was the substance of a volley of letters exchanged between the Jesuit Provincial in Portugal and Company leaders in Rome in the 1550s and 1560s. Many recruits in Portugal, Miguel da Torres advised, were

[83] O'Malley, *The First Jesuits*, 7–8. Not only the educational curriculum but even the final contents of the *Constitutions* – the document that defined what Ignatius Loyola described as the Jesuit "way of proceeding" – had yet to be worked out. A first version was promulgated in 1552 and it was approved for print with minor changes in 1558–1559 in the course of the meeting of the First General Congregation of the Company, convened to elect Loyola's successor (he died in 1556).

[84] O'Malley, *The First Jesuits*, 202–215. Polanco, as secretary, composed and circulated a letter explaining the official position to the Provincial of Portugal in 1551, encouraging him to open schools there.

[85] O'Malley, *The First Jesuits*, 200–232; the quoted passage appears on 227.

poor teachers and even poorer administrators, and their Latin was frequently found wanting.[86] Even among Jesuit priests, it seemed to Torres,
some men were notably better suited to the Company's work than others.
Thanks in part to its educational endeavors, capable Jesuits were too few
and too many of them had bad Latin.

From the perspective of Nóbrega in Brazil, the demands of apostolic
work in the empire exacerbated these problems. Most members of the
Company bound for work in Portugal's overseas dominions hoped to be
posted to Goa or elsewhere in Portuguese Asia, not to settlements in
Portuguese America. And it was to India or China, rather than to Brazil,
that the most talented Jesuits were sent. Once there, some Jesuits who had
been fortunate enough to find their way to the Asian apostolate succumbed to the temptations of wealth and found their way out of the
Company altogether, disappearing into the lucrative world of maritime
trade. Juan Rojo was a signal example. He had been assigned to Angola,
asked to go to India instead, was granted the request, and then left the
Company a few years after he landed in Goa.[87]

The Brazilian missions faced nearly the opposite problem. It was
harder to attract Jesuits to Portuguese America. The hardships of mission
life, which were materially poor, combined with intermittent outbreaks of
disease made it hard to keep the missionaries who came. The young
Cipione Comitoli, an Italian Jesuit bound for Brazil, barely survived a
fever while sailing along the Gulf of Guinea only to develop a severe case
of gout in Brazil. In Bahia, he made good progress in his Tupí lessons.
But the gout finally convinced him to flee – which he did with a number of
other Jesuits and against explicit instructions from then Jesuit Superior
(Nóbrega's successor) Luís de Grã.[88] That would not be the last time that
acute illness led a Jesuit to abandon the Brazilian apostolate.[89]

These were issues with which Nóbrega was all too aware. He had
entered the novitiate in Portugal during its early, formative years. He
had been privy to the concerns weighing on Company leaders. And he
had faced disappointment when his own hopes for an assignment to Goa

---

[86] As suggested in letters to Loyola in 1553 and again to Laínes in 1564.

[87] *MB* vol. 3, 303, and n. 31.

[88] *MB* vol. 3, 486–488, and 488, n. 41. Comitoli had been assigned to the Asian apostolate
and only disembarked in Brazil because he had grown too ill at sea.

[89] This was only one of many reasons why the would-be missionary António de Gouveia
earned the attention of religious authorities on both sides of the Atlantic in the early
1560s. See ANTT, TSO, IL, 028, 05158.

were dashed – and that in part because Company leaders harbored doubts about Nóbrega's intellectual prowess.[90]

In Brazil, Nóbrega's decision to stress linguistic expertise as the kind of knowledge most critical for Company success there reflected his understanding of the Company's increasing entanglement with Portuguese imperial ambitions. When in 1561 he wrote to the Provincial Torres explaining his policies over the last decade, Nóbrega left no doubt that it was a question about knowledge – about the production and deployment of a particular kind of expertise – that he was deciding. When he wrote of "the language of the land" as being "the principal" and "most necessary" kind of "knowledge," he spoke not of learning in general but of "scientia."[91] For Nóbrega as for every other Jesuit priest, that Latin term meant something rather precise: certain knowledge derived from first principles in proper Aristotelian fashion. It referred especially to the domain of knowledge demarcated by natural philosophy, which was concerned with claims about ultimate causes and the inner-workings of the cosmos. Natural philosophy was propaedeutic for both medicine and law, and (the highest faculty) theology – the learning that every Jesuit had to acquire before ordination.[92]

That was why, when Miguel da Torres read Nóbrega's letter in Lisbon in June of 1561, he could not have missed the implication. Language and rhetoric – the very areas of knowledge that Nóbrega argued were critical for the Brazil missions – were not really *scientia* at all. Nóbrega had purposefully misused of the term. It was intentionally ironic – a tongue-in-cheek reference to students who were judged either unsuited to the priesthood or unlikely to accede to it. He might well have had in mind other men like himself – faithful, determined, but perhaps underestimated.

Regardless, it was a strategic attempt to lower the qualifications for service in Brazil. He hoped to convince the Company's leadership that the lackluster neophytes crowding into Jesuit colleges should be admitted to the missions in Brazil not simply despite their shortcomings but because of them. As Nóbrega put it, the Brazilian apostolate called for no more than "a little theology and a little Latin."[93] Senior Jesuit colleagues in Brazil

---

[90] Cohen, *Fire of Tongues*, 15–16.   [91] *MB* vol. 3, 363.
[92] For a discussion of these issues, see Rivka Feldhay, "Knowledge and Salvation in Jesuit Culture," *Science in Context* 2 (1987): 195–213; and Peter Dear, "Jesuit Mathematical Science and the Reconstitution of Experience in the Early Seventeenth Century," *Studies in History and Philosophy of Science* 18 (1987): 133–175.
[93] *MB* vol. 4, 368–369.

agreed. António Pires insisted that young Jesuits bound for Brazil need not worry if their studies were left unfinished. In Brazil, he urged his young readers in Lisbon, "your learning" (*vossas letras*), was unnecessary. There were no gripping theological questions to dispute, no doubts about the faith that needed elaborate philosophical treatment. Unlike in Goa – where, as I have shown, the Jesuits saw highly public battles of wit between authoritative representatives of competing faiths as indispensable to the work of spiritual and bodily health – Jesuits in Brazil, Pires explained, would be busy imitating the apostles. According Pires, poverty would define their circumstances and preaching would occupy their time.[94]

Nor was it necessary to be a sterling preacher. So low were expectations for performance in the pulpit that by the late 1550s the sermons of some Jesuits in Brazil had begun to inspire sarcasm. According to one Jesuit, Francisco Pires was so bad that his colleagues wondered whether those who heard him "would want to go to heaven after all."[95]

It was this same competition for missionaries among distant theaters of empire, combined with the simultaneous pursuit of patronage among metropolitan leaders, that patterned Jesuit reports of Brazilian nature and disease. It was in order to meet those demands on Company resources (at once human, intellectual, and linguistic) that Jesuits began to advocate the view that Brazil was healthy and that its nature was of dubious therapeutic value.

Shortly after his arrival in 1549, Nóbrega had written to his superiors about the prospects for Amerindian conversion. On the health of the continent that lay before him, Nóbrega was emphatic: "there are no fevers here," he wrote.[96] It was precisely the kind of appraisal that his Jesuit superiors and João III anticipated – a terse reiteration of the points made in Caminha's letter from the Brazilian coast fifty years earlier. In 1549, Nóbrega's report reflected a combination of Caminha's imagery and the accumulation of rumor and opinion that had begun to circulate across the Atlantic in the intervening half-century.[97] It also drew an important distinction between Portuguese America and the now notoriously debilitating environment of Portuguese Africa. But by 1560, from

---

[94] *MB* vol. 3, 308.   [95] *MB* vol. 3, Nobrega to Sousa July 1559, and n. 79.

[96] Manuel da Nóbrega, *Cartas do Brasil e mais escritos do P. Manuel da Nóbrega*, ed. Serafim Leite (Coimbra: Universidade de Coimbra, 1955), 89.

[97] Laura de Mello e Souza, *The Devil in the Land of the Holy Cross: Witchcraft, Slavery, and Popular Religion in Colonial Brazil*, trans. Diane Grosklaus Whitty (Austin, TX: University of Texas Press), 3–44.

the vantage point of either side of that ocean, Nóbrega's pronouncement must have looked strikingly naïve.

The journey across the Atlantic was the first test of a missionary's constitution. Of life "at sea," Lourenço do Vale reflected, there were simply "those who have it in them and those who don't; and the latter suffer dearly" (*tem quem tem; e quem não padece*).[98] On the ground in Brazil, even when good health prevailed among indigenous converts, sickness often reigned among the Jesuits. In Lisbon, accounts of debilitating illness among the missionaries in Brazil – stories about men like the absconding Comitoli and his several companions – had begun to accumulate almost immediately. Both José de Anchieta and Vicente Rodriguez wrote of lingering afflictions during their first years in Brazil in the early 1550s.[99] Reports of Nóbrega's ill-health were legion. By 1557, after an evaluation in Bahia by a *medico*, one Licenciado Jorge Fernandes, Nóbrega was told he suffered from a cryptic assortment of broken blood vessels – "now in my head, now in my chest," he mused ironically. It was not a broken blood vessel that worried him but an affliction he judged far more serious: "what I most feel is the fever wasting me away little by little."[100]

In Bahia, once the epidemic of dysentery and fever subsided in 1559 (it had spread northward from Espírito Santo), and once daily affairs had begun "proceeding according to the rules again" as Rui Pereira put it, the fate of the missionaries remained uncertain. For "where things corporeal were concerned" (*quanto ao corporal*), the situation remained dire. The Jesuit Rodrigues, in the outlying aldeia of Bom Jesus, was often too weak to leave his seat in the church.[101] The faithful in search of baptism would have to come to him. Similar circumstances obtained elsewhere. João de Mello in Salvador and Brás Lourenço in Espírito Santo both complained of the fevers that plagued them.[102] From Piratininga, in March 1562 Anchieta wrote that the lay brothers were frequently visited with a combination of fevers, chest pain, and diarrhea.[103] And from Bahia, Lourenço do Vale groused that fevers seemed to afflict the missionaries even more than their indigenous charges.[104]

Doubts harbored by Jesuits about the meaning of disease among their charges were matched by doubts about the causes of their own afflictions and about what exactly they should do about them. "Especially in this

---

[98] *MB* vol. 3, 486.   [99] *MB* vol. 1, 352.   [100] *MB* vol. 2, 404, n. 14.
[101] *MB* vol. 3, 296–298, 389.   [102] *MB* vol. 3 281, 284. See also *MB* vol. 2, 225.
[103] *MB* vol. 3, 452.   [104] *MB* vol. 4, 505.

land," Anchieta found, Jesuits were frequently "vexed with diverse infirmities, whether they be of the head or the stomach, whether they be of fevers or other pains."[105] "It seems there is no *medico*," Anchieta concluded, "who knows how the treat [this long list of illnesses]."[106] Beset with enigmatic afflictions, even university-trained physicians were of little use to Jesuit missionaries in Brazil.

So pervasive were diseases of many kinds among the missionaries and so consistently did they figure into their letters that Jesuits in Brazil began to worry they would turn their colleagues away from the colony. If the apparent riches and apostolic prestige of Asia were enough to shrink concern for its evident epidemiological perils, that was not true for Brazil. The image of Portuguese America needed burnishing. It was to this epistolary labor that many a missionary pen was put in the 1550s and 1560s, in letters composed in Brazil for metropolitan audiences.[107] Company members developed a range of discursive tactics to draw their colleagues out to the Brazilian apostolate. Some countered the image of colonial poverty with visions of valuable commodities. In a letter to fellow Jesuits in the Lisbon college of São Roque in 1562, Lorenzo do Vale insisted at some length that "those who come to Brazil should be as happy as those sent to India" precisely because Brazil, too, contained riches of its own. India had "wars and spices" (the stuff of glory and wealth), Vale conceded, but Brazil had "sugar, cotton, brazilwood, amber, and slaves," which was more than sufficient to sustain a prosperous missionary enterprise.[108]

Considerably more ink went to the question of colonial health. After having complained of his own ailments, Rui Pereira asked his fellow Jesuits to ignore reports like his own. They should not do what Pereira himself confessed to having done and "think the land unhealthy." It was "easy [for his companions] to be there, far away, and to imagine the worst things," especially since they were "surrounded by people who have never

---

[105] *MB* vol. 3, 380. Relief from so many afflictions came occasionally from the most unexpected of places. Pereira's doctor told him to sleep in a hammock "in the air, between two trees," rather "like a bunch of grapes." To his surprise, it worked. Pereira said he would "never look at a mattress again." See *MB* vol. 3, 297–298.

[106] *MB* vol. 3, 379–380. Similar comments about the dubious value of learned medicine and the confusion among physicians were common. See for example *MB* vol. 2, 158–159, 404 and n. 14; and *MB* vol. 3, 18, n. 2, 289.

[107] And this amid the growing insistence of Company leaders that missionary letters be composed with edification in mind. See Luke Clossey, *Salvation and Globalization in the Early Jesuit Missions* (New York: Cambridge University Press, 2011), ch. 3.

[108] *MB* vol. 3, 486.

been [to Brazil]" and who therefore share such an [unfortunate] opinion."[109] Vale explained why reports of disease among Company missionaries might have seemed so common. The problem was not that Portugal's South American colonies were unhealthy but that the hardships and poverty of the colonies combined with constant travel, preaching, and language study were so taxing. Ill-health became a testament to the zeal and selflessness of the Company's men. Their poverty and suffering were but imitations of the life of Christ, in whose name they laboured.[110] The climate of Brazil, these Jesuits insisted, was perfectly healthy. Pereira went so far as to compare Brazil to paradise on earth – "if," that is, "there were such a place at all."[111] And what of the ills that they so often complained about? Pires, Anchieta, and Pereira variously insisted that they had carried their afflictions with them from Portugal.[112] Company members touted Portuguese America as the ideal place to convalesce.[113] Ailments that in the kingdom had proven chronic could in Brazil be cured.[114] In all of its salubrious splendour, Brazil was well-suited for priests and brothers with overseas ambitions but without the health to match. Portuguese America became the ideal mission field for Jesuits who were weak in mind or body or both.

Nature was recruited to this vision of Brazil in similarly contradictory ways. Nóbrega had first praised Brazilian nature. But the initial decades of Jesuit activity produced letters that were much more ambiguous – and even disparaging – in their estimation of Brazilian nature. Brazil was not the source of wondrous nature but a site for the production and harvest of well-known and valuable commodities. Hence the list that Vale cited in an effort to assuage his companions' concerns that Brazil had little to offer: sugar, cotton, brazilwood, amber, and slaves. An unremarkable nature – splendid but useless – also made the experience of disease more comprehensible and accounts of it in the face of abundance more convincing. Brazil might be healthy but its drugs were of dubious quality and of uncertain use, which was why members of the Company in Brazil asked their companions in Lisbon to ship medicines to them.[115]

Such an attitude might have been difficult to square with Loyola's early insistence that outbound Jesuits take careful note of the new worlds that unfolded before them. But Loyola's directive had been no less considered and strategic from a metropolitan perspective than was Nóbrega's for the

---

[109] *MB* vol. 3, 296–297. [110] *MB* vol. 3, 486; *MB* vol. 4, 83, 189, 215.
[111] *MB* vol. 3, 296. [112] *MB* vol. 3, 285, 307. [113] *MB* vol. 3, 289, 296–297.
[114] *MB* vol. 2, 158–159. [115] *MB* vol. 1, 356.

Jesuits in Brazil. When Loyola instructed Company men to give careful attention to rare and exotic plants and animals, it was meant for missionaries on their way to Asia. The Company founder had Asian *naturalia* in mind. His interest lay not in medicine but patronage – not in *materia medica* but *mirabilia*. At the Roman curia and elsewhere, the splendor of Asian *naturalia* sent by missionaries in the Estado da Índia would be strategically gifted to patrons actual and potential to serve Company interests.[116] Like so many of their contemporaries, members of the Company trafficked in exotica but in a very particular way. Ambiguous attitudes toward Brazilian flora were so common in metropolitan circles early on (recall the comments of Vespucci and Scaliger) that they made them less valuable in the early modern gift economy. Ambivalence became self-reinforcing.

Nóbrega's vision of the Company's way of proceeding in Brazil did not go uncontested. Quite the opposite: his plan to recruit and teach native children was perhaps the single most internally divisive issue that the Company faced during its first two decades in Portuguese America. It pit Nóbrega against fellow Jesuit Luís de Grã, and sparked an acrimonious transatlantic debate that drew in everyone from the bishop of Lisbon to the Jesuit Provincial in Portugal, and the presiding Father General of the Company, Diego Laínes, in Rome. It ended only in 1560, when Grã unceremoniously replaced Nóbrega as mission Superior in Brazil. Nóbrega was a cantankerous figure and, once Grã suceeded him, it was not only Nóbrega's poor health but his temper that got him a lasting assignment back in São Vicente – about as far away from the colonial capital as it was possible to be.[117]

Nóbrega was nevertheless an astute and ultimately influential observer. He may have been replaced as Superior but his plan for the instruction of native children became policy. His decision to recruit less-distinguished Jesuits for the Brazilian missions had a lasting impact. Surveying the composition of the Company at the end of the sixteenth century, Charlotte de Castelnau-L'Estoile identifies precisely these as the characteristics that by 1598 had come to characterize the Company. And while Castelnau-L'Estoile is concerned with the period beginning in the 1570s and focuses on Company policy under Gouveia, my reading of the earlier

---

[116] *MB* vol. 2, 99–113 and 256, n. 54.

[117] The policy debate and the debate surrounding Nóbrega's leadership more generally were separate issues. They nevertheless grew entwined in internal discussions of Company policy. Much of this can be traced through a volley of letters between the Brazilian captaincies of Bahia and São Vicente to Lisbon and Rome. See *MB* vol. 3, 22–367.

sources indicates that in fact these patterns grew from concerns among the first generation of Jesuits in Brazil.[118] Meanwhile images of Brazil as at once healthy but possessed of a dubious natural world circulated widely. They found their way into successive editions of the *Nuovi Avisi* – collections of letters authored by Jesuits spread across Portugal's empire, which were translated into Italian and periodically printed in Venice, and bound into fine leather volumes. Interspersed among accounts of fickle Indians and "marvelous" conversions were Nóbrega's descriptions of unremarkable plants, Anchieta's accounts of rampant fever among way-ward converts, and Rui Pereira's contradictory descriptions of Brazilian health, missionaries taken ill, and the consequent confusion of physicians (*medicos*) at the Jesuit college in Salvador.[119] According to Laura de Mello e Souza that ambiguity would be among the Jesuits' lasting contri-bution to metropolitan views of Portuguese America.[120] I have argued that it had particular consequences for the study of nature and disease in sixteenth-century Brazil.

Yet in the middle of the sixteenth century, their colonial contemporar-ies continued to harbor profound doubts about Jesuit claims of the cause and treatment of illness. The contradictory claims about disease, together with the consequent uncertainty and confusion they caused within the Company, also seeped beyond it. Relationships between the Jesuits, their indigenous charges, native shamans, and many other colonial inhabitants grew increasingly fraught. Both the widespread experience of epidemic disease and Jesuits' early claims that it derived from forces unseen would prove formative in ways that served to undermine their authority rather than enhance it.

SHAMANISM

Relegating disease to the category of the spiritual and approaching it as a consequence of moral failing helped Nóbrega reconcile competing demands on Company resources on either side of the Atlantic and across Portugal's empire. But in Brazil the emphasis on language, speaking, and preaching as a way to manage the challenge of epidemic disease created

---

[118] Charlotte de Castelnau-L'Estoile, *Les Ouvriers d'une vigne stérile: Les Jésuites et la conversion des Indiens au Brésil 1580–1620* (Paris: Centre Culturel Calouste Gulben-kian, 2000), part 3.

[119] The publication and circulation of these are noted by the editors in, respectively, *MB* vol. 1, 155–156 and 273–275; and *MB* vol. 3, 246–247, 285–286, and 367–368.

[120] Souza, *The Devil in the Land of the Holy Cross.*

tensions and ambiguities of its own. Perambulation and prognostication were the quotidian activities of Tupí *pajés*. Itinerant speechmaking was one of the primary ways in which these powerful shamanic figures commanded the unseen forces that, among other things, caused illness. The more eloquent they were, the greater was their capacity to command those forces. Hence Pires's description of a Tupí shaman in Salvador: he was above all a "man of speech" (*señor de la habla*).[121] In the matter of healing no less than in the matter of faith, Nóbrega once remarked that native shamans were the "greatest opponents we have."[122]

Despite Jesuit assaults – they harangued pajés, threatened them with violence, and said their rituals were little more than "acts against nature" (*estranhas à natureza*)[123] – and in part because of uncontrolled epidemics, shamanic knowledge not only retained authority but drew growing numbers of adherents. Over the late sixteenth century, disease and famine thrust growing numbers of colonial inhabitants into the multiplying *santidade* movements. Variously interpreted as millenarian movements, or as collectivities formed out of an explicit rejection of either missionary demands or the violence and coercion of the plantations, they drew Indians and *mamelucos* – slave and free – along with Portuguese colonists and persons of African descent. Transcripts from the inquiry into what was perhaps the largest and best known of them, the santidade of Jaguaripe, reveal that the shamanic knowledge of the Tupí gave substance and credibility to the claims of the group's leaders – as, for instance, their promise of a "land without evil." [124]

As the proliferation of santidade movements suggest, even as the Jesuits insisted on the superiority of their faith, their evident inability to direct the forces of life and death counteracted the work of conversion and limited Jesuit influence both within their mission field and beyond it.[125] The movement also demonstrated just how promiscuous and open-ended shamanic power might be. In Jaguaripe, the leaders were mestiço.

Through their clever imitation of shamanic ritual, the Jesuits would attempt to convey to their indigenous listeners that they, too, had shamanic power. Perhaps no Jesuit in the sixteenth century was more

---

[121] *MB* vol. 3, 408, n. 20.   [122] *MB* vol. 1, 152.   [123] *MB* vol. 2, 112.

[124] Alida C. Metcalf, "Millenarian Slaves? The Santidade de Jaguaripe and Slave Resistance in the Americas," *American Historical Review* 104 (1999): 1531–1559; and Ronaldo Vainfas, *A heresia dos Indios: Catolicismo e rebeldia no Brasil colonial* (São Paulo: Companhia das Letras, 1995). Metcalf develops the link between famine and instability further in Metcalf, *Go-Betweens*, 127–129.

[125] *MB* vol. 3, 404.

successful at the cultivation of a shamanic persona than José de Anchieta. He would be remembered – even mythologized – for assuming the attributes of the Tupí *pajé*.[126] In eloquent speech of his own, Anchieta communicated across the boundaries of bodily form that structured the overlapping cosmologies of Tupí and Guaraní peoples.[127] He conversed with monkeys when it suited him, commanded serpents in moments of danger, and summoned fish in times of famine.[128] And when he, Nóbrega, and Grã had foundered at sea amid a pitched battle with the French in July of 1557, it was Anchieta who summoned the whale that saved them.[129] The colony's native birds – flocks of ibis, parrots, macaws, and swallows – were often the subject these tales. For the Tupí, these birds had special significance.[130] Ibis chicks in particular were the objects of Tupí dye work. Their multicolored feathers were cultivated, carefully colored, and woven into ornate capes used for shamanic rituals.[131] By the seventeenth century, Anchieta's power over a flock of ibis had become one of the best-known stories about him. It was a short, simple tale: rowing from Bertioga toward Santos, Anchieta and his native oarsmen had begun to grow bored, tired, and suffered greatly beneath a glaring sun. Anchieta simply summoned a flock of ibis to shade his party. Evidently the feat could be seen all along the coast. Decades later, witnesses swore to it – several could still recall the number of oarsmen ("seven or eight" they said).[132] Anchieta's rhetorical skill went well beyond

---

[126] He was finally sainted in the spring of 2014.

[127] Eduardo Viveiros de Castro, "Cosmological Deixis and Amerindian Perspectivism," *Journal of the Royal Anthropological Institute* 4 (1998): 469–488.

[128] Simão de Vasconcelos, *Vida do veneravel Padre Ioseph de Anchieta da Companhia de Iesu, Taumaturgo do Novo Mundo, na Provincia do Brasil* (Lisbon: João da Costa, 1672), 189, 275, 280.

[129] Vasconcelos, *Vida*, 122–124 (although in hindsight the chronicler Vasconcelos wondered if perhaps it were not a more mythical sea serpent instead).

[130] Vasconcelos, *Vida*, 87–88, 137–138, 204, 210–211, 275, 281, 333–334. Adoption of, communication with, and command over birds like the parrot, ibis, and macaw, were characteristic of the Tupí. So too was the use these feathers for the objects and dress required for war (weapons and shields) and ritual (caps and capes). Both of the chroniclers of France Antarctique – Jean de Léry and André Thevet – described these practices in detail. So did Anchieta shortly after his arrival. For a discussion of these issues more broadly see Marcy Norton, "The Chicken or the *legue*: Human-Animal Relationships and the Columbian Exchange," *American Historical Review* 120 (2015): 28–60.

[131] Amy Buono, "Crafts of Color: Tupi Tapirage in Early Colonial Brazil," *The Materiality of Color: The Production, Circulation, and Application of Dyes and Pigments, 1400–1800* (2012), 235–246.

[132] Vasconcelos, *Vida*, 204.

communication with the creatures of Brazil. With ritual pronouncements he healed the sick, foretold deaths, freed captives, resuscitated the dead, and managed a storied conversion of the Maramonís.[133]

As it turned out, Anchieta's work slipped rather too easily back and forth across the colonial confessional divide. It was that facet of his missionary work that made trouble for his hagiographer, Simão de Vasconcelos. Late in the seventeenth century, Vasconellos compiled an account of Anchieta's life, the *Vida do veneravel Padre Ioseph de Anchieta*. That Anchieta summoned creatures, spoke to them, and that they, in turn, obeyed him seemed to demonstrate well enough Anchieta's "dominion over animals."[134] But as with the oft-repeated account of the cloud of ibis, Anchieta's communion with nature was achieved neither in polished Latin nor even in good Portuguese but in the "lingua Brasilica."[135] Anchieta mastered natured in Tupí. While Vasconcelos offered plenty of evidence that his god favored Anchieta, and although he insisted that the Jesuit had been "Adam for this New World paradise,"[136] he also hedged his claims about Anchieta's accomplishments. He assured readers that if in his exposition, he used words like "saint, martyr, prophet, miraculous, and other similar expressions," he meant them only "according to the style common among writers of history"[137] – only, that is, as a reflection of how Anchieta was remembered in the Piratininga missions, on the streets of Santos, shipboard along the Brazilian coast, and in the Jesuits colleges of Bahia and Espírito Santo. But Vasconcelos would not – or could not – vouchsafe the precise spiritual register in which Anchieta had worked.

If Anchieta's turn to shamanic performance was a way of tending to Jesuit failings. It was also further testament to them. The Jesuits could

---

[133] Vasconcelos, *Vida*, 207, 203, 164, 215–216, 317.

[134] Vasconcelos, *Vida*, 137–138, 190.

[135] Vasconcelos, *Vida*, 204; the quote is from 275.   [136] Vasconcelos, *Vida*, 34.

[137] Vasconellos, *Vida*, ***iij. Note that for the front matter of the *Vida* the publisher used this somewhat unusual pagination. Here Vasconcelos has become entangled a wider debate. By the late seventeenth century, the question of what exactly constituted "history" was itself a matter of debate – and the Jesuits themselves were often at the center of it. Questions like whether history should principally be about people or events, about how best to assess the veracity of historical claims, and whether it was appropriate for authors to concern themselves with the causes of events (causes usually fell within the domain of philosophy, rather than history) were all very much open to question. See Anthony Grafton, *Defenders of the Text: The Traditions of Scholarship in an Age of Science, 1450–1800* (Cambridge, MA: Harvard University Press, 1991); and, for colonial Latin America and the Atlantic, Cañizares-Esguerra, *How to Write the History of the New World*.

never have hoped to monopolize the art of faith healing and prognostication. Epidemic disease – inexplicable and unstoppable as it was – meant that pajés remained indispensable to Amerindian communities coping with it. Intercession with the animal world on behalf of the human, skill at divination and faith healing, and rhetorical eloquence: so well had Anchieta assumed the attributes of the pajé that by the time of his death in 1597 he was widely regarded not as a priest who enjoyed the particular favor of God in the heavens but as a *pajéguaçu* – a "great pajé."[138]

It was in those terms that, according to Vasconcelos, so many of the colony's inhabitants lamented his death.[139] Even the frontispiece of Vasconcelos's *Vida* registered the ambiguity (Figure 6.2).

In the plain woodcut illustration, Anchieta stands amid an abundant coastal landscape. A powerful but tamed natural world is to hand. But the symbols of edenic mastery are not the familiar Old World animals. Anchieta is surrounded by jaguars, a macaw, and a monkey. In the background is a vignette of that oft-told tale about Anchieta and the ibis: a boat plies the coastal waters beneath a beaming sun but shaded by a cloud of nurturing fowl. In the colony as on the page: it was not at all clear whether it was the Company's god or shamanic knowledge that commanded nature.

PATTERNS OF INQUIRY

At the end of the sixteenth century, the persistence of an ambiguous vision of Brazil was far from inevitable. As university courses on *materia medica* became common and as natural history had begun to emerge as a domain of knowledge apart from therapeutics, emergent accounts of Brazilian nature like those by the Jesuit Fernão Cardim might have insinuated Brazilian nature more thoroughly into the catalog of imported therapeutics getting newfound attention in medical curricula. But events especially in Lisbon and Rome combined to push the Company's intellectual work within metropolitan Europe not toward some aspect of medicine or the study of nature but toward mixed mathematics and cosmology. In Portugal, the Crown relied increasingly on Jesuit instruction to train pilots in navigation, instrumentation, and practical mathematics.[140]

---

[138] Vasconcelos, *Vida*, 202–203.   [139] Vasconcelos, *Vida*, 202–203.

[140] Luis de Albuquerque, "A 'aula de esfera' do Colêgio de Santo Antão no século XVII," in *Anais da Academia Portuguesa de História* 21 (1972): 337–391; Henrique Leitão "Jesuit Mathematical Practice in Portugal, 1540–1759" in *The New Science and Jesuit Science: Seventeenth Century Perspectives*, ed. Mordechai Feingold (Dordecht: Kluwer Academic Publishers, 2003), 229–247.

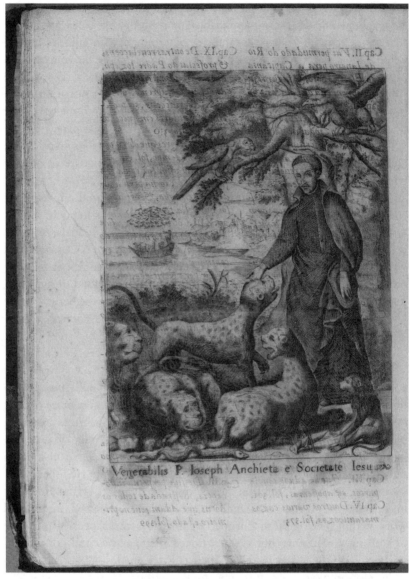

FIGURE 6.2 Missionary Performance, Shamanic Expertise. The Jesuit José de Anchieta in the frontispiece from Simão de Vasconcellos, *Vida do veneravel Padre Ioseph de Anchieta da Companhia de Iesu, Taumaturgo do Novo Mundo, na Provincia do Brasil* (Lisbon: João da Costa, 1672).
Courtesy of the John Carter Brown Library at Brown University.

Especially at the Roman curia but also across early modern Europe, the Company's pursuit of patronage and influence turned in part on questions in fields ranging from theoretical mathematics to observational astronomy.[141] Meanwhile, the Jesuit Christopher Clavius's influential work in cosmography and mathematics, the successes of Matteo Ricci and later Jesuits in China, and (in the early seventeenth century) the growing debate over heliocentrism all helped consolidate a privileged position for mathematics and allied fields within the intellectual life of the Company.[142] These, much more than medicine or natural history, would be the focus of Jesuit inquiry and publication. Both within metropolitan Europe and in the prestigious Asian apostolate. Natural history would always retain a marginal place in Jesuit intellectual work and would remain a small proportion of total Jesuits publications until the suppression of the order in middle of the eighteenth century.[143]

But among members of the Company in Brazil, natural inquiry took a different course. By placing disease within the domain of shamanic knowledge, Jesuits did not gain control over healing. They merely consented to the terms in which the contest for clinical primacy would be waged – terms already set by the Tupí and Guaraní themselves. That disease in Portugal's American colonies was, foremost, a consequence of forces unseen, and that tending to disease meant managing those forces, had by the late sixteenth century become a matter of fact with lasting

---

[141] See the survey by Rivka Feldhay, "The Cultural Field of Jesuit Science," in *The Jesuits: Cultures, Sciences, and the Arts, 1540–1773*, 2 vols., eds. John W. O'Malley, S.J., Gauvin Alexander Bailey, Steven J. Harris, and T. Frank Kennedy, S.J. (Toronto: University of Toronto Press, 1999), vol. 1, 107–130.

[142] James M. Lattis, *Between Copernicus and Galileo: Christoph Clavius and the Collapse of Ptolemaic Cosmology* (Chicago: University of Chicago Press, 1994); Ugo Baldini, "The Academy of Mathematics of the Collegio Romano from 1553 to 1612," in Feingold, ed., *Jesuit Science*, 47–98; and Edward Grant, "The Partial Transformation of Medieval Cosmology by Jesuits in the Sixteenth and Seventeenth Centuries," in Feingold, ed., *Jesuit Science*, 127–155. On the prominence of the Asian missions, see Ugo Baldini and Bernardino Fernandes, "As Assistências ibéricas da Companhia de Jesus e a actividade científica nas missões asiáticas (1578–1650)," *Revista Portuguesa de Filosofia* 54 (1998): 195–246; and on the Jesuits in China, see Jonathan D. Spence, *The Memory Palace of Matteo Ricci* (New York: Penguin, 1984); and Florence C. Hsia, *Sojourners in a Strange Land: Jesuits and Their Scientific Missions in Late Imperial China* (Chicago: University of Chicago Press, 2009).

[143] Graphs of Jesuit publications over time and by field are presented in Steve J. Harris, "Transposing the Merton Thesis: Apostolic Spirituality and the Establishment of the Jesuit Scientific Tradition," *Science in Context* 3 (1989): 29–65.

clinical significance. Who best manipulated those forces was open-ended and defined in multiple ways.

Not only medical expertise but expertise over the inner-workings of the natural world more broadly was as open as it had ever been. Just as cultural, religious, and political affiliations ramified, so too did authority over explaining and treating disease and, more generally explaining events in nature.[144] The precedent for a dynamic but embattled medical heterodoxy had been set just as enslaved Africans and their diverse knowledges had begun to arrive in increasing number and frequency. Portuguese colonialism in Brazil helped give rise to a profusion of approaches to disease and the study of nature. And that in turn would pattern natural inquiry in important ways over the next century, when shamanism would remain integral as a way to mitigate not only the loss of life but also the erosion of Jesuit influence in the missions.[145]

Yet at the same time, and increasingly as the sixteenth century drew to a close, members of the Company would find that they could no longer ignore the bodily aspects of disease among would-be adherents to Catholicism. Taking the pulse and blood-letting were common practices by 1560.[146] Jesuit letters discussing disease both among members of the Company and within their mission settlements gave increasingly detailed accounts of the afflictions they witnessed. What in the early 1550s were nondescript accounts of illness[147] increasingly became stories of fever, dysentery, and pox; by the early 1560s Jesuits took care to distinguish among particular fevers with terms like "tertian" and "quartan."[148] And, increasingly, they began to speak of their work in the mission field in distinctly medical

---

[144] The transatlantic roots of religious syncretism are traced in Ronaldo Vainfas, *Trópico dos pecados: Moral, sexualidade, e inquisição no Brasil* (Rio de Janeiro: Campus, 1989); Souza, *The Devil and the Land of the Holy Cross*; and James H. Sweet, *Recreating Africa: Culture, Kinship, and Religion in the African-Portuguese World, 1441–1770* (Chapel Hill, NC: University of North Carolina Press, 2003).

[145] Charlotte de Castelnau-L'Estoile, "The Uses of Shamanism: Evangelizing Strategies and Missionary Models in Seventeenth Century Brazil," in O'Malley et al., eds., *The Jesuits*, vol. 2, 616–637. In some parts of the colonies, native peoples began to refer to any Jesuits and then any Christians as *caraíbas*. See *MB* vol. 2, 133–134, n. 17.

[146] *MB* vol. 3, 249–255, 293, 379–381, 454.

[147] *MB* vol. 1, 302–305, 379, 395–396, and 428–429; and *MB* vol. 2, 83–84, 108, 209.

[148] *MB* vol. 2, 392–395; *MB* vol. 3, 18, n. 2, 19, 60, 101, 266–268, 283–284, 291, 379–381, 397, 404, 416, 453, and 505; and *MB* vol. 4, 273. See also Metcalf, *Go-Betweens*, ch. 5.

terms.[149] In the seventeenth century, António Vieira (perhaps the most influential Jesuit of the seventeenth-century Portuguese world) would embrace medicine and greater clinical care for the body as indispensable to the Company's missionary endeavor in Brazil.[150] Subsequent bioprospecting in the colony would, over the course of the seventeenth century, earn the Jesuits their reputation as naturalists and field medics. The Jesuit emphasis first on faith healing and then on *materia medica* were learned, pragmatic adjustments to the exigencies of fieldwork on the ground out in empire.

[149] *MB* vol. 2, 158–159; *MB* vol. 3, 250–253, 291, 357, 379–381, 454, and 548; and *MB* vol. 4, 163–164, 179–181, and 272.
[150] Cohen, *Fire of Tongues*, 205.

7

Split Decisions

Anything is credible no matter how strange it may seem, for not all of the secrets of nature were revealed to mankind, such that no one can reasonably deny and take as impossible the things which they have not seen and of which they have no news.

Pero de Magalhães Gândavo[1]

THE VIEW FROM LISBON

In Lisbon, on a sunlit day in June 1515, in a yard alongside the Casa da Índia, an Asian elephant and a rhinoceros from Cambay squared off to the delight of Manuel I, his court, and a festive crowd. To believe contemporary engravings of such beastly encounters, the duel was vigorous and heated. In one moment, the elephant bent its left foreleg, lunged with its right, and drove a tusk at the head of its stocky opponent. The rhino dropped low. The tusk flew wide of its mark (Figure 7.1).

It would not be a match to the death – not, at least, on this occasion. The spectacle ended when the elephant fled the yard, plunged headlong into the narrow streets of the imperial capital, and found its way northward, back to the calm of the royal stables in Rossio. It was probably in good company. More than a dozen elephants ambled ashore across Lisbon's wharves in the sixteenth century. On ceremonial occasions – as in a parade surely calculated to reflect the might of the Crown and the reach of its empire – D. Manuel mounted his favorite pachyderm to lead a

[1] Gândavo, *História*, 32.

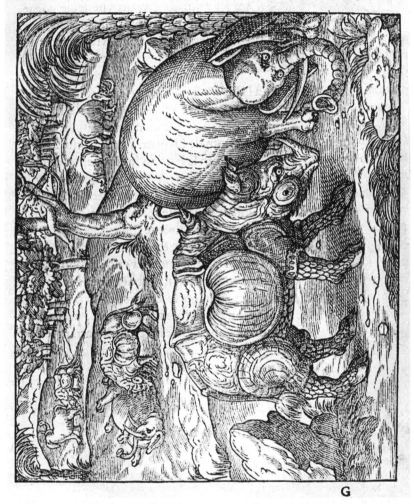

DE LA LICORNE, 25

FIGVRE DV COMBAT DV RHINOCEROS
contre l'Elephant.

G

FIGURE 7.1 An Elephant and a Rhino Square Off. An image from Ambroise Paré, *Discours d'Ambroise Pare ... a savoir, de la mumie, de la licorne, des venins, et de la peste, avec une table des plus notables matieres contenues esdit discours* (Paris: Gabriel Buon, 1582).
Courtesy of the John Carter Brown Library at Brown University.

procession from the Paço da Ribeira up the winding streets to Lisbon's cathedral.[2] This was a fitting performance for a ruling family that at the time claimed dominion over "either side of the sea in Africa" and styled itself "Lord of Guinea, and of the Conquest, Navigation, and Commerce of Ethiopia, Arabia, Persia, and India."[3]

With global networks, Lisbon in the sixteenth and seventeenth centuries swelled with the rare, the exotic, and the marvelous. Observers like the poet Diogo Velha da Chancelaria, wondered at the enormous variety of things natural and artificial – the "monsters, talking birds, diamonds, and porcelain" – that so inundated the imperial capital that they came to seem "quite common."[4] Across early modern Europe, too, cabinets of wonders filled. Collections of curiosities multiplied. Exotic beasts proliferated. Orta's liquid amber, unicorn horns from Africa, Asian bezoars, a fish-skin shield from Cambay, Tupí featherwork, the bill of a Brazilian toucan, and the mottled green eggs of an Australian emu were all part of the flood of exotica that made its way from Lisbon to points scattered between Antwerp, Brussels, Milan, and Rome.[5] The victorious rhino of 1515 was gifted to Pope Leo X. And though it sank with its ship while crossing the Mediterranean, many other creatures – an African zebra, a snow leopard, a Persian horse, and a succession of elephants (most famously, a white elephant named Hanno) – had more felicitous metropolitan itineraries.[6]

[2] Bits and pieces of the episode appear in Lach, *Asia in the Making of Europe*, vol. 2, bk. 1, 162–164; and Annemarie Jordan Gschwend, "A Procura Portuguesa por Animais Exóticos/The Portuguese Demand for Exotic Animals," in *Cortejo Triunfal com Girafas: animais exóticos ao service do poder/Triumphal Procession with Giraffes: exotic animals at the service of power* (Lisbon: N.p., n.d.), 33–77.

[3] Vasco da Gama, *Em Nome de Deus: The Journal of the First Voyage of Vasco da Gama to Índia*, trans. Glenn J. Ames (Leiden: Brill, 2009), 157.

[4] Silvio A. Bedini, *The Popes Elephant* (Nashville, TN: J.S. Sanders Company, 1998), 161.

[5] Daston and Park, *Wonders*, 154–155; Buono, "Crafts of Color: 240–242; Novoa, "Unicorns and Bezoars"; A. Pérez de Tudela and Annemarie Jordan Gschwend, "Luxury Goods for Royal Collectors: Exotica, princely gifts, and rare animals exchanged between the Iberian courts and Central Europe in the Renaissance (1560–1612)," in *Exotica. Portugals Entdeckungen im Spiegel fürstlicher Kunst- und Wunderkammern der Renaissance. Die Beiträge des am 19, und 20. Mai 2000 vom Kunsthistorischen Museum Wien veranstalteten Symposiums, Jahrbuch des Kunsthistorischen Museums Wien* 3, eds. H. Trnek and S. Haag (Mainz: P. von Zabern, 2001), 1–127.

[6] Lach, *Asia in the Making of Europe*, vol. 2, bk. 1, 17–33, 144–146; and Almudena Pérez de Tudela and Annemarie Jordan Gschwend, "Renaissance Menageries: Exotic Animals and Pets at the Habsburg Courts in Iberia and Central Europe," in *Early Modern Zoology: The Construction of Animals in Science, Literature and the Visual Arts*, eds. Karl A. E. Enenkel and Paul J. Smith (Boston: Brill, 2007), 419–445.

Not only strange nature but unanticipated diseases, too, seemed pervasive. As the ill-fated rhino sank at sea, its would-be papal master contemplated the creation of a new hospital in Rome – one for victims of what some said was an entirely new illness. The great pox, what university-trained physicians often referred to as the French disease (*morbo gallico*) and most modern historians as venereal syphilis, sparked debate among physicians scattered from Ferrara to Leipzig, London to Lisbon. The great pox joined the plague and, together with afflictions more localized but no less inexplicable (a mysterious sweating sickness in England, a fever that ravaged southern Spain), these became subjects of profound and pressing interest. What caused them, whether they were known to Hippocrates or Galen, and which, if any, of the medicines described by Dioscorides or Pliny could be used to treat them: these had all become matters of grave concern and speculation.[7]

The consequences of metropolitan encounters with the strange and the unexpected in the sixteenth century were profound and lasting. The most prominent European naturalists of Orta's generation had, like Orta himself, been university-trained physicians.[8] At home and abroad, they had focused their investigations largely on flora with presumed medicinal value – an endeavor that variously incorporated text and experience and that unfolded with distinct chronologies throughout Portugal's empire, from the Guinea Coast to Goa and Portuguese America. By 1600, much had changed. European physicians had an enlarged catalog of diseases that demanded theoretical elaboration. Treatises on plague and pox now kept printers busy. Tracts on fever would soon do the same.[9] Metropolitan physicians in London, Lisbon, Seville, and Paris had begun to ask their seafaring contemporaries for reports of strange symptoms and anomalous afflictions.[10] Naturalists, meanwhile, were a diversifying lot

---

[7] Arrizabalaga, Henderson, and French, *The Great Pox*; Hays, *The Burdens of Disease: Epidemics and Human Response in Western History* (New Brunswick, NJ: Rutgers University Press, 1998), 63–72; and Hamlin, *More than Hot*, 62–69. For shifts in Portuguese medical literature, see Chapter 8 and *BL* vol. 1, 760–762; *BL* vol. 3, 320; and *BL*, vol. 4, 52, and 235.

[8] Ogilvie, *Science of Describing*, 30–39; Cook, "The New Philosophy and Medicine"; and Maclean, *Learning*, ch. 13.

[9] Arrizabalaga, Henderson, and French, *The Great Pox*, ch. 10; Hays, *Burdens of Disease*, 63–74; Hamlin, *More Than Hot*, 62–87.

[10] Joan-Pau Rubiés, "Instructions for Travellers: Teaching the Eye to See," *History and Anthropology* 9 (1996): 139–190; Daston and Park, *Wonders*, 238–239; Mundy, *Mapping New Spain*, ch. 3.

with interests of their own. If in the sixteenth century the most influential naturalists had been physicians, that was no longer the case. Many naturalists continued to dabble in *materia medica* but a shrinking proportion of them had any formal medical training at all. Confronted with a natural world of unknown variability, a more motley community of naturalists increasingly thought nature worthy of study quite apart from any prospective therapeutic use it might have had. Well-to-do patrons and benefactors agreed. Natural inquiry was taken up by members of newly founded private academies and state-sponsored societies. As the preoccupations of the physician and the naturalist diverged, medicine and natural history parted ways.[11] And indeed, their histories are often told in isolation.[12]

Yet by the turn of the seventeenth century, both medicine and natural history shared a set of essential philosophical quandaries. And if metropolitan Portuguese observers had become acutely aware of the open-ended variety of nature earlier than most of their contemporaries,[13] they nonetheless confronted these challenges along with everyone else in the closing decades of the sixteenth century. Writing in Lisbon in 1576, and in the wake of a global itinerary that had taken him to India and Brazil, Pero de Magalhães Gândavo summed up the situation: "Anything is credible, he mused, "no matter how strange it may seem, for not all of the secrets of nature were revealed to mankind." Consequently, he thought, "no one" could "reasonably deny and take as impossible the things which they have not seen and of which they have no news."[14]

What might be said to exist in nature (ontology) and upon what basis it might be possible to know those things (epistemology): these were heady philosophical issues indeed. Grappling with them now meant not only greater skepticism toward the authority of ancient texts and the embrace of experience as an epistemic tool (a preoccupation, as I have shown,

---

[11] Findlen, *Possessing Nature*, chs 6 and 7; Daston and Park, *Wonders*, 158–159, and 217–218; and Ogilvie *Science of Describing*, 28–49.

[12] Siraisi, "Medicine, 1450–1620, and the History of Science."

[13] In previous chapters, I have charted an intellectual genealogy that links Duarte Pacheco Pereira to Tomé Pires, Simão Álvares, and Garcia de Orta. Onésimo Teotonio de Almeida offers additional examples, though with a different argument in mind, in "Portugal and the Dawn of Modern Science."

[14] Gândavo, *História*, 32. Considerable uncertainty surrounds Gândavo's itinerary, on which see Vasco Graça Moura, *Sobre Camões, Gândavo e Outras Personagens* (Lisbon: Campo das Letras, 2000), 117–141.

common in various forms among Portuguese from the Gulf of Guinea to the wharves of Goa and the coast of Brazil); it meant as well the deliberate suspension of disbelief in fanciful claims and a widening of the grounds on which an account of nature might be judged credible. That Gândavo – professor of grammar and sometime statesmen but by no means a natural philosopher – so readily identified these deep interpretive dilemmas suggests just how pervasive such questions now were in some quarters of imperial Lisbon. If nature seemed evermore boundless – evermore pregnant with possibility – then the rules for constituting knowledge about it would have to be rewritten.[15]

Two pieces of writing – one little known, the other largely ignored – dramatize the peculiar ways in which Portuguese in the Atlantic began to do just that, participating in the multifaceted transformations in medicine and natural history then enveloping early modern Europe. The physician Aleixo de Abreu and the sugar-planter Ambrósio Fernandes Brandão probably never knew one another personally. But by the turn of the seventeenth century, both men had ties to imperial administrators in Lisbon, both had criss-crossed the Atlantic, and both the physician and the planter confronted first-hand the unsettling combination of enigmatic disease and unanticipated nature. Removed from the court, the cabinet of curiosities, the academy, the university, and the state-chartered society (all of which had become institutions vital to natural inquiry elsewhere in Europe[16]), they were insinuated instead into the networks of patronage and commerce that had come to characterize Portugal's Atlantic empire at the turn of the seventeenth century.

Abreu's *Tratado de las siete enfermedades*, composed in Lisbon in the early 1620s, was the first book written and published by a physician who had spent time on both sides of the intertropical Atlantic. And though he took up the problem of several diseases, his *Tratado* focused centrally on fever. Abreu's *Tratado* reveals what happened when diagnostic categories fashioned in the ancient and medieval Mediterranean were finally brought to bear on the fevers that plagued Portuguese settlements in the Atlantic. From front to back, the *Tratado* is marked by the inescapable tension between Abreu's effort to explore the development and

[15] Here I follow the reasoning in Daston and Park, *Wonders*.
[16] See the chapters contained in "Part II. Personae and Sites of Natural Knowledge," in Katharine Park and Lorraine Daston, eds., *The Cambridge History of Science, Volume 3: Early Modern Science* (New York: Cambridge University Press, 2003).

interrelationship of unfamiliar diseases within the body – which was inherently speculative – and the book's self-consciously didactic aim, which demanded that Abreu assume authority and draw firm conclusions about the identity of distinct illnesses. As a discussion of medical curiosities encountered overseas (which, I will argue, is what certain kinds of fever were for Abreu), the *Tratado* illustrates the increasingly dubious value of novelty in metropolitan circles, and especially for a practicing physician. As a medical treatise, the book presented a genuinely Atlantic perspective – a medical instantiation of the politically, socially, and geographically unified system of production and reproduction detailed by Luís Felipe de Alencastro.[17] Although largely forgotten by historians of medicine,[18] Abreu's work would prove formative. By the end of the seventeenth century it would help give Portuguese debates over fever in the Atlantic greater clarity and definition, and would ultimately become a point of reference for physicians wishing to reformulate metropolitan visions of health and disease not only in the Atlantic but throughout the intertropical world.

Ambrósio Fernandes Brandão, too, had much to say on the question of fever and a number of other afflictions. But in Brandão's *Diálogos das grandezas do Brasil* it was the dizzying diversity of Brazilian nature, not the causes and treatment of a diversifying range of enigmatic Atlantic diseases, that drew most of his attention. Through accounts like Brandão's *Diálogos*, much of Brazil's unfamiliar nature finally emerged as a potentially exploitable resource in metropolitan medical and commercial imaginations. Written in Brazil around 1618 but never published, the fictive conversations in Brandão's *Diálogos* offer a glimpse into the social and cultural relations that gave shape and texture to natural inquiry as it was practiced in Brazil at the turn of the seventeenth century.

After nearly two centuries of colonial activity in the region known to antiquity as the torrid zone, the environmental and epidemiological

---

[17] Luis Felipe de Alencastro, *O Trato dos Viventes: Formação do Brasil no Atlântico Sul, séculos XVI e XVII* (São Paulo: Companhia das Letras, 2000).

[18] This is partly a consequence of the marginal place of Portugal in the historiography but partly, I would suggest, a result of the vital manuscript culture that persisted in Lisbon, which stands in contrast to the print culture on which so many seventeenth-century studies focus. On the historiographical predicament, see Palmira Fontes da Costa, "Identity and the Construction of Memory in Representations of Garcia de Orta," in Costa, ed., *Medicine, Trade and Empire*, 237–265. On manuscript culture in Lisbon, see Chapter 8.

coherence of intertropical latitudes had yet to take shape. But, taken together, the work of Abreu and Brandão reveals the outlines of an emerging debate over climate, nature, and disease in Brazil, the Atlantic, and the intertropical world more broadly. Abreu's *Tratado* and Brandão's *Diálogos* demonstrate that by the opening of the seventeenth century, the once-indisputable good health of Brazil had been thrown into question. The pathologization of Brazil had begun. As that happened, the idea of the tropics became a possibility.

FEVER AND AN ATLANTIC EPIDEMIOLOGY

Inexplicably – in a metropolitan capital with ties to medical outposts on three continents and faced with what many have claimed was a dramatic shortage of trained physicians[19] – Abreu failed to find work in Lisbon. He decided instead to seek an appointment overseas. And for that he turned to his father, a friend of the Count of Merino, for help. Beyond Lisbon, the location of his posting was less important to Abreu than the salary he could expect once he got there. Abreu wanted, as he put it, "to become rich, as all men desire to do."[20] When family connections finally got him the post of personal physician to João Furtado de Mendonça, the sixth governor of Angola (1594–1602), Abreu took it. That was how the son of a well-to-do Old Christian family with a newly minted medical degree from Coimbra (where he studied on a royal stipend) found his way to one of the least desirable spots on Portugal's imperial map.[21] Not until 1606 did Abreu finally return to the kingdom, establish a private practice, and get the kind of royal patronage he had long hoped for: in 1612 he became personal physician to the Portuguese exchequer and in 1616 was appointed a physician of the royal chamber of the future Philip III (1621–1640).

Those positions were made possible by his work over twelve long years, from 1594 to 1606, in the Atlantic. During that time, his

---

[19] See, for example, Mário Sérgio Farelo, "On Portuguese Medical Students and Masters Travelling Abroad: An Overview from the Early Modern Period to the Enlightenment," In *Centers of Medical Excellence? Medical Travel and Education in Europe, 1500–1789*, eds. Ole Peter Grell, Andrew Cunningham, and Jon Arrizabalaga (New York: Routledge, 2010), 125–147.

[20] Abreu, *Tratado*, [unnumbered page 11].

[21] Even the Company of Jesus struggled to establish a presence there. See Alden, *The Making of an Enterprise*, 75–76.

preference for an illustrious career in the imperial capital and his dependence upon his gubernatorial patrons would effectively align his investigative priorities with their political and economic interests. Of course,
physicians had always been concerned with the body. But in the aftermath
of encounters on three continents, surrounded by the unanticipated variety of nature, and well acquainted with the courtly interest in exotica that
prevailed in Lisbon, Abreu could choose where to focus his investigative
efforts. If, in Portuguese Asia, commodified plants were the focus of
profitable commerce and hence natural inquiry, the same was not true
in the Portuguese Atlantic. There, individual and imperial fortunes hinged
on the transoceanic commerce in commodified bodies. Their value as
instruments of productivity made them valuable objects of natural
inquiry. In this way, the imperial exigencies of the Atlantic endowed
Abreu's work with a particular geographical perspective and precise
investigative focus.

The slave trade and the treatment of disease had become increasingly
intertwined and evermore central to imperial policy in West Central
Africa in the years leading up to Abreu's arrival. Luanda – port to one
of Portugal's earliest sub-Saharan mission fields[22] but otherwise little
more than a way station for India-bound ships – attracted increased
attention in the late sixteenth century for a number of reasons. Rumors
of silver mines in the interior sparked early interest and led to the
creation of a governorship there after 1570. In the years before the union
of the Crowns, this was a move taken by D. Sebastião (1557–1578) not
only to enrich the empire but also to match the wealth that Spain now
drew from mines in Zacatecas, Potosí, and elsewhere in the Americas,
and to counter Spanish influence among members of the Portuguese
nobility in Lisbon. In Luanda, meanwhile, a series of dynastic wars
eventually involving the Portuguese helped give their agents easy access
to captives taken in war and reduced to slavery.[23] The devastating
population loss among native peoples in Portuguese America coupled
with (and substantially caused by) the expansion of plantation agriculture there drove the growing demand for slave labor from the African

---

[22] John Thornton, "The Development of an African Catholic Church in the Kingdom of
Kongo, 1491–1750," *Journal of African History* 25 (1984): 147–167.
[23] See the chapter on "Slavery and the Slave Trade" in John K. Thornton, *Africa and
Africans in the Making of the Atlantic World, 1450–1800* (New York: Cambridge
University Press, 1998).

coast. Luanda's slave markets were by the 1590s among the most heavily trafficked in the transatlantic trade.[24]

When in 1580 Portugal and its empire became part of the Spanish Hapsburg domain, it was in the strengthening of plantations and slavery that Philip I took a particular interest. Faced with a half-century of demographic catastrophe in Brazil and a total failure to find the fabled silver mines in Angola, Philip turned to one Domingos de Abreu e Brito for a report and recommendations on his newly won Atlantic interests. Brito visited Angola in 1590 and 1591. His report, the *Inquérito à vida administrativa e economica de Angola e do Brasil* (*Inquiry into the Administrative and Economic Affairs of Angola and Brazil*) appeared in 1592. In the year or so before Mendonça and Abreu left Lisbon for Luanda, it was Brito's inquiry that had become a point of reference for discussions of policy in the Portuguese Atlantic.[25] Brito had argued that plantation agriculture be extended to the Luandan hinterland from the island of São Tomé, just as it had been to Brazil from Madeira earlier. He argued that ready access to slaves at Luanda made his plan both feasible and prudent. But the key to making Angola a profitable venture, so thought Brito, still lay in the search for those elusive mines. He urged their discovery.

And yet, as Brito put it, if any of these plans were "to have any effect," there were more basic problems that needed attention.[26] The Crown would have to attend to issues of health and disease in the colony. "Principally," at least in Brito's view, that meant an "apothecary" with "all the necessary medicines." It also meant "physicians and surgeons" who had "knowledge of these medicines."[27] Besides that, Brito was notably vague. Like Tomé Pires in India at the beginning of the century, Brito complained of the sad state of medicines that arrived to the colony from the kingdom. They were "corrupt and old," he wrote, and did no more than "consume the lives of ... poor conquistadors." Unlike Pires earlier, what he did not say was precisely which medicines and precisely what knowledge was, as he put it, "necessary."[28]

Brito's report did, however, at least imply a solution. As I argued earlier, Portuguese apothecaries in Indian Ocean Asia were awash in

[24] Sweet, *Recreating Africa*, 15–22.
[25] Domingos Abreu e Brito, *Inquérito à vida administrative e economica de Angola e do Brasil* (Coimbra: Imprensa da Universidade, 1933 [1592]).
[26] References to the problem of ill health peppered his report. Brito, *Inquérito*, 10, 16, 21, 27, 37.
[27] Brito, *Inquérito*, 21. [28] Brito, *Inquérito*, 21.

materia medica that were generally familiar, even if the names under which they traded, and the condition in which they were shipped, were not. In Luanda the case was different. The problems of ill health generally and fever in particular were by now all too familiar. Its *materia medica* were not – at least not to newcomers like Brito. But he stated in his report that he had spoken to persons "with experience of the land," and that those exchanges led him to believe that local therapeutics could solve the problem.[29] He was vague about what, exactly, he had in mind but promised to provide a list of these medicines "should it become necessary" (*quando necessario for*).[30] Whether or not he ever found it necessary to send that list in unclear. What is clear, at least based on Brito's comments, is that by the 1590s Luanda had become home to a thriving medical culture of its own – one in which Portuguese sailors, Luso-African traders, and a succession of Crown-appointed governors all participated.[31]

Governor João Furtado de Mendonça, with the physician Abreu in tow, partly followed Brito's recommendations. Once in Luanda in 1594, Mendonça took measures to strengthen the transatlantic slave trade, including a series of wars to that end, and commissioned a hospital to care for the growing number of sailors and soldiers coming to Luanda. Mendonça ignored the mines. Under his governorship, enslavement and the trans-Atlantic trade took precedence over inland conquest and pursuit of the elusive metal. When Mendonça's successor resumed the mineral search and in 1605 finally managed to reach the Cambambe Hills where the mines were supposed to be, he found exactly nothing: no silver whatsoever. Luanda was and would remain principally a slave port for plantations on the far side of the ocean.[32]

By 1605, Abreu had crossed the Atlantic. But his time in Luanda, roughly eight years between 1594 and 1602, had been formative. Abreu's medical work (like that of Orta in Goa earlier) almost certainly involved him in the affairs of the hospital. It would have been in keeping with the

---

[29] Brito, *Inquérito*, 21.   [30] Brito, *Inquérito*, 21.

[31] BNP Res. Cod. 3794; and the documents gathered into Luciano Cordeiro, ed., *Memorias do ultramar: Viagens, explorações e conquistas dos Portuguezes. Producções, commercio e governo do Congo e de Angola segundo Manuel Vogado Sotomaior, Antonio Diniz, Bento Banha Cardoso, e Antonio Beserra Fajarado, 1620–1629* (Lisbon: Imprensa Nacional, 1881), especially 15–18.

[32] David Birmingham, *Trade and Conflict in Angola: The Mbundu and Their Neighbors under the Influence of the Portuguese, 1483–1790* (Oxford: Clarendon Press, 1966); and Alencastro, *Trato dos Viventes*.

post of personal physician to the governor for Abreu to have overseen its operation, and especially the treatment of cases of acute disease. And although no documentation confirms that he supervised the hospital, Abreu referenced his observation of both sailors and slaves in Luanda as the premise for his conclusions in the *Tratado*.[33] These were not merely medical exams of the living. With the help of two surgeons and a Spaniard serving as nurse, he performed postmortem dissections, which became the basis of his comments on afflictions he termed *mal de Luanda* and *mal del guzano* (respectively, the "disease of Luanda" and "disease of the worm").[34] He, like Brito, said little about local *materia medica*, though he noted that the manual operations for treating certain other maladies (one, a worm that grew in the legs; another, an odd looking creature that afflicteded the soles of the feet) were masterfully performed by many in the colony.

If in Luanda Abreu's work was marked by an emphasis on the bodies of people in transit and a general ignorance of indigenous *materia medica*, his experience in Brazil under Diogo Botelho would reinforce both tendencies. Precisely how he got the appointment to Diogo Botelho, Brazil's incoming governor (1602–1608), is unclear.[35] Abreu arrived in Portuguese America directly from Luanda in 1602, was appointed to Botelho's service in 1603, and would not return to Portugal for a few years yet (until 1606). Had Abreu established a reputation that made its way back to Lisbon even while he was in Angola? Had Botelho heard of Abreu's work among the slaves and sailors moving in and out of Luanda? The autobiographical sketch that opened the *Tratado* (which is virtually the only source of information about Abreu) answered none of these questions. What is clear is that Botelho shared Mendonça's interest in slave labor and Abreu's claims to penury – once complaining that all he wanted for himself in Brazil was merely "to earn a living, for the colony is very expensive."[36] He was also (much like Sousa in Goa some six decades earlier) an unusually controversial figure – the first in a string of governors concerned as much with defense and territorial conquest as with colonial

---

[33] Abreu, *Tratado*, [unnumbered page 13].
[34] These are now identified as scurvy and guinea worm, respectively. See Abreu, *Tratado*, 154v; and Guerra, "Aleixo de Abreu," 67. Roxanne Nelson, "The Last Worm: A dreaded Tropical Disease Is on the Verge of Eradication," *Scientific American* 307 (2012): 24.
[35] His tenure ended in 1605 but his successor was not named until 1607 and did not arrive until 1608. See Guerra, "Aleixo de Abreu."
[36] Diogo Botelho to the Count of Linhares, ANTT, CJ, mç. 8, doc. 129; quoted in Schwartz, *Sovereignty and Society*, 194.

administration. His handling of the intertwined issues of the slave trade, policies toward Brazil's indigenous peoples, and epidemic disease were key points of contention.[37]

When Botelho left Lisbon for the South American colonies, he headed not for the capital of Salvador – which was expected since it remained the administrative capital of the colonies – but, in a move that earned him censure from the Crown, went straight to Pernambuco, still the wealthiest captaincy in Portuguese America. Personal connections with the local treasurer, temporary donatarial absence, ongoing conflict with the fugitive slaves of Palmares, and a thriving coastal market all gave Botelho easy access to slaves – both newly subjugated Potiguar and Aimoré from the interior (where skirmishes to that end continued), recaptured slaves from Palmares, and Africans (largely from either Kongo or Ndongo) newly arrived from Luanda.[38] Because of the captaincy's unmatched productivity, labor costs were particularly high and Botelho made the most of his Pernambuco detour. It earned him, among other things, charges of price fixing and of interfering in public slave auctions. Those in turn ensnared him two separate formal inquiries into his gubernatorial affairs, the first of which was innocuous but the second proved inconclusive only because someone, it seems, made off with the report.[39]

Under Botelho, conflict with the Jesuits came to head, too, over what was widely perceived as the missionaries' near-monopoly on access to Amerindian labor. The governor wanted to put the missions into the hands of the secular clergy and loosen the restrictions on Amerindian enslavement – changes in line with recent shifts in Crown policy. Jesuit faculty in the coastal colleges at Olinda and Salvador opposed those changes. They claimed that the colonists wrongly enslaved the natives and that secular clergy and officials like Botelho failed to protect both native communities and Jesuit mission villages from planter depredations. Jesuits repeatedly cited the mistreatment, ill-health, and death that was sure to befall the enslaved workers in cane fields and at the sugar mills.[40]

---

[37] Schwartz, *Sovereignty and Society*, 125, 193–194.

[38] Thornton, *Cultural History*, 296.

[39] Schwartz, *Sovereignty and Society*, 195; Francis A. Dutra, "A New Look into Diogo Botelho's Stay in Pernambuco, 1602–1603," *Luso-Brazilian Review* 4 (1967): 27–34; Hemming, *Red Gold*, 172–173; John K. Thornton, "Les États de l'Angola et la formation de Palmares (Brésil)," *Annales* 63 (2008): 769–797.

[40] Schwartz, *Sovereignty and Society*, 132; Hemming, *Red Gold*, 148–149, 208–210. To make matters worse – in an episode that evinced Botelho's similarly antagonistic stance toward the regular clergy and which reflected the growing conflict between secular and

The rancour and factionalism were only exacerbated by tensions arising from a spate of epidemics that afflicted the captaincies of the northeast in these years. Botelho's governorship began in the immediate aftermath of a series of pox epidemics. Memories of the one in 1585 in Ilhéus, south of Bahia and far to the south of Pernambuco, may have begun to fade. But cutaneous afflictions hit much closer to home in 1597 in Rio Grande do Norte and then again in Pernambuco itself in 1599.[41] The fact that pox and fevers alike afflicted not only Brazil's indigenous peoples but everyone in the colony led to multiple competing explanations. By now, the most prominent of these was that African slaves brought pox to the colonies. So pronounced had the anxiety over pox in particular now become, and so indelible the association between it and slave cargoes, that it was in precisely these years around the turn of the century that the municipal councils of both Salvador and Recife instituted their first quarantine measures.[42]

Learned medicine, meanwhile, was increasingly recruited to the service of the Atlantic slave trade. In the very years that Abreu was in Brazil, fear that African bodies somehow spread disease brought slaves under the purview of colonial physicians. When councilors suspected slave cargoes of harboring what some observers described as "contagious disease," they enlisted the learned eye of university-trained physicians. Procedures of bodily invigilation grew tighter.[43] Disease in Brazil was now undeniably a persistent and widespread problem. Epidemics endangered plantation agriculture and exacerbated factionalism and intra-colonial strife. Nearly everyone in any of Portugal's coastal enclaves on either side of the South Atlantic had an interest in solving the puzzle of disease.[44]

---

ecclesiastical influence in the colony – the governor was embroiled in a protracted struggle with the local bishop over the order of procession on feast days. See Stuart B. Schwartz, "The King's Processions: Municipal and Royal Authority and the Hierarchies of Power in Colonial Salvador," in *Portuguese Colonial Cities in the Early Modern World*, ed. Liam Matthew Brockey (Burlington, VT: Ashgate, 2008), 177–203.

[41] Dauril Alden and Joseph C. Miller, "Out of Africa: The Slave Trade and the Transmission of Smallpox to Brazil, 1560–1831," *The Journal of Interdisciplinary History* 18 (1987): 200; Schwartz, "Indian Labor," 52.

[42] *DHAM-AC*, vol. 1, 39–40. The filth of the city as a cause of disease was itself of growing concern as evinced in *DHAM-AC*, vol. 1, 7, 19, 22, and 315–316; and *DHAM-AC*, vol. 5, 78.

[43] And violators who attempted to evade such inspections paid a penalty of 40 cruzados. On these shifts see *DHAM-AC*, vol. 1, 39–40; and *DHAM-AC*, vol. 6, 22–30.

[44] Joseph C. Miller, *Way of Death: Merchant Capitalism and the Angolan Slave Trade, 1730–1830* (Madison, WI: University of Wisconsin Press, 1988), especially 418–425; Alden and Miller, "Out of Africa"; and Hemming, *Red Gold*, 148–149.

Abreu's *Tratado de las siete enfermedades* spoke to their multiple, overlapping concerns. Abreu wrote it as a guidebook. Part field manual (in Spanish), part learned treatise (in Latin), he addressed it to those most in need of it and best able to use it: medically untrained but literate laypersons having to sort out diseases and treat them on their own – not only slave traders, Jesuits, and *senhores de engenho* but many people on either side of the Iberian Atlantic – as well as university trained physicians eager to learn what one of Abreu's supporters described as "things of medicine very particular and necessary in order to avoid the gravest illnesses."[45] Abreu delivered. In some five hundred pages of printed text, his *Tratado* identified with approximate precision some nine distinct afflictions – more, even, that the title *Tratado de las siete enfermedaades* (or *Treatise of Seven Diseases*) promised (Figure 7.2).

Abreu based all of this on a careful reading of ancient texts (he dealt at length with Galen and Avicenna), and on his own investigations of the afflicted. In the pages of the *Tratado* – under the discipline of Galenic medicine – the bodies and fluids of the living and the entrails of the dead came under close scrutiny. Although at once bookish and diligent in his clinical work, Abreu would not escape the shadow of ontological and epistemological uncertainty that Gândavo had identified so very presciently.

Taken together, five infirmities constituted the heart of the *Tratado* and comprised its principal case study. Each of these afflictions was related and they all began with a single humoral imbalance that Abreu described as a corruption of the bile located principally in the liver and in "its neighboring parts."[46] The "inflammation" of the liver spread by way of the veins to the omentum, pyloris, and kidneys, and collectively comprised a condition that Abreu termed "universal inflammation" (because it was generalized throughout the abdominal cavity). In the course of treatment – and, as Abreu was wont to point out on several occasions, especially when treated improperly – the original illness ("universal inflammation") could undergo a succession of "transmutations" (to use Abreu's preferred term).[47] These material changes in the illness itself led to a cascade of subsequent and overlapping afflictions. Abreu identified two such transmutations. The first led to the disease of "satyriasis" (an uncontrollable yearning for sex). The second resulted to the condition

---

[45] Abreu, *Tratado*, [unnumbered page 3].   [46] Abreu, *Tratado*, 17.

[47] He repeated it often. See, for example, Abreu, *Tratado*, 23, 88v, 90, 91v, 116v, 234, 388, 450v.

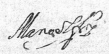

TRATADO DE LAS
SIETE ENFERMEDADES,

De la inflammacion vniuerſal del Higado, Zirbo,
Pyloron, y Riñones, y de la obſtrucion, de la
Satiriaſi, de la Terciana y febre maligna,
y paſsion Hipocondriaca.

Lleua otros tres Tratados, del mal de Loanda, del Guzano,
y de las Fuentes y Sedales.

Dirigido al Reuerendiſsimò Señor P. Fr. Antonio de Soto
Mayor, Confeſſor de la Real y Catholica Mageſtad del
Rey Don Philippe IIII. nueſtro Señor, Rey de
las Eſpañas, y ~~de Portugal.~~

Autor el Licenciado Alexo de Abreu, Medico del miſmo Señor, y de
los Miniſtros, y Officiales del Conſejo de Hazienda, y de los
Cuentos del Reyno y caſa de Portugal.

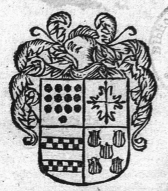

Con licencia de la S. Inquiſicion, Ordinario, y Rey.

En Lisboa, por Pedro Craesbeeck Impreſſor del Rey. Año 1623.
¶ A coſta del Autor. ¶ Vendeſe en caſa de

FIGURE 7.2 Emblem of Medical Uncertainty. The title page from physician
Aleixo de Abreu's *Tratado de las siete enfermedades* (Lisbon: Pedro
Craesbeeck, 1623).
Courtesy of the Biblioteca Nacional de Portugal.

of "hypochondria" (by which Abreu and his contemporaries meant a deep and lasting melancholy). Hence from a single illness could come many.

Curiosity was important to the reception of Abreu's book. In language indicative of the appeal that the *Tratado* had to metropolitan readers generally, one Inquisitorial censor insisted that Abreu had "ingeniously and learnedly" suggested "many particularities and curiosities not commonly known." Abreu's documentation of four afflictions "unknown to ... ancient [authors]" was symptomatic of the generalized metropolitan interest in novelty, and suggestive of the way in which it continued to propel medical inquiry.[48] Indeed, two of the four novel diseases – mal de Luanda and mal del guzano – each received an essay of its own.[49]

But in Lisbon by the 1620s, a focus on curiosities was especially problematic for a physician in Abreu's position. The issue was twofold. First, curiosities themselves had begun to lose some of their cache. They were now, as the poet Chancelaria put it decades earlier, "quite common." Other aspects of natural inquiry, however, had grown in importance. For audiences in metropolitan Lisbon in the early seventeenth century, new knowledge was increasingly valued for its potential contribution to the common weal.[50] Abreu was well aware of these shifts and composed his book accordingly – an aspect of the *Tratado* not lost on Inquisitorial censors. Its treatments, one noted, appeared "learned and tried (*experimentado*) by the author." Given such proofs of its utility, the reviewer continued, the "printing [of the *Tratado*] would serve the common good."[51]

The second problem with novelty was that, apart from the quality of novelty itself, the reportage of seemingly new diseases was (much like that

---

[48] Abreu, *Tratado*, 199v.

[49] These were inserted separately and at the end of the *Tratado*. Mal de Luanda (meaning "the disease of Luanda"), which was characterized by chest pain, weak legs, and lethargy, with dark, painful, suppurating gums and foul breath; mal del guzano ("disease of the worm") was identified as the consequence of the rotting of the internal organs and typified by the appearance of countless small worms along the intestines to the rectum and anus. Two others remained unnamed, were buried deep within the main text of the *Tratado*, and were afforded no therapeutic attention at all. One resulted in a worm that resembled a small flea and that grew between the toes and in the soles of the feet of its victims. Another gave rise to worms that grew "in the legs of men." See Abreu, *Tratado*, 161, 199v–200. On the modern diagnosis of these, see below and 219, n. 34 above.

[50] This was an increasingly common refrain throughout Europe. See, for example, the discussion in Daston and Park, *Wonders*, 231–239.

[51] Abreu, *Tratado*, [unnumbered page 3].

of novel *materia medica*) of dubious clinical value. Their causes (or, in the case of plants, their curative properties) lay in a tangle of occult influences. There could be no certain knowledge about them. And it was certain knowledge – *scientia* – that underwrote the medical corpus in which Abreu had been schooled. Also, (and again, much like novel plants), unusual diseases were exceedingly difficult to fit within the Hippocratic-Galenic textual tradition, and yet the practice of commentary and debate in dialogue with claims of that tradition were a hallmark of learned medicine.[52]

Medical curiosities *qua* curiosities neither served the interests of public utility nor satisfied the demands of professional medicine. Abreu had to approach the afflictions of the Atlantic in a way that reconciled both the needs of patrons and laypersons (who prioritized useful recommendations for the treatment of disease) and the demands of his profession (for which nuanced explorations of the cause and transformation of disease remained vital). Abreu's solution was to focus the *Tratado* on the problem of fever, and especially tertian fever. It was at once a confounding and eminently useful affliction.

Running throughout the entire *Tratado* – uniting its principle case study (the tripartite account of the transmutation of the universal inflammation first into satyriasis and then into hypochondria) and the coverage of both mal de Luanda and mal del guzano – was an abiding concern for tertian fever. Tertian fever occurred simultaneously with each of the other afflictions discussed in the *Tratado* and it persisted despite their successive transmutations. To Abreu, it was not at all clear that the tertian fever that accompanied each of these successive ailments was in fact the same fever. In an aside placed awkwardly within his principal case study, he elaborated on what he determined were three different kinds of tertian fever. One was a standard tertian fever characterized by febrile paroxysms that occurred regularly on every third day. This fever, he was sure, accompanied the panoply of diseases that began with liver inflammation and led to hypochondria. Yet there was also a more unusual kind of fever – one that Abreu believed to be, in fact, two overlapping but nevertheless distinct fevers. One, a malignant fever, was constant but grew progressively more

---

[52] The failure of learned medicine, wedded as it was to those practices and that corpus, to satisfactorily handle novel diseases increasingly undermined its credibility within Europe in this period. See Roger French, *Medicine before Science: The Business of Medicine from the Middle Ages to the Enlightenment* (New York: Cambridge University Press, 2003), 150–153, and 157–164.

severe. The other was similar to the standard tertian fever but was more erratic. Abreu called it "semi-tertian."[53]

Three fevers were at issue. Two were tertian. These were promiscuous and evasive but ubiquitous. According to Abreu, a tertian fever of one kind or another was always involved in the infirmities whose courses he chronicled and whose treatments he prescribed. As a matter of practical medicine, an extended exploration of tertian fever and its related afflictions had at least one major shortcoming. It was pox, not fever, that posed the greatest danger to the sugar economy in Brazil. Given Abreu's transatlantic itinerary and his years at work in both Angola and Pernambuco, the physician well knew that it was an abiding concern for pox that repeatedly led to the practices of quarantine, triage, and the bodily inspection of the enslaved. Pox, however, as a fashionable topic of learned medical debate had begun to wane in metropolitan medical circles. That made it correspondingly less useful in Abreu's pursuit of notoriety and professional advancement in Lisbon – where, after all, pox seemed to pose rather little threat. But even if he had thought pox still worthy of extended discussion, it was also true that Abreu – whose claims to authority in the *Tratado* and whose hopes for promotion in metropolitan Lisbon rested firmly on his overseas tenure and on his intimate knowledge of the bodies of the afflicted – had not been personally privy to a pox epidemic. Pox coursed through the Atlantic system and erupted with particular fury in Brazil both before and after Abreu's tenure, but not during the four years in which Abreu was actually there.[54] Hence, despite so much concern for pox in Brazil, not one single page in the *Tratado* was given over to an account of it.

By contrast, as an intellectual problem, fever – and especially tertian fever – had several advantages. Whereas pox seemed to threaten health and prosperity only in Brazil, tertian fever seemed to occur throughout the Atlantic. Abreu found that tertian fever was common to Lisbon, Luanda, and Brazil alike. That made tertian fever an immanently useful topic of inquiry, for it was relevant to all of the principal locations of Portugal's Atlantic empire.

Tertian fever and the associated trifecta of inflammation, satyriasis, and hypochondria were also ideal topics of inquiry and disquisition because they held distinct advantages both epistemic and therapeutic. Abreu personally suffered from each of these ailments. He could claim

---

[53] Abreu, *Tratado*, 72v–73v.
[54] This according to the chronology given in Alden and Miller, "Out of Africa."

to have observed them with utmost immediacy. Abreu's own most enduring and debilitating diseases were thus also his surest source of knowledge. And indeed, in the *Tratado* Abreu took himself and his own experience with tertian fever and its affiliated illnesses as the case study upon which he built his analysis.

It was also true that fevers, though pervasive, were rather ethereal entities. They were well suited to theoretical discussion but not for practical medicine. This gave Abreu no small amount of liberty. For he could discuss this principal malady but not actually worry about treating it. For a treatise designed to establish Abreu's reputation in both philosophical and clinical circles, tertian fever was the perfect affliction. And in fact, apart from the intermittent theoretical discussion in Latin aimed at peer physicians, Abreu frequently noted the presence of tertian fever but rarely discussed the treatment of it directly. Instead, Abreu focused the *Tratado* on rather less arcane and rather more definite and tangible matter: organs, *materia medica*, recipes, and the day-to-day business of bedside care.

What made tertian fever most useful was that fevers in general and intermittent fevers in particular had a long and distinguished pedigree. They were among the most prominent topics in the corpus of medical learning long required of university-trained physicians in Portugal.[55] As Abreu would have learned as a medical student in Coimbra, each intermittent fever was supposed to have a distinct prognosis. A quartan fever, for example, was often deadly. A tertian fever, by contrast, was more benign and could be expected to pass. Its victims would live. Exploration and settlement carried that framework and its attendant expectations into the Atlantic, where – as among the Jesuit missionaries in Brazil – such terms as *quartãs* and *terças* ("quartan" and "tertian" respectively) remained indispensable to the interpretation of fever.[56]

---

[55] James D. Goodyear, "Agents of Empire: Portuguese Doctors in Colonial Brazil and the Idea of Tropical Disease" (PhD diss., Johns Hopkins University, 1985), 74–78, and 118–119, discusses Coimbra's medical curriculum in this period. Relevant to my discussion here are the Hippocratic texts (in Latin or Portuguese) including *Aforismos, De ratione victus* and *Epidemicos e prognosticos* and – crucially – those by Galen or that were heavily Galenic: *Tegne e de locis affectis, De morbo et symptomate, De diferentiis febrium, De simplicibus, De usu partium, De methodo medendi, De sanguinis missione, Ars curtiva ad Glauconem, Quos et quandro purgare conveniat, De crisibus, De diebus criticis, De naturalibus facultatibus, De pulsibus ad tirones* and *De inaequali intemperie*. To these were added two essays by Avicenna and one from Rhazes.

[56] See Chapter 6 and also Metcalf, *Go-Betweens*, ch. 5. These terms are pervasive in Jesuit letters from Brazil in the middle and late sixteenth century.

Contact with the intertropical Atlantic gave those distinctions new meaning. A bit of modern malariology helps set Abreu's interpretive dilemma in high relief. Of the four strains of malaria that affect humans, two of them – *Plasmodium vivax* and *Plasmodium malariae* – had been endemic throughout the Mediterranean since antiquity. *P. vivax* caused a tertian fever that was unpleasant but often benign. The quartan fever, by contrast, was the result of *P. malariae* and was more dangerous. Along the Guinea Coast, a third strain of malaria predominated. This was *P. falciparum*; it mimicked the tertian fever of *P. vivax* but was much more virulent than either of the Mediterranean variants.[57] When the Portuguese and other Europeans ventured southward into the Atlantic, they did so with the understanding that quartan fevers were deadly but that tertian fevers, if treated properly, would subside.[58] With exposure to *P. falciparum*, tertian fever became a much more ambiguous and often more virulent affliction. Of course, neither ancient authors nor their early modern readers – including Abreu – interpreted intermittent fevers (be they tertian or quartan) as symptoms of the bodily invasion of malarial protozoa. They knew them as distinct ailments signalled by the unique periodicity of the fevers themselves.

As a diagnostic category, tertian fever had been thrown into disarray. With seafaring and settlement in the African Atlantic – it had become the ambiguous marker of a far deadlier affliction. Even if it did not necessarily pose the most pronounced threat to any single theatre of colonial activity (as pox did in Brazil), fever was nevertheless valuable to Abreu because it was an enigmatic and distinctly pan-Atlantic affliction. Not only were theoretical investigations of fever a staple in the textual practices of scholarly physicians (which made it professionally useful), but – because it could now be so much more lethal – identifying and treating tertian fever had become a much more urgent concern. Tertain fever was a practical and professional asset.

As Abreu explained to his readers, observational discipline was the surest way out of the epidemiological morass. Outlasting any of the maladies linked to tertian fever – and, by extension, surviving in

---

[57] Frederick L. Dunn, "Malaria," in Kiple, ed., *Cambridge World History of Human Disease*, 855–862; Webb, *Humanity's Burden*, 20–41. The fourth strain, *P. ovalae*, does not figure prominently in the historiography of this period so I do not discuss it here. In all cases the observed periodicity of each fever is the consequence of the reproductive cycle of the parasite.

[58] See the discussion in Robert Sallares, *Malaria and Rome: A History of Malaria in Ancient Italy* (New York: Oxford, 2002), 17–22.

Portugal's Atlantic colonies – meant properly identifying the disease in question and matching it with its remedy. Abreu's readers were to learn how to do the former and concoct the latter. Only with the proper signs read and a proper diagnosis achieved could the most effective remedy be put to good use. For that reason, in a medical sense, Abreu taught his readers to see what they otherwise could not: the invisible inner-workings of the body. He laid out the most important indices of humoral activity up front: the pulse, stools, urine, sleep and dreams.[59] A direct somatic engagement with these – when considered together, not in isolation – would allow even the uninitiated young missionary or unseasoned seaman (were he literate) to envision and interpret the inner-workings of the body, things which were not themselves susceptible to direct experience.

To support this kind of "reading" (my word, not Abreu's), the doctor offered a discussion of the internal organs of the body's central cavity. And in a metaphor that serves as a reminder of the kind of gendered milieu in which medicine was taught, learned, and practiced, Abreu explained why it was that he referred to the initial infirmity as an "inflammation of the liver," even as he explained at length that the principal humoral imbalance shifted between the liver, kidneys, and "neighbouring parts":

As it is common among learned men when in the house of someone taken ill, be that person one of the children or the wife or any other person living therein, although the man of the house be not taken ill, it is said for that reason [his being the head of the household] that it is he who is taken ill, then so too with infirmities: because just as the man is the principal of the home, when the neighboring parts of the liver are affected, whatever they may be, it is called the inflammation of the liver.[60]

Patriarchy, it seems, had a knack for investing even the body with an intelligible order. The most invisible bodily recesses – though rank and fetid – were susceptible to its metaphor.[61] Ideas of household order helped make medical sense of the body. That they could do so was critical for Abreu's treatise to get the readership he wanted and which – again, according to his Inquisitorial censors – the empire badly needed.

---

[59] Abreu, *Tratado*, [unnumbered page 19].   [60] Abreu, *Tratado*, 26.

[61] Here I take inspiration from the discussions of both Linnaean botany and the origins of the taxonomic category of "mammalia" in Londa Schiebinger, *Nature's Body: Gender in the Making of Modern Science*, 2nd edn. (New Brunswick, NJ: Rutgers University Press, 2004), chs 1 and 2.

A penetrating gaze was not enough. The external signs of internal bodily activity still had to be accumulated, collated, and interpreted. Especially for a disease that might undertake an endless series of permutations (Abreu, after all, never claimed to have exhausted all possible outcomes), momentary measures of humoral imbalance were simply inadequate. What the physician needed was an elaboration of humoral change across roughly standard measures of time. Most of the *Tratado* was given over to a lengthy case study of the original disease and what Abreu referred to as its successive "transmutations" – from liver inflammation (*inflamación del higado*), to excessive sexual excitation (*satiriasi*), and finally deep depression (*hypochondria*).

Throughout the *Tratado*, Abreu modeled the kind of observational discipline and interpretive prudence he thought necessary to discern the transformations of one sickness into another. He kept a record of daily assessments that included both the day's date and the total number of days since the onset of a given illness. He noted in particular those days when symptoms ("accidents") grew more or less severe, more or less erratic. He built his argument for the development of distinct diseases and drew distinctions between them based on these observations. In this way, the *Tratado* taught its readers how to envision and interpret the body, read its effluvia and excrescences, distinguish between maladies, and determine the moments in which they were transformed.

No practical manual such as this would have been complete without guidance on the treatment of the various afflictions it described. Abreu packed the *Tratado* with medicinal recipes for what seemed to him to be every conceivable eventuality. Limiting his recommendations to only the recipes that were, in his words, "most effective as judged by my own experience," he drew on an imperial pharmacopoeia that bore all of the signs of the Asian trade that helped produce it, and little of the plant matter native to sub-Saharan Africa or South America that remained marginal within it.[62] Indeed, the *Tratado* was a veritable index of the extent to which the *materia medica* featured in Orta's *Coloquios* dominated an imperial curative repertoire common to Lisbon, Luanda, and the coast of Brazil. Abreu's recipes required cinnamon, rhubarb, neem, cardamom, opium, red and white sandal, ginger grass, tamarind, and aloes.[63] But it said nothing of such things as the balamban described by

---

[62] I discuss these in the following chapter.

[63] Abreu, *Tratado*, 47, 78–78v. According to Carney and Rosomoff, *Shadow of Slavery*, 24 and 33, tamarind was actually of sub-Saharan African provenance.

Pereira in the Atlantic (discussed in Chapter 1) or tobacco, the "holy herb" (*erva santa*) described by Jesuits and many others in Brazil (see the discussion in Chapter 6 and the notes there).[64]

So what, after all, did those who consult the *Tratado* learn about disease in the sprawling Iberian empire that had been bound together by the union of the Crowns? They saw that the Atlantic, rather than a more expansive intertropical world, constituted a coherent epidemiological region. Its most debilitating characteristic diseases were all linked to tertian fever. In practice however, diagnostic and therapeutic labor focused on organs and humors. Despite Abreu's tenure in Brazil and despite that region's evident natural abundance and economic importance, therapeutics from Portuguese America were conspicuous in the *Tratado* only by their absence. Treatment drew on an imperial pharmacopoeia of European and Asian origin.

By Abreu's own admission, the product of his efforts was less than convincing. Even after so much disciplined observation of his own, Abreu harbored severe doubts about the distinctions he had drawn. He opened the *Tratado* with an almost apologetic discussion of the "difficulties of writing a book."[65] Even great minds failed, he reminded his readers: "Homer, too, occasionally fell asleep."[66] This should be read neither as a sheepish introduction to an otherwise sly critique of authoritative medical authors, nor as an instance of the time-honored tactic of obfuscation for the sake of plausible deniability and the protection of his own medical reputation.[67] Rather, deeply aware that his evident confusion laid the *Tratado* open to sharp criticism or, worse still, outright dismissal, Abreu outfitted his treatise with a lengthy discussion on the proper conduct of physicians when faced with such uncertainty and divided in opinion. It was to remain a guarded secret – something that was best kept between specialists and altogether beyond the view of the patient.

There could hardly have been a more pointed testament to the seemingly enigmatic nature of fevers in the Atlantic and the uncertainty of learned medicine in the face of them. Far from a text precociously inaugurating the field of tropical medicine, Abreu's book remained confusingly imprecise to generations of readers. In the *Tratado de las siete*

---

[64] On the shifting impressions of tobacco for the period, see Norton, *Sacred Gifts*, especially 47–61 and 114–120.

[65] Abreu, *Tratado*, [unnumbered pages 8–20].

[66] Abreu, *Tratado*, [unnumbered page 13].

[67] McVaugh, *Medicine before the Plague*, 136–144 and 166–189; French, *Medicine before Science*, 99–107.

enfermedades, the author seemed to promise his readers precisely that – a discussion of *seven* illnesses. The title page appeared to articulate precisely which infirmities were under discussion. Yet the grammar and syntax of the original title itself were none too clear. How these diseases were to be counted was anything but certain. So confounding were the title and text that one nineteenth-century Spanish reader finally dismissed the whole book as mere "gibberish."[68]

Although I have here divided *the Tratado* in such a way as to render seven plausibly distinct illnesses, these are not exactly the divisions that Abreu drew within the text itself, and according to which he organized his book. Where the author was surest of his findings – as with hypochondria and mal de Luanda – he assigned individual maladies their own self-contained chapter.[69] But with most illnesses the chapters overlapped. The discussion of ostensibly distinct ailments were split. He argued that liver and kidney inflammations were part of a single malady and treated the nondescript "obstruction" as one of a number of factors leading to satyriasis. He said almost nothing at all of the tertian fever that accompanied the initial inflammation of the liver (the exception being a single stray comment about day forty-two). Unsure of whether or not the tertian and (constant) malignant fevers were in fact distinct infirmities (in what circumstances a patient might suffer from two fevers simultaneously was a longstanding point of discussion[70]), Abreu included them together in a single chapter and offered the same recipes for their treatment. The tertian fever that Abreu thought provoked the development of small worms in the rectal cavity – the affliction of mal del guzano – was treated both as a possible transformation of the original liver inflammation (in his first chapter) *and* as a separate illness (later in Chapter 8). Whereas in the earlier mention he argued for their interconnection and referred readers to the latter section, when he finally took up the discussion in the latter section he did so without any reference at all to the originating illness or the tertian fever. Precisely where many of these illnesses were located was no less a matter of uncertainty. That metaphor equating the liver with the head of a household only served to elide Abreu's evident confusion about which organ might actually house the inflammation. To buttress his claim that a clearer distinction was inessential, he launched into a lengthy

---

[68] Bartolome Jose Gallardo, *Ensayo de una Biblioteca Española de libros raros y curiosos … aumentados por … M. R. Zarco del Valle y J. Sancho Rayón*, 4 vols. (Madrid: M. Rivadaneyra, 1863–1889), quoted in Guerra, "Aleixo de Abreu, 57.
[69] Abreu, *Tratado*, 201–213v.   [70] Hamlin, *More than Hot*, 125–148.

discussion of why that was so and concluded – in concurrence with Galen – that "so many distinctions are not pertinent."[71]

GEOGRAPHIES OF MEDICAL AUTHORITY

Ambrósio Fernandes Brandão almost certainly never read Abreu's work. The physician and the sugar planter ran in the same imperial circles (Brandão counted the imperial treasurer among his friends; Abreu would later become his personal physician) but they sailed the Atlantic in different directions. In 1583, as Abreu was finishing his medical studies at Coimbra, Brandão was preparing to set out for Brazil as a collector of taxes. By 1594, when Abreu made passage to Luanda, Brandão had become a prosperous merchant, led a militia of his peers in the conquest of Paraíba (north of Pernambuco), and battled against native Tupí in the Brazilian interior. In Pernambuco, Brandão held titles to land and owned the *engenho* of São Bento in the parish of São Lourenço da Mata. He also maintained a household in Olinda. Abreu was still in Luanda when, in 1597, Brandão returned to Lisbon. By the time Abreu returned to the imperial capital in 1606, Brandão had made a successful living there as a civil servant. He had managed to cultivate relationships with the treasurer of Lisbon, the bishop of Coimbra, a number of Portuguese governors, and the royal treasurer. If the two met at all, it would have been in Lisbon in 1606 or 1607. Whether Abreu had begun writing the *Tratado* by then or had yet begun to reflect upon and talk openly about his pan-Atlantic observations, is unclear. By the time Abreu's manuscript had begun to change hands in Lisbon (although perhaps only among censors) in 1621, Brandão had long since returned to Pernambuco (probably in 1608). He penned the *Diálogos* there in the first half of 1618.[72]

Had Brandão met Abreu, discussed diseases in the Atlantic with him, or read some part of Abreu's treatise, Brandão would have found much to agree with. The afflictions that Brandão thought characteristic of Brazil were almost identical to those of Abreu. He identified tertian and quartan fevers, *mal do bicho* (mal del guzano), pox, and the oddly shaped creature that seemed to infest the feet, and added a gastro-intestinal affliction – a mild form of the dysentery (*mordexim*) that he knew to afflict Goa as well

[71] Abreu, *Tratado*, 93v.
[72] Brandão's biography is carefully reconstructed by José Antonio Gonsalves de Mello, ed., *Diálogos das Grandezas do Brasil*, 2nd edn. (Recife: Imprensa Universitária, 1966), x–xx.

and which, in Brazil as in Goa, was accompanied by fever, abdominal pain, and frequent diarrhea. Mild fever and chills, Brandão explained, "tested" anyone who came to Portuguese America. Anyone who stayed was likely to grapple as well with tertian and quartan fevers – agues "common to everyone," and which varied in intensity, Brandão explained, according to one's peculiar "nature and constitution." Those fevers and the occasional dysentery were the result of the climate of the colonies but were never severe. Suffering them constituted a process of acclimation. But these passed with ease and posed a far smaller threat than Abreu would have suggested. According to Brandão, Brazil enjoyed distinctly "auspicious skies and [a] good climate."[73]

Like Abreu, Brandão debated the possibility of the epidemiological and environmental coherence of the Atlantic, not of the intertropical world. But he did so in way that refuted even the coherence of the intertropical Atlantic. Abreu's vision of the Atlantic as a unified and internally consistent epidemiological region elided what Brandão argued were crucial differences that distinguished one side of the Atlantic from the other. Local climatic variations brought by wind and rain produced distinct landscapes and made even the intertropical Atlantic environmentally and epidemiologically heterogeneous. For Brandão, the Atlantic was a region of undeniable complexity.[74] To explain how that was so, Brandão mustered the same collection of texts – among them Ptolemy, Albertus Magnus, Sacrobosco: all dissenters from the Aristotelian vision of the torrid zone – that I have argued were crucial points of reference for observers of the first sub-Saharan voyages in the fifteenth-century. The entire region between the Tropic of Cancer and the Tropic of Capricorn, Brandão explained in the *Diálogos*, may be subject to the extreme heat of the sun. But South America was bathed by cool breezes that blew in from the Atlantic. They brought moisture and tempered the heat of the sun. On the African side, Brandão surmised, the winds arrived in western Africa only after traversing an expansive and scorching continental interior.[75] The air was thereby rendered hot and dry. Those qualities made the air more pernicious and the whole region less healthy.

---

[73] Rodolfo Garcia, ed., *Diálogos das grandezas do Brasil* (Rio de Janeiro: Tecnoprint Gráfica, 1968), 132–150, and especially 133–134, 143, 145–146.

[74] See the discussion in Chapter 1 and the notes there.

[75] Brandão may have known that contemporary reports identified that landscape as characteristic of much of the interior of southern Africa, as had, for example Brito, *Inquérito*.

Those regional differences in the Atlantic were foundational for Brandão's account of disease in Brazil. Southern African winds, he argued, produced South American epidemics. They deposited pernicious substances upon the bodies of the inhabitants, which came with enslaved Africans across Atlantic. Brandão called these entities "seeds" (*sementes*). And it was these seeds that produced the various kinds of pox (*bexigas* and *sarampo*) and the "burning fevers" that Brandão counted as the most dangerous afflictions in Portuguese America.

The competing accounts of disease that Abreu and Brandão offered their readers highlights an important dynamic usually left out of histories of medicine and natural history in this period. In their explanations of disease, the physician and the planter staked out divergent positions both supported by the Hippocratic-Galenic medical corpus. Abreu's explanation of disease emphasized humors to the near exclusion of environmental factors. His was a deeply Galenic theoretical orientation that focused on the nonnaturals (especially exertion) and medicine to restore humoral balalnce. Brandão was much more eclectic. His account emphasized environmental determinants of disease and ignored any discussion of their humoral aspects. His references to climate and exertion were consonant with the Hippocratic-Galenic framework. But his claim that disease was brought as seeds and invaded susceptible bodies – that it was external and communicable – amounted to a theory of contagion. These divergent explanations accurately reflected the wider field of contemporary medical debate. Brandão's explanation was not an escape of Galenism but a resort to one of Galen's minor works – one that had been resuscitated in the debates over plague and pox in the early sixteenth century.

What makes all of this so striking is that Brandão, of course, was not a physician. The most careful examination of his life to date has suggested that he had little formal education at all.[76] In the world of learned medicine, Brandão was an interloper. He could not have participated in the kind of line-by-line commentary that consumed so much of Abreu's energy (and so many pages of the *Tratado*). And yet his tenure in the Atlantic had emboldened him to claim authority on some of the finer points of medical theory. Just as the enigma of nature drew physicians and a growing contingent of others to its study, so the enigma of disease

---

[76] See Mello, ed., *Diálogos*, x–xx.

enabled non-specialists to participate increasingly in the very discursive practices – debate over competing, textually-grounded, theoretically informed explanations – that university-trained physicians had insisted for centuries distinguished and elevated the medicine they proffered.[77] In the Atlantic, authority even on matters of canonical medical theory was up for grabs. Indeed, Brandão made no secret of his disdain of physicians in Brazil who stumbled through diagnosis and treatment in a hollow attempt to "secure a learned reputation" (*por serem reputados por cientes*).[78]

COSMOPOLITANISM, NATIVE SECRETS, AND THE PLANTER-NATURALIST

It was not disease but the plants and animals of Portuguese America that were Brandão's principal interest. A propagandist of the colony, Brandão's unwavering insistence on Brazilian health was an extension of earlier claims inaugurated by Caminha and reinforced by the Jesuit reportage I explored in the last chapter. Much else that Brandão wrote in the *Diálogos* would challenge what now constituted conventional wisdom concerning Brazil. Brazilian nature had been ignored for the better part of the sixteenth century. Brandão sought to change that. Most fundamentally, his extended advocacy of both the wonder and utility of Brazilian nature challenged the prevailing colonial emphasis on sugar production. Brandão wanted to draw metropolitan attention beyond the narrow focus on a single imported crop, to expand it so that it encompassed the whole blooming, buzzing, confusing, natural world of Portuguese America. This was the world that Brandão had in mind when he referred to the majesty – the "great things" (*grandezas*) – of Brazil. "Wherever I look," he wrote, beckoning to his readers, "I see leafy trees, dense forests, tangled woods, and inviting fields." "The eye," he insisted, simply "could not comprehend it all."[79]

In the *Diálogos*, Brandão wanted to help his readers do just that: more fully comprehend the therapeutic and commercial value of Brazilian nature. It would not be easy. Like both Orta in Goa and Abreu in the Atlantic, Brandão would have to undertake considerable representational

---

[77] McVaugh, *Medicine before the Plague*; French, *Medicine before Science*; and the excellent discussion in Green, *Making Women's Medicine Masculine*, ch. 1.

[78] Garcia, ed., *Diálogos*, 137, 139, 301.   [79] Garcia, ed., *Diálogos*, 197.

labor to make his claims about Brazil both meaningful and valuable to metropolitan contemporaries. But for Brandão this entailed challenges that neither of those physicians had to face. First, unlike either Orta or Abreu, Brandão had little in the way of a textual canon to orient his inquiries and vouchsafe his claims. *Maracujá* (passion fruit), to take but one example, was not among the plants discussed by Dioscorides.[80] And whereas Orta could ignore or gloss over novelties (as he did with such things as neem) in favor of things like pepper and cinnamon that were more recognizably valuable to his readers, Brandão clearly could not. The sugar planter had to make things that were once unknown to his audience and frequently denigrated by metropolitan contemporaries seem, on the contrary, indispensable to their ends – whatever those ends may be. For Brandão this would entail the elaboration of an epistemology that would embrace, rather than dismiss, esoteric knowledge of the occult forces believed by many to permeate Brazilian nature. Much as with the Jesuits – and in contrast to the dominant interpretation that insists that New World encounters and the commodification of its flora and fauna pro-pelled the disenchantment of nature – esoteric knowledge and a command of occult forces were indispensable to Brandão's natural history. They were every bit as important as the evidence of the senses in the transform-ation of New World nature into global commodities.[81]

In order to highlight the wealth, splendour, and utility of Brazilian nature, Brandão would not only have to improvise an epistemology but he would also have to cultivate a novel investigative persona. Brandão, aftera all, was a *fazendeiro*; he made his living as a sugar planter and mill owner. That occupation defined not only what a person did but what one did not do – and sugar planters, to quote a classic and still indispensable study by one of the foremost authorities of colonial Brazil, "were not much given to intellectual pursuits." Planters like Brandão were "great orators" but they were "not often friends of the pen."[82] This character-ization of the fazendeiros's *habitus* continues to resonate in scholarship on colonial Brazilian cultural and intellectual life. Yet Brandão's example

---

[80] Garcia, ed., *Diálogos*, 197, 235–262.

[81] Bauer, "New World of Secrets"; Norton, *Sacred Gifts*; Gómez, *Experiential Caribbean*. Representative of the range of alternative approaches are Anthony Pagden, *European Encounters with the New World: From Renaissance to Romanticism* (New Haven, CT: Yale University Press, 1993); Barrera-Osorio, *Experiencing Nature*; Walker, "Medicines Trade"; and Bleichmar, *Visible Empire*.

[82] Schwartz, *Sugar Plantations*, 286.

suggests that this longstanding thesis needs some qualification.[83] By the early seventeenth century, the intellectual life and investigative endeavours of sugar planters had perhaps become more dynamic and diverse than historians have recognized.

The study of nature and the cultivation of a persona I call the planter-naturalist would be an asset for Brandão. It would ultimately allow him to bridge the divergent views of wealth, status, and honour that distinguished the world of colonial sugar planters from that of their Habsburg contemporaries in metropolitan Spain and Portugal. Much like his near-contemporary Johann Joachim Becher at the Habsburg courts of northern Europe, Brandão's knowledge of New World nature made it possible for him to mediate between the heady world of merchant capital (which underwrote the development of plantation agriculture that he knew so well) and the court culture cultivated by the Habsburgs and their allies in Lisbon, to which he was an outsider and which took a rather dim view of such commercial wealth.[84]

In the *Diálogos*, Brandão began by explaining what he thought were principal challenges now facing the empire. Asian trade was faltering and, consequently, the royal purse was shrinking. Brandão's explanation and his solution were straightforward. The Crown laid out monies to cover shipbuilding, payments and privileges, stowage allowances, tax exemptions, and the housing, feeding, and equipping of soldiers to garrison the forts meant to keep the pepper trade in particular in Portuguese hulls. Brandão quoted expenses and earnings to the effect that the Crown sometimes made a little money on its Asian enterprise but that it often lost a lot more. In the face of what he saw as the declining and costly Asian trade, Brandão argued that valuable Asian plants should be cultivated instead in Brazil, where they could be more cheaply harvested and shipped.[85] The Crown, he argued, could do better in Brazil without, in Brandão's estimation, spending "one single cent."

Imperial profits, however, lay not in Asian spices alone. According to Brandão, Brazil's had a vast array of resources of its own that the Crown had yet to exploit. These resources were of two kinds. Nature abounded in the colony and its countless uses challenged the imagination. But in

---

[83] Hence the "rural planter ethos," referred to in Sweet, *Domingos Álvares*, 104.

[84] Pamela H. Smith, *The Business of Alchemy: Science and Culture in the Holy Roman Empire* (Princeton, NJ: Princeton University Press, 1994), uses Becher to explore this tension in the Habsburg dominions of northern Europe.

[85] Garcia, ed., *Diálogos*, 166–170 and 186–196.

addition to its natural resources Brazil was also possessed of untapped intellectual resources. It was true, Brandão conceded, that with so few "good apothecaries" the medicinal and other properties and the range of possible uses of so much Brazilian *naturalia* remained unknown to his metropolitan contemporaries and even to most of his peers in Brazil.[86] But theirs was not the only kind of expertise to which Brandão and his contemporaries had recourse.

Though it remained materially poor (and Brandão pointedly referenced that persistent feature of colonial life) it had otherwise become a cosmopolitan hive of intellectual and cultural exchange. That at least is the impression that Brandão gave in the *Diálogos*. He spoke of Brazil as a "public academy," a place where one could easily cultivate "all manner of civility, learn to speak well and honourably, do good business, and other such valuable things."[87] And while, in the *Diálogos*, Brandão gave little detail to support his assertions, they are a fair estimation of the kind of colony that surfaces in other parts of the documentary record for Brazil at the turn of the seventeenth century. Colonists came from diverse distant origins: enclaves like Mazagão or Arzila in North Africa, the Dutch city of Antwerp, the English Channel port of Dieppe, or Mediterranean cities like Genoa, Naples, and Smyrna. Others had itineraries still more circuitous, with pan-Atlantic travels that had taken them to Terçeira, to Lisbon and Angola, to Mexico and Madeira.[88] From Brazil, merchants in particular maintained contacts (family, friends, and co-religionists, both Christian and Jewish) that extended throughout the Atlantic to the Indian Ocean, and across the Pacific.[89] Books added heft to the baggage they brought to Brazil. Jesuit colleges kept libraries.[90] But so, too, did some sugar planters. Up and down the Brazilian coast, banned books – from a vernacular Portuguese Bible to popular romantic fiction – traded hands.[91] Clues to this traffic surfaced in testimonies

---

[86] Brandão is particularly pointed on this issue in Garcia, ed., *Diálogos*, 198–201.

[87] Garcia, ed., *Diálogos*, 184–185.

[88] AHU, ACL, CU 015, Cx. 10, doc. 926; AHU, ACL, CU 017, Cx. 3, doc. 238; *PVBC* 56, 70, 91–93, 134, 152; *PVBD* 292; *PVPC* 12, 35–38, 126–128, 141–144; *SVB*, 376, 457–458, 509–511.

[89] Subrahmanyam, *Portuguese Empire*, ch. 6; and Studnicki-Gizbert, *Nation*, ch. 4.

[90] Mark L. Grover, "The Book and the Conquest: Jesuit Libraries in Colonial Brazil," *Libraries and Culture* 28 (1993): 266–283.

[91] *PVBC* 45–46; *PVBD* 319–320; *SVB* 356–357. The book was Jorge de Montemayor, *Los siete livros de Diana* (Granada: Rene Rabut, 1564 [1559]). At least two people appeared before the first Inquisitorial and confessed having read it before passing it on. *PVBC* 44; on Domingos, Gomes Pimentel said he read it in collusion with a Jesuit friend; see *PVBC*

before the Holy Office. Jesuit Inquisitors, keen to know more, pressed for details: An author's name? Was the text printed or in manuscript? And what of the size of its leaves: Was it a standard folio, a quarto, or an octavo perhaps?[92]

The colonies teemed with natural knowledge. The authors cited by Brandão in his defense of the health of Brazil (Ptolemy, for example) would not have been out of place in a naturalist's library on either side of the Atlantic. University graduates, sugar planters, merchants, and factors alike debated such grand ideas as the diameter of the globe, its true circumference, the nature of the celestial spheres, and the meaning of the equinoctial line.[93] One of the most pronounced expressions of this cultural and intellectual ferment were the cultures of inquiry and practice that centered on the body. These were not monolithic and stable but rather dynamic and interconnected. Jesuits such as Francisco Pinto continued the tradition of missionary faith healing inaugurated in the colony by Anchieta.[94] Other Jesuits had begun the bioprospecting that would earn the Company a small fortune and a reputation as Brazil's foremost colonial naturalists.[95] Tupí shamans remained central to colonial therapeutic practices. Forms of *santidade* persisted.[96] It may have been true, as Brandão claimed, that few apothecaries had yet come to Brazil. But a number of physicians had.[97] Surgeons were legion in the seventeenth century – employed by municipalities, colonial officials, individual planters, and especially in the regiments that came to fight the fugitive slaves of Palmares in the interior and to

---

98–99. That it circulated Spanish posed little problem and in fact may indicate that a Jesuit was the source of the book. See Eduardo Javier Alonso Romo, "Português e Castelhano no Brasil Quinhentista: À Volta dos Jesuítas," *Revista de Indias* 65 (2005): 491–510.

[92] *SVB* 356–357.

[93] *PVBC* 44; *PVBC* 288–289; Garcia, ed., *Diálogos*, 98–99; *PVPC* 12–13. Literacy was imperative for keeping accounts. *Fazendeiros* like Pernambuco's Bento Teixeira opened a school "de primeiras letras."

[94] Castelnau-L'Estoile, "The Uses of Shamanism," 616–637.

[95] Serafim Leite, "Serviços de Saúde"; Asúa, "Los Jesuítas"; Walker, "Medicines Trade."

[96] Castelnau-L'Estoile, "The Uses of Shamanism"; Schwartz, *All Can be Saved*, 187.

[97] Their stories have scarcely come to light but they surface in the following documents: AHU, ACL, CU 014, Cx. 3, doc. 189; AHU, ACL, CU 015, Cx. 3, doc. 185; AHU, ACL, CU 015, Cx. 3, doc. 252; AHU, ACL, CU 015, Cx. 12, doc. 1220; AHU, ACL, CU 015, Cx. 14, doc. 1372; AHU, ACL, CU 017, Cx. 1, doc. 63; AHU, ACL, CU 017, Cx. 1, doc. 76; AHU, ACL, CU 018, Cx. 1, doc. 47.

defend against the Dutch along the coast.[98] Folk-healers – men and women, free and slave, Portuguese, African, Amerindian, or of mixed ancestry – were the healers of first resort for most colonial inhabitants.[99] Women of African descent in particular treated the pox and fevers that repeatedly pulsed through the colonies.[100] And not only did Portuguese and others depend upon African healers but so too did African-descended communities turn to university trained Portuguese physicians. In 1682 the university-trained physician João de Quintanilha was sufficiently emboldened by his work among the inhabitants of the fugitive slave settlement of Palmares to ask for recompense from the Crown.[101]

The assemblage of overlapping curative knowledges from among persons of varied combinations of indigenous, African, and European descent and identity had by the early seventeenth century, given rise to a distinctly eclectic pharmacopoeia.[102] The most knowledgeable healers according to Brandão drew on imported African and native Tupí therapeutics. And it was by virtue of the expertise of native and African-descended healers that Brandão learned what he knew of the curative properties of Brazilian nature. Potatoes and pine nuts made good purgatives. Sarsaparilla was good for the "bubonic humor" (*humor boubático*). The oil of the *copaiva* was good for dysenteries (*mordexim*) both mild and severe, and had become an object of intracolonial trade. Brandão claimed it was no being exported to Lisbon as well.[103] And just as certain drugs were assimilated into Portuguese pharmacopoeia and bought and

---

[98] AHU, ACL, CU 005, Cx. 1 doc. 36; AHU, ACL, CU 009, Cx. 2, doc. 163; AHU, ACL, CU 009, Cx. 5, doc. 618; AHU, ACL, CU 009, Cx. 6, doc. 692; AHU, ACL, CU 009, Cx. 8, doc. 829; AHU, ACL, CU 013, Cx. 1, doc. 32; AHU, ACL, CU 017, Cx. 3, doc. 238; AHU, ACL, CU 017, Cx. 5, doc. 501. They also surface in a number of Inquisition files: *PVBD* 281, 301, 323; *PVPC* 16; *SVB* 460.

[99] Souza, *The Devil in the Land of the Holy Cross*, 103–105; Sweet, *Recreating Africa*, 139–160; Timothy D. Walker, "The Role and Practices of the Female Folk Healer in the Early Modern Portuguese Atlantic World," in *Women of the Iberian Atlantic*, eds. Sarah E. Owens and Jane E. Mangan (Baton Rouge, LA: Louisiana State University Press), 148–173.

[100] Simão Pinheiro Morão, *Queixas repetidas em ecos dos arrecifes de Pernambuco contra os abusos medicos que nas suas capitanias se observam tanto em dano das vidas de seus habitants*, ed. Jaime Walter (Lisbon: Junta de Investigações do Ultramar, 1965 [1677]); Walker, "The Role and Practices."

[101] *SVB*, 453–455; AHU, ACL, CU 015, Cx. 12, doc. 1220. On the timing, see Thornton, *Cultural History*, 297.

[102] The situation parallels that described for the Caribbean in the same period by Gómez, *Experiential Caribbean*, ch. 5.

[103] Garcia, ed., *Diálogos*, 141–147.

sold in Lisbon apothecary shops, so, too, were imported flora from Europe and Africa incorporated into the curative repertoire of the native persons whom Brandão referenced so frequently. From Luanda came both *guandu* and guinea peas. In Brazil, they found their way into recipes culinary and curative.[104]

From this eclectic "academy" of natural knowledge, Brandão learned that many of the fruits, leaves, stems, or seeds that were part of the enigmatic array of Brazilian nature "possessed within themselves the greatest powers and occult qualities."[105] His appreciation for such esoteric knowledge of nature's hidden powers did not end there. But it was not unequivocal either. More than any other aspect of his *Diálogos*, Brandão's handling of indigenous place myths evinced the ambiguity toward such knowledge that suffused his account. He dismissed rumors that certain caves deep within Pernambuco would kill any Portuguese who entered. But he would not go so far as to "put [those rumors] to the test."[106] And when he heard of the carvings that adorned a certain cave along the Araçuagipe River in Paraíba, he would neither dismiss them as a sign of diabolical ritual nor as the unintelligible product of a savage mind. Instead, he confessed, the markings were enigmatic, indecipherable, and best left for "those with greater understanding."[107] The unseen forces at work within Tupí ritual sites could neither be confirmed, as pajés might insist nor denied as Jesuit missionaries were so often wont to do. Place myths, and the hidden forces that well might inhabit them, were best left untested.[108]

Attention to so much natural knowledge – the consequence of a certain cosmopolitan curiosity that, in the *Diálogos*, Brandão attempted to model – could fill a tome more valuable than that of Dioscorides himself. This was a "public academy" indeed. Both colonial inhabitants and metropolitan collectors had, in different ways, borne witness to indigenous ingenuity. Manioc would prove poisonous were it not for the manipulations of native women. Brightly-colored plumed capes like the one that adorned the cabinet of Manfredo Settala in Milan would have been distinctly monochromatic were it not for the technique of

---

[104] Garcia, ed., *Diálogos*, 235–239.   [105] Garcia, ed., *Diálogos*, 197.
[106] Garcia, ed., *Diálogos*, 77.   [107] Garcia, ed., *Diálogos*, 72–73.
[108] Nor was credence in the hidden powers of New World nature in this period a uniquely Iberian affair. See Cañizares-Esguerra, *Puritan Conquistadors*, ch. 4; and Parrish, *American Curiosity*, ch. 7.

tapirage, by which skilled Tupí cultivated variously colored feathers on the backs of live birds.[109] Brandão noted both.[110]

The implications were not to be missed. Turning poison into food was an ambition of the alchemist. Art that imitated nature was an achievement of the skilled artisan, painter, or sculptor.[111] These were useful skills indeed.

Yet to say so much in Portuguese America in these years was particularly dangerous. It was on this point that Brandão's efforts put him in a tenuous position. It amounted to giving quarter to the very kinds of knowledge that, as I argued in the last chapter, was at issue in the duels between Jesuit missionaries and Tupí pajés. Brandão readily conceded the "savagery" (*barbaridade*) of many of Brazil's natives and he revisited what was now a common set of accusations.[112] They lacked any proper kind of religion, law, or politics; "if they worshiped anything at all," he quipped, it was "the devil."[113] They were not only lascivious but the ritual of couvade, in which postpartum women nurtured their men, was an especially unexpected and unsettling subversion of the gender norms that structured the world of Brandão and his countrymen. The natives were vindictive by nature, killed with brutish violence, and ritually feasted on human flesh, and they strung the teeth of their victims on necklaces grown weighty with victory and death.

And yet along with so much depravity, Brandão insisted, there was also virtue. If some were lascivious, others were chaste. Through the couvade, women displayed humility and resignation. Brazil's native communities were riven with factionalism, yes, but they could also be compassionate and fiercely loyal to one another.[114] Brandão vigorously advocated the view that the occult knowledge of African and especially

---

[109] Amy Buono, "Crafts of Color," 235–246. On the circuits that channeled such items to Italy see also Novoa, "Unicorns and Bezoars."

[110] Garcia, ed., *Diálogos*, 278–279.

[111] William R. Newman, *Promethean Ambitions: Alchemy and the Quest to Perfect Nature* (Chicago: University of Chicago Press, 2004); Lawrence M. Principe, *The Secrets of Alchemy* (Chicago: University of Chicago Press, 2013); Smith, *The Body of the Artisan*; Daston and Park, *Wonders*, ch. 7.

[112] Garcia, ed., *Diálogos*, 359.

[113] Garcia, ed., *Diálogos*, 333. Here Brandão also recited the commonplace quip that the language of the natives lacked the letters "f," "l," and "r," signifying the absences of *fe*, *lei*, and *rei*: faith (meaning religion), law, or king.

[114] Garcia, ed., *Diálogos*, 345–361; and for a concise explanation of the couvade see Frederick Holden Hall, William F. Harrison, and Dorothy Winters Welker, trans. and eds., *Dialogues of the Great Things of Brazil* (Albuquerque, NM: University of New Mexico Press, 1987), 330, n. 23.

native persons deserved more attention than was sanctioned by authorities. Most important – and breaking as much with the claims of a succession of more recent historians as with many of his contemporaries in Brazil – was their "keenness of sense."[115] Their search for natural omens may have been misguided but, Brandão conceded, it endowed them with a curiosity of their own. They had learned to read the signs of nature. They tracked their human quarry with diligence, precision, and deadly accuracy. They judged the changing seasons by the ripening of fruit. And they knew the stars in the heavens as well as any astrologer might. Amid abundance, they did not live in a golden age but understood the inner workings of nature and could make it do their bidding.[116]

By now, of course, Brandão was on dangerous footing. He had insisted that, in contrast to the claims of so many Jesuits, many of Brazil's native peoples were not simply in a pact with a devil nor had they been naively fooled by the fiendish trickery of his henchmen. Rather, the Tupí could reason intelligently about observable phenomena. In short, the natives may have been culturally deficient but that should not be taken as a measure of intellectual incapacity. Just as savagery did not characterize the totality of Amerindian culture, nor could it sustain the dismissal *in toto* of their knowledge of nature.

Here was the crux. What Brandão had to explain was why, if these people could reason and manipulate the forces of nature, were they culturally aberrant in so many other ways. On his ability to render this claim intellectually defensible hung the credibility of his *Diálogos* (and possibly, for all he knew, the fate of his reform proposals and his prospects for patronage and promotion). He handled this apparent contradiction by with a defence that not even Jesuit inquisitors could reject. He claimed that the natives of Brazil had learned bad habits from their ancestors.[117] So much deviant and even immoral behaviour was vestigial cultural artifice and did not – or at least should not – diminish their evident intellectual acuity when it came to matters of nature.

This very same claim had become a standard refrain among the accused in hearings before the Inquisition. It was a subtle but brilliant manoeuvre, for this was a defence that, as Brandão well knew, the

---

[115] Garcia, ed., *Diálogos*, 348. Prominent arguments that the natives could not manipulate the natural world include Todorov, *Conquest*.
[116] Garcia, ed., *Diálogos*, 357–361.   [117] Garcia, ed., *Diálogos*, 336.

Inquisition was quite likely to accept. The first visitation of the Holy Office to Brazil occurred in Bahia and Pernambuco between 1591 and 1595 – the very place and the very years in which Brandão's plantation-based fortunes were in the ascendant.[118] The forms of religious deviance that so preoccupied these inquisitors were not the disturbing habits of mind and body among the unconverted natives. They had not accepted Catholicism and could hardly be subject to the strict application of ecclesiastical law, much less accused of heresy.

Rather, when it came to suspicion of religious heterodoxy and accounts of heresy, the group in question was the New Christians. Among the practices that had become common in Brazil and which drew suspicion and accusations of crypto-Judaism were the refusal to abide by ritual fasting on Fridays and the disposal of seemingly clean water after a birth or death in the family, and sometimes for no apparent reason at all. The former had become one of the most common ways of signaling Catholic belonging in the colony; the latter raised suspicion of the ritual bathing required of adherents to Judaism. When New Christians appeared before Inquisitorial officials – some to confess, others for having been denounced – their pleas for mercy were predicated on their claim that they were good and faithful Christians who undertook the incriminating practices merely because they had learned them from their parents and grandparents before them. Otherwise, confessants and defendants would claim, they had no knowledge of why it was done and had not intended it as a subversive act. Much less was it a habit sustained by the secret practice of heretical beliefs and accidentally observed by the prying eyes of neighbors. Often enough, these claims led to exoneration or manageable forms of atonement.[119]

Inquisitorial investigations into human relations had dramatized a certain highly useful exculpatory tool. Brandão would put it to use in the service of natural inquiry. Brandão, himself a New Christian, had surely heard accounts of Inquisitorial proceedings from friends, family, and neighbors.[120] His Atlantic crossings were propelled by two

---

[118] Mello, ed., *Diálogos*, x–xx.

[119] *PVBC* 23, 31–32, 130–131, 136, 156, 173; *PVBD* 243–244; *PVPC*, 102–104, 106–107, 117–118.

[120] Inga Clendinnen, *Ambivalent Conquests: Maya and Spaniard in Yucatan* (New York: Cambridge University Press, 1987), ch. 9, masterfully explores the dynamic by which those called before the Inquisition developed shared strategies for evading conviction and punishment.

Inquisitorial investigations undertaken into his own affairs – the first in Pernambuco in 1595, the second in Lisbon in 1607. He was acquitted both times, but the process must have made him think carefully about the kinds of claims that were permissible before ecclesiastical authorities. Those were the same authorities that were most likely to grow suspicious of the networks and epistemology that underwrote Brandão's investigative work in the colony. And so, in defense of his claims, Brandão imported a strategy from ecclesiastical inquiry into colonial natural history.[121]

Brandão may have given a serviceable defense of his reliance on esoteric colonial knowledge. But that he had engaged in natural inquiry at all might itself appear remarkable. Many things should have mitigated against it. What precisely were these things? And why, and by what means, would a planter become a naturalist?

By the time Brandão first stepped ashore in Pernambuco toward the end of 1583, the practice of natural history had come to revolve around a distinct set of institutions and practices that appear to have been wanting in Brazil. The experience of nature entailed the first-hand observation of particulars, the creation of a written record of whether, where, and by whom particular plants or other unusual objects had been described before. It also entailed the communication of those findings in conversation, correspondence, print, and illustration. Travel, gardens, herbaria, menageries and cabinets, notebooks, printed texts, and pictures were all techniques for keeping account of collectively accumulated observations. Brandão's metropolitan contemporaries shuffled back and forth between the library, the cabinet, the printer's shop, the wharf, and the countryside.[122]

In the colony, things were different. Planters perhaps had relatively few books. They had no press at all. Publication was possible only in metropolitan Portugal and under the imperious eyes of Inquisitorial censors. There were no universities either. The sons of prosperous planters took university degrees at Coimbra or Evora.[123]

Also more problematic in Brazil were the peripatetic inclinations of the early modern naturalist. Brandão's contemporaries – Orta's translator

---

[121] Daston and Park, *Wonders*, ch. 6, have identified an epistemological borrowing from ecclesiastical practice to the investigation of nature, too, but of a different kind.

[122] Here I rely principally on Ogilvie, *Science of Describing*, ch. 4.

[123] Stuart B. Schwartz, ed., *A Governor and His Image in Baroque Brazil: The Funereal Eulogy of Afonso Furtado de Castro do Rio de Mondonça by Juan Lopes Sierra*, trans. Ruth Jones (Minneapolis, MN: University of Minnesota Press, 1979).

Clusius was among them (he died in 1609) – might make their way through the outskirts of Paris, the German countryside, or the Alps risking thieves and cutthroats. But in Brazil, not only were such meandering itineraries fraught with physical danger; they were also freighted with moral ambiguity.[124] Those who wandered through the colonial backlands and lived to tell their tale had often changed their food and dress, joined in native rituals, ignored Catholic ones, and frequently tattooed their bodies. Savagery, heresy, and bodily mutilation: those were the kinds of stories that interested ecclesiastical officials, and which populated the records of the Inquisition. Metropolitan travels rarely implied such personal transformation or moral transgression.[125]

Yet the most fundamental barrier to natural inquiry in the colony would appear to have been the apparent tension between the habitus of the metropolitan naturalist and that of the colonial sugar planter. The very thing naturalists spent much of their time doing – frequently and diligently examining all manner of *naturalia* – was by many accounts precisely what colonial sugar planters hoped to avoid. Naturalists got their hands dirty; planters did not.[126] These attitudes were surely strengthened at the very time that Brandão was preparing to sail for Brazil. In Portugal, the cultural influence of the Spanish Habsburgs had begun in the 1520s and deepened with the union of the Crowns in 1580. It brought, among other things, an aversion to trade, speculation, and the emergent practices of market-oriented merchant capitalism – all of which were viewed as undignified and ignoble – and instead emphasized land as the proper source of noble wealth.[127]

---

[124] In his comparison, Ogilvie, *Science of Describing*, dramatically oversimplifies the differences that marked the peripatetic adventures of European naturalists at home and in the colonies.

[125] This was perhaps particularly true for Portugal, were there were no witch hunts. See José Pedro Paiva, *Bruxaria e superstição num país sem 'caça às bruxas: Portugal, 1600–1774* (Lisbon: Editorial Notícias, 1997).

[126] The comments of Gândavo, *Tratado*, at the end of the sixteenth century; Brandão, *Diálogos*, at the beginning of the seventeenth century; and Andre João Antonil, *Cultura e opulência do Brasil por suas drogas e minas* (Lisbon: Officina Real Deslandesiana, 1711), at the beginning of the eighteenth century, each reflect this common colonial sensibility.

[127] Subrahmanyam, *Portuguese Empire*, 32–37. When the House of Aviz came to power late in the fourteenth century, merchants and master craftsmen were among its staunchest supporters. The lasting importance of seaborne trade gave early modern Lisbon a distinctly maritime orientation and the House of Aviz a commercial sensibility. By the time that Abreu and Brandão inhabited the imperial capital nearly all of its most important buildings – not just the Casa da Índia and the Paço da Ribeira but even the

Institutional poverty, moral ambiguity, and a preoccupation with the accouterments of a landed nobility would all seem to have mitigated against the emergence of a shared culture of natural inquiry in the colony. Yet the prevailing depiction of colonial Brazil as bereft of an inquisitive culture is overdrawn, the limits to intellectual inquiry overstated, and planter interest in the study of nature underestimated. By the turn of the seventeenth century, both the ever-uncertain fortunes of colonial agriculture, a Habsburg interest in collection and display, and a preoccupation with the perceived dangers of commercial wealth all combined to make the practice of colonial natural inquiry and the ownership of natural knowledge assets in ways that they had not previously been. This convergence of economic, political, and cultural shifts enabled the fashioning of a new investigative persona: the planter-naturalist. Brandão's *Diálogos* suggests how and why such a persona took shape.

If for most of the sixteenth-century planters had worried much less about cultivating natural knowledge and far more about cultivating sugarcane and a respectable public image, it was for good reason. As a group, sugar planters dominated the colonial economy and the most prosperous among them strongly influenced colonial politics. But the position of individual planter families was often tenuous. Most were from the distinctly undistinguished classes of merchants, craftsmen, or cane farmers (*lavradores de cana*). They were newly moneyed and new to the ranks of the landed elite.

In a colony without legal titles of nobility, they continually risked losing both. The brutality of chattel slavery led to everyday forms of resistance and subversion among the enslaved, and, among fazendeiros, the persistent fear of violent insurrection. Then there were the uncertainties and expenses of the business itself. Fire and drought were almost constant threats, while the contracts for resources like wood and cane – indispensable for the milling of sugar and always signed in advance of the

royal opera house – lined the Tagus. Well-to-do merchants and nobles came and went on launches. Comparisons to Venice were common. Habsburgs, by contrast, tended to see merchants as parasites who drove up prices (as middlemen) or drained wealth (as importers and moneylenders) from their domains. They produced neither craft nor agriculture but dealt in money alone. As a form of wealth, money could sustain only itself. Anathema to both the cooperative world of the guild and the communal world of the peasant, a merchant's wealth – money – was purely individualist. True nobility avoided such unseemly entanglements. See Smith, *The Business of Alchemy*, ch. 1, and the sources cited there.

harvest – were in effect high-stakes bets about what the future might hold.[128] Sugar planters were often heavily indebted, bankruptcy was common, and plantations regularly changed hands.[129] I argued in the last chapter that epidemiological uncertainty in the colonies helped fuel therapeutic diversity, including medical prognostication. Laura de Mello e Souza has similarly argued that the instability and financial uncertainty of the sugar economy in Brazil led to a particular fascination with magic, and especially divination.[130] In either case – epidemic disease or financial misfortune – only occult influences at the very limits of human perception and intervention seemed to explain such sudden and profound changes of circumstance. Brandão agreed. But he put it more simply: "Wealth," he wrote, "is little more than a matter of luck."[131]

Luck, certainly, but friends and connections surely helped. Financial survival depended on credit. And credit depended on interpersonal relationships and the moral estimations of one's peers. Public reputation (*fama publica*) had real, material implications. In financial terms, it was a matter of life and death.[132] Participation in natural inquiry and the possession of natural (especially esoteric) knowledge provided a hedge against financial insecurity. The same families that were vital sources of colonial credit were also among the most expansive collectors in early modern Europe. Banking and merchant families like the Fuggers and the Schetzes were not only critical to the financing of plantation agriculture in Brazil but accumulated enormous collections of objects natural and artificial. Unchecked, Hans Jacob Fugger's penchant for collecting exotica from Brazil and throughout Portugal's was so costly that it helped bankrupt the family (ironically leaving Fugger to manage the accounts of his wealthier peers).[133] Participation in the act of collecting and gifting

---

[128] And these were all exacerbated by the structure of the colonial sugar market itself. See Schwartz, *Sugar Plantations*, ch. 7.

[129] Schwartz, *Sugar Plantations*, 202–241.

[130] Souza, *The Devil in the Land of the Holy Cross*.   [131] Garcia, ed., *Diálogos*, 195.

[132] The point is underscored by Wadsworth, *Agents of Orthodoxy*, ch. 5, who explores how failure in the rigorous applications process for familiars of the Inquisition alone could damage a carefully cultivated reputation and lead to real material costs and, potentially, to financial ruin.

[133] Mark A. Meadow, "Merchants and Marvels: Hans Jacob Fugger and the Origins of the Wunderkammer," in Smith and Findlen, eds., *Merchants and Marvels*, 182–200; Stefan Halikowski Smith, "Demystifying a Change in Taste: Spices, Space, and Social Hierarchy in Europe, 1380–1750," *The International History Review* 29 (2007): 240 [237–257]; and Iain Buchanan, "The Collection of Niclaes Jongelinck: II. The 'Months' by Pieter Bruegel the Elder," *The Burlington Magazine* 132 (1990): 547.

could link colonial planters to metropolitan collectors and would-be patrons, easing access to badly needed credit.[134] Indeed, with the union of the Crowns, collection and display – the cultural components of an aspirational Habsburg Universal Monarchy – grew more pronounced in Lisbon.[135]

As European princes found their fortunes increasingly tied to the ignoble pursuits of commerce and trade, opportunities opened for those who could master both courtly sociability and natural inquiry, thereby tempering the perceived contradictions between disparate notions of wealth and propriety.[136] And ultimately, for the sake of his own fortune, that is precisely what Brandão attempted to do in the *Diálogos*. The document was an artifact of both calculated natural inquiry and the strategic deployment of natural knowledge. Brandão's familiarity with colonial finance was the basis of his exchanges with the royal treasurer. But it was his knowledge of colonial nature that brought him into conversation with a member of the Austrian nobility in Lisbon.

Planters were creatures of commerce. However much they might nurse their pretensions to titled nobility, theirs was a world of merchant capital. Brandão's explanations of the vagaries of the sugar economy – as exemplified by a discussion of the deep capital investment required to start and maintain a mill – conveyed in no uncertain terms just how crucial speculative investment was to the enterprise.[137] Yet when he pitched his plan for imperial reform, Brandão was well aware that he spoke in terms of commerce, investment, and trade with a nobility who understood wealth in terms of land. He couched his proposals for imperial reform within a rhetoric that made the values and wealth of planters appear entirely consonant with the values of a landed nobility. The similarity, although partial, was surely genuine: planters repeatedly advocated that titles be extended to Brazil.[138] Brandão argued that wealth derived from Brazil was superior in kind to that derived from trade in Asia. The riches of Asia yielded only moveable wealth, which was why the most prosperous Portuguese in Asia could return home to newly built mansions. Brandão argued that, like their metropolitan counterparts whose ranks they hoped

---

[134] See the essays in Smith and Findlen, eds., *Merchants and Marvels.*

[135] Annemarie Jordan, "Diplomata e dealer de arte," *L+arte* 20 (2006): 58–60; Juan Pimentel, "The Iberian Vision: Science and Empire in the Framework of a Universal Monarchy, 1500–1800," *Osiris*, 2nd ser., 15 (2000): 17–30.

[136] Smith, *Business of Alchemy.*   [137] Garcia, ed., *Diálogos*, 168–181.

[138] Schwartz, *Sugar Plantations*, 274.

to join, Brazilian sugar planters derived their wealth from the land. The sugar planter – as a planter-naturalist – bridged oceans, social ranks, and disparate notions of wealth that were at the time part of a global Habsburg empire.

ATLANTIC ITINERARIES, IMPERIAL TRANSFORMATIONS

Abreu's *Tratado* has remained a source of considerable debate. In a bid to clarify Abreu's work and refurbish his reputation, Francisco Guerra took to the pages of the *Journal of Tropical Medicine and Hygiene*, arguing that Abreu was the author of "the earliest book on tropical medicine." Guerra convincingly made the case that Abreu had indeed – however unknowingly – described the bodily effects of a number of pathogenic afflictions (amoebiasis, malaria, typhoid fever, scurvy, yellow fever, dracontiasis, trichuriasis, and tungiasis) in disparate passages scattered throughout the *Tratado*.[139] But, as I have shown, Guerra's essay was wrong in one very substantial way. Abreu's treatise was not so much a founding text of tropical medicine, as it was a rejection of the idea of the tropics itself. As far as Abreu was concerned, such a thing did not yet exist – not, at least, in a medically meaningful way. For Abeu, the Atlantic rather than the tropics, defined a region of medical coherence. By the end of the seventeenth century, Abreu's Atlantic itinerary would help draw attention to imperial service in the far-flung empire as a pathway to employment in the innermost chambers of some of imperial Lisbon's most powerful households. His *Tratado*, the intellectual prestige accorded to fevers, and their frequency and distribution in the Atlantic would all make fevers – and especially tertian fevers – prominent objects of inquiry among a growing number of metropolitan physicians as the seventeenth century unfolded.

The medical conjectures of Brandão suggest something of the way in which the uncertainties attending natural inquiry had opened up even medical theory to the incursions of the nonspecialist. His *Diálogos* illustrates some of the ways by which Brazilian nature finally made its way into metropolitan pharmacopoia and natural history more broadly. His efforts as a naturalist challenged dominant historical interpretations of the cultural and intellectual life of the colonial sugar planter. Yet the *Diálogos* is probably more historiographically revealing now than it was

---

[139] Guerra, "Aleixo de Abreu."

intellectually influential in its time. The manuscript remained unpublished throughout the period in question. Two copies have survived. But whether there were ever more than these remains uncertain. The extant copies provide few clues as to their circulation. It is nearly impossible to tell just how widely read the *Diálogos* might have been. But one measure may be the influence of the Dutch. During their occupation of Pernambuco (1630–1654), the Dutch physician Willem Piso and German naturalist Georg Marcgraff cataloged the flora and fauna of Brazil's northeastern littoral,[140] and it was their work, rather than that of Gândavo, Cardim, Sousa, or Brandão, that became the essential reference for Portuguese on either side of the Atlantic. Portuguese administrators would rely on it; Portuguese physicians would reference it.

The tropics had not yet come into being. As the divergent opinions of Abreu and Brandão illustrate, observers could still look out across the intertropical field of Portuguese imperial activity and conceive of multiple regions defined by varied environmental and epidemiological conditions. Where Aristotle and his strictest adherents had seen uniformity, Abreu, Brandão, and their contemporaries saw complexity. Yet changes were afoot. Even as Aristotle's claims about the nature of the region between the two iconic parallels of Cancer and Capricorn were increasingly discredited, sixteenth-century maritime competition made latitude in general evermore central to Iberian imperial perspectives. Maritime and terrestrial geographies alike had now been rearranged.[141] At the beginning of the sixteenth century, the apothecaries Pires and Alvares described the labyrinthine configuration of island Southeast Asia in terms that mirrored itinerary maps and maritime rudders.[142] Only decades later, Brazil was plotted across a Ptolemaic graticule, ordered by fixed lines rather than wayfaring itineraries. By 1600 latitude more thoroughly calibrated administrative perspectives and structured colonial reportage: when the colonies finally became the subject of sustained natural inquiry, Gandavo and his contemporaries began their accounts by introducing each captaincy according to the precise latitudes it occupied. In the *Diálogos*, Brandão followed suit.

---

[140] Willem Piso and Georg Marcgraff, *Historia naturalis Brasiliae* (Leiden: Franciscum Hackium and Lud. Elzevirium, 1648).

[141] Alison Sandman, "Mirroring the World: Sea Charts, Navigation, and Territorial Claims in Sixteenth-Century Spain," in Smith and Findlen, eds., *Merchants and Marvels*, 83–108.

[142] Padron, *Spacious Word*, explores this at length for early Spanish exploration in the Caribbean.

Until about the turn of the seventeenth century, the distinctions between West Africa and Brazil posed *intra*-tropical epidemiological distinctions in their sharpest form. Yet few could still claim as Caminha had that Brazil was uniformly healthy and only the uninitiated would aver, as Nóbrega had, that Brazil was without fevers or other diseases. As the work of Abreu and Brandão reveal, explanations for the occurrence of fever and pox were now ensnared in the wider medical debate over the causes of disease in general and the nature of contagion in particular. Over the course of the seventeenth century, epidemics of fever and pox would increasingly be associated with life in Brazil. By the turn of the eighteenth century, metropolitan opinions of Brazil would undergo the same kind of shift they had for West Africa two centuries earlier. Brazil by 1700 would be seen as perilously riddled with fever and pox.

Finally, with the pathologization of Brazil, it would be possible to see not only prodigious nature but debilitating fevers as common across the intertropical world. Events both within metropolitan Portugal and throughout its empire would over the late seventeenth century make it advantageous for metropolitan physicians and imperial policymakers to conceive of the that world in both ways simultaneously. That story begins not in Portugal or its colonies but with a disenchanted diplomat at the court of Louis XIV.

8

Fault Lines

From the ardent tropic ...

Pascual Ribeiro Coutinho

THE ACCIDENTAL NATURALIST

Duarte Ribeiro de Macedo, special Portuguese envoy to the court of Louis
XIV, found little to admire about France. Shuffling between Paris,
St. Cloud, St. Germain, and Versailles, he thought the winters too cold
and damp, the summers too hot and humid, and Paris – though notably
clean and well-lit – too gray and gloomy. Rumor and intrigue at court
were rampant and "it was suspected by some," Macedo confided to a
friend, that the frequent "parties and dances" were the product of
unspoken "political machinations."[1] French aristocratic sociability also
troubled him. He thought French women were too "libertine," French
men too "lenient," and husbands too easily cuckolded by their wives. To
make matters worse, dispatches from Lisbon – including his salary, official correspondence, and other news – arrived late or not at all.[2] Macedo
repeatedly complained that he was kept not simply poor but poorly
informed. Poverty and isolation, combined with the uncomfortable
seasons, decadent social life, and disorderly households of France left
Macedo eager to return home.[3]

---

[1] BNP Res. Cod. 1549, f. 17.   [2] BNP Res. Cod. 1549, ff. 18–19.
[3] Virginia Rau, *Política Economica e Mercantilismo na Correspondência de Duarte Ribeiro
de Macedo (1668–1676)* (Lisbon: N.p., 1968), 7–10. Ribeiro has been the subject of a

Yet when in the spring of 1668 he was asked to represent Portuguese interests at the French court, Macedo had hurried to make his departure. At issue were pressing matters of state. The union of the Crowns – the sixty-years in which the Spanish Habsburgs ruled Portugal and its empire – had ended in 1640 with a palace revolt that inaugurated almost three decades of intermittent war between the two Iberian kingdoms. By 1668, much of the countryside that stretched along their shared border had been ravaged, its population depleted, its agriculture exhausted. The Portuguese royal treasury had been ruined to the point of public embarrassment, and was an object of mockery and laughter even among shopkeepers in distant Rome.[4]

The Treaty of Madrid put an end to the Iberian conflict. The problem then – and the reason why Macedo left for France – was that peace with the Spanish risked conflict with the French. The Treaty of Madrid violated certain terms of an agreement that prince regent D. Pedro (soon to be Pedro II) had reached with Louis XIV a year earlier.[5] Macedo was in France to mend damaged relations. No sooner had the Madrid treaty been announced than Macedo departed. When affairs were settled to his satisfaction the following year, he petitioned to return home. The request was denied. Macedo, who in 1668 had been certain that his was "unlikely to be a long stay," remained in France for the next eight years.

Those years at the French court were transformative – for France, for Macedo, and ultimately for conceptions of nature and disease in Portugal's empire. As I argued in the last chapter, ideas about disease, medicine, the health of Brazil, and the place of Brazilian nature in the empire had all begun to change in the early seventeenth century. The physician Abreu and the planter-naturalist Brandão disagreed about the causes and severity of the fevers and dysenteries that plagued Brazil. But the Jesuit Nóbrega's earlier claim that there were no fevers in Brazil had become clearly untenable. Brazil seemed to share not only the intertropical situation of

recent biography as well: Ana Maria Homem Leal de Faria, *Duarte Ribeiro de Macedo: Um Diplomata Moderno (1618–1680)* (Lisbon: Biblioteca Diplomática do Ministério dos Negócios Estrangeiros, 2005).

[4] António Vieira, *Cartas do Padre Antonio Vieyra da Companhia de Jesus a Duarte Ribeiro de Macedo* (Lisbon: Eugenio August, 1827), 166.

[5] The terms had stipulated that, among other things, Portugal and France would jointly pursue war against Spain, and that neither Portugal nor France would negotiate peace without the consent of other, which was precisely what the Prince Regent Pedro had done anyway. The political machinations on all sides are revealed in Edgar Prestage, *As relações diplomáticas de Portugal com a França, Inglaterra e Holanda, de 1640 a 1668* (Coimbra: Imprensa da Universidade, 1928), especially 106–108.

Portuguese settlements in West Africa, India, and Angola but many of the bodily afflictions common to those areas as well.

Until the late seventeenth century, questions about nature and illness in Portugal's colonies were the subject of investigation and debate chiefly among members of disparate cultures of natural inquiry resident in those same colonies.[6] But in seventeenth-century Lisbon, assertive and increasingly influential university-trained physicians – some had worked overseas and returned but many had never left the imperial capital – began to draw attention to apparent intertropical commonalities in ways that they had not done before. Some made claims of intertropical coherence in terms at once environmental and epidemiological. These would inspire new approaches to colonial health and medicine. They would help change the relationship between nature and empire and, consequently, between naturalists and imperial policy. The accumulation of knowledge about colonial nature increasingly became the focus of metropolitan observers, the work of metropolitan institutions, and the subject of concerted investigative effort. In these transformations, the disenchanted diplomat Macedo was influential.

There was perhaps no better place in late-seventeenth-century Europe to debate the merits of state-coordinated projects that were botanical in focus and imperial in scale than the French court of Louis XIV. Neither was there a more likely place for Macedo – jurist and ambassador – to develop a keen interest in the natural world. Yet Macedo was a most unlikely, even accidental, naturalist. Unlike Cadamosto, Pereira, and Barros in the African Atlantic, or the apothecaries Pires and Álvares, the pilot Rodrigues, and the physician Orta in Asia, or the physician Abreu and the planter Brandão in Brazil, Macedo never traveled beyond the shores of Europe and rarely corresponded directly with anyone who had. Nor did he keep or collect exotic plants, inspect or sketch unusual animals. His familiarity with what many contemporary naturalists might have considered canonical authors – Aristotle or Pliny – was probably general and (especially in the case of Pliny) superficial at best, drawn from readings and lectures required of him as a young student. Yet at European courts, as aboard ship at sea, within colonial households, in overseas missions, and on colonial plantations, the study of nature and who could participate in it remained open. Courtly sociability made metropolitan apartments, drawing rooms, salons, and dining halls into venues for the

---

[6] Harrison, *Medicine in an Age of Commerce and Empire*, has observed a similar pattern in the British empire.

exchange not only of imperial ambitions or political intrigue but of ontological claims and epistemological sensibilities.[7]

Thanks in part to the initiative of Jean-Baptiste Colbert, the French court was a hive of natural inquiry. The very years Macedo spent there happened to be a momentous and deeply formative period in the history of French natural history.[8] Everyone at court spoke of plants and empire – from the son of the prominent Dutch jurist Hugo Grotius to Lord Ralph Montagu, a member of the Royal Society whose London mansion would later house the British Museum. With this motley cast, Macedo traded schemes of imperial-botanical brinksmanship. He learned of the undertakings of the Académie Royale des Sciences and of the Royal Society of London. He read about them too. Macedo thumbed through the *Histoires de l'Académie Royale des Sciences*, "the journal of the savants of Paris" (citing a paper dated June 3, 1675). He read extracts of the Royal Society's *Philosophical Transactions* (material from volume 5) and he absorbed "with great curiosity" a French copy of Thomas Spratt's *History of the Royal Society* (translated but a few years earlier).[9] In these volumes, plants figured prominently – and so too did an abiding preoccupation with climate, environment, and global measurement. From these courtly encounters – with French ministers, the texts of learned societies, and an ensemble of European ambassadors – Macedo drew the outlines of his own plans for the renewal of Portugal and its empire.

It was Colbert who most immediately impressed the Portuguese diplomat. French economic policy under Colbert – an industrial mercantilism predicated on interventionist Crown policies – had begun to enlarge both the value of French manufacturing and the power of the French state. Macedo was inspired. He assembled a series of his own policy ideas into an economic brief penned in Paris in 1675 and sent straightaway to Lisbon. The "Discurso sobre a introdução das artes no Reino" was a pointed defense of bullionism, a blueprint for the development of Portuguese manufacturing (*industria*), and a statement of what Macedo believed was the centrality of Crown policy to both. Within metropolitan

---

[7] Daston and Park, *Wonders*, especially 265–276; Findlen, *Possessing Nature*, 9, 352–354, 398; Biagioli, *Galileo, Courtier*.

[8] James E. McClellan III and François Regourd, *The Colonial Machine: French Science and Overseas Expansion in the Old Regime* (Turnhout: Brepols, 2011).

[9] BNP Res. Cod. 11377 ff. 74–76v; and Thomas Sprat, *The History of the Royal Society of London for the Improvement of Natural Knowledge* (London: N.p., 1734 [1667]); and Spratt, *L'Histoire de la Societe Royale de Londres* (Geneva: Jean Herman Widerhold, 1669).

Portugal, the "Discurso" was widely influential – not least because Mace-do's friend and fellow statesmen, Dom Luis de Meneses, the Count of Ericeira, had only that same year been appointed Portuguese Lord of the Treasury. Macedo's ideas informed initiatives that ranged widely from Portuguese wool and silk manufacturing to a proposal to illuminate the streets of Lisbon. Many of those policies were enacted but short lived and of dubious consequence. Macedo nevertheless was (and is still considered) one of the most influential economic thinkers of late-seventeenth-century Portugal.[10]

It was Macedo's plans for the empire – a set of proposals all but forgotten by historians[11] – that would help redefine the intertropical world. The union of the Crowns had led to deepening imperial turmoil that neither good relations with the French nor peace with the Spanish could resolve. Not only had the religious, commercial, and administrative affairs of the two Iberian powers become entangled but new lines of alliance and aggression had been drawn, and imperial relations recon-figured. Portugal and its empire had been swept into contests between the Spanish Habsburgs and their more northern rivals. Those conflicts per-sisted long after the Portuguese Restoration of 1640 and peace with the Spanish in 1668. No European empire posed a greater threat to Portu-guese interests overseas than the Dutch. Their East India Company captured Malacca in 1641, laid siege to Colombo in 1655, forced its capitulation (and gained control of its cinnamon) in 1656, and then took both Cochin and Cannanore (long the principal ports of the Portuguese pepper trade) in 1663. By the time Macedo left for Paris five years later, the Portuguese Estado da Índia had withered. Most of the Asian spices bound for Europe traveled in East India Company hulls – including mace and nutmeg, which the Portuguese never managed to control as the Dutch now did.[12]

---

[10] Faria, *Duarte Ribeiro de Macedo*, 311–390; and Carl A. Hanson, *Economy and Society in Baroque Portugal, 1668–1703* (Minneapolis, MN: University of Minnesota Press, 1981), 161–176, 182; Rau, *Política Economica*.

[11] Which is to say that they are mentioned only on occasion and only as part of his overall economic agenda as in the case of Hanson, *Economy*; and Rau, *Política Economica*. Faria, *Duarte Ribeiro de Macedo*, 353–355, 361–366; is the exception that proves the rule.

[12] The Dutch also captured, among other ports, São Tomé de Meliapor in 1662, which as the resting place of St. Thomas. Home to private Portuguese traders, it was foremost perhaps a symbolic loss. See Meilink-Roelofsz, *Asian Trade*; Subrahmanyam, *Portuguese Empire*; Ernst Van Veen, *Decay or Defeat?: An Inquiry into the Portuguese Decline in*

In the Atlantic, the Dutch West India Company sacked Bahia in 1624 and 1625 and then captured, settled, and ruled Pernambuco from 1630 to 1654. Along the African littoral, the Dutch captured both Luanda and Benguela – the major Portuguese slave ports of West Central African – along with the island of São Tomé in 1641. If Macedo's countrymen had managed to retake Pernambuco, Luanda, and Benguela, the loss (however temporary) of Brazil's wealthiest and most productive captaincy was a devastating blow to an export-oriented agricultural economy that had already shown signs of trouble.[13] Although retaken, its sugar estates lay in ruins, its mills destroyed, their fires snuffed out – "fogo morto" in the language of Macedo's contemporaries. The geography of sugar cultivation and the profits derived from it had shifted decidedly northward. Sugar especially from English and French plantations in the Caribbean had begun to replace Portuguese sugar from Brazil on European markets. Lisbon warehouses that would have held payloads awaiting trans-shipment to Amsterdam and elsewhere became instead storehouses piled high with crates that could not be sold and therefore could not be taxed. Without pepper or cinnamon, nutmeg, cloves, or mace, with its treasury empty and its warehouses full, Portugal and its empire were in crisis.[14]

That was the situation Macedo observed from Paris. As he saw it, there were two basic problems: the losses in the Indian Ocean, which he thought were irretrievable in the short term, and flagging Brazilian agri-culture, which he thought could be quickly reversed. In a policy brief titled "Observações sobre a transplantação dos fructose da Índia ao Brasil" – penned at about the same time as the "Discurso" – Macedo offered his solution for imperial reform. To shore up Asian trade and strengthen the Portuguese hold on Brazil Macedo proposed nothing less than a concerted imperial effort to transfer the most profitably traded plants from the East Indies to Brazil, where they would be grown and

Asia, 1580–1645 (Leiden: Research School of Asian, African, and Amerindian Studies of the University of Leiden: 2000).
[13] Stuart B. Schwartz, "A Commonwealth within Itself: The Early Brazilian Sugar Industry, 1550–1670," in *Tropical Babylons: Sugar and the Making of the Atlantic World, 1450–1680*, ed. Stuart B. Schwartz (Chapel Hill, NC: University of North Carolina Press, 2004), 158–200.
[14] Hanson, *Economy*, especially ch. 6.

exported to Lisbon and elsewhere in Europe.[15] The plan was ambitious, even visionary, but also contentious and deeply problematic. To generate consensus around it, Macedo had to tend to three central issues: How could he possibly think that a strategy amounting to the near abandonment of the Estado da Índia might actually return it to Portuguese control? What made him so sure that Asian flora could thrive in Brazil? And how could Portuguese carry it off especially given what Macedo increasingly understood as the distinctly dispersed geography of natural knowledge in Portugal's empire? If the first was a question of imperial strategy, the latter two were fundamentally questions about the inner workings of the natural world and about the accumulation and deployment of expertise about that world. Macedo's "Observações" tended to all three.

Macedo's proposal depended on his own idiosyncratic, contentious, but ultimately defensible conception of the region that lay between the Tropic of Cancer and the Tropic of Capricorn. As every Portuguese imperial minister since at least the creation of the pilfered Cantino atlas understood, India lay above the equinoctial line in the east while Brazil lay below it in the west. When Macedo claimed that the drugs and spices of South and Southeast Asia would grow with equal vigor when transplanted to Brazil, he did not merely stake out a position about the similarities in climate and environment that he believed characterized those particular places. He instead made a claim about climate and environment across the entire region of the terraqueous globe that stretched from the Tropic of Cancer north of the equator to the Tropic of Capricorn in the south. Macedo argued that Asian plants would do well in Brazil because this vast intertropical constituted a single, coherent, and internally consistent global region. In a climatic and environmental sense disparate locations throughout the intertropical world – from north to south and from east to west – were interchangeable. Macedo allowed for qualifications and exceptions but that was his contention. It was a sweeping one. It stood in stark contrast with the Aristotelian torrid zone. And it would help reformulate metropolitan visions of the intertropical world. But for Macedo's view of intertropical environmental coherence to have any sway among his peers and colleagues in Lisbon – which was indispensable if his scheme for the

---

[15] Spratt, *History of the Royal Society*, 86–87, had already insisted that his countrymen investigate whether it might be possible to transplant "Eastern spices and other useful Vegetables" to England's "Western Plantations" in the Caribbean.

*intra*tropical transplantation of drugs and spices were to ever get off the ground – Macedo had some convincing to do.

COCONUT PALMS AND GLOBAL MEASURES

Macedo justified his plan to bring Asian flora to South America in ways calibrated precisely to the strengths and weaknesses of Portugal's empire. When Macedo justified his proposal he addressed explicitly the challenges posed by the Dutch. He also dealt implicitly with the issue of Caribbean sugar as well as with a range of concerns that increasingly troubled late-seventeenth-century metropolitan statesmen and policymakers – the pervasive shortage of ships and personnel, lasting divisions over the break with Spain, and questions over the place of precious metals in the imperial economy.

"There is no doubt," Macedo urged, "that if Brazil were to produce cloves, pepper, cinnamon, and all of the other plants that nature produces and that are cultivated in the East," and if those spices were sold in metropolitan Lisbon, they would prove to be "an asset more useful and less costly than the mines of Potosí or Sofala." This was, he explained, a single solution to several problems. Because Brazil was scarcely two months sailing from Portugal, the profitably traded fruits, seeds, leaves, stems, and roots that it produced would arrive for sale in Lisbon "purer, in better condition, and cheaper" than if they had shipped from India.[16] Producing Asian spices in Brazil for sale in Lisbon meant that "all nations of Europe" wishing to enjoy the spices of "the East" would descend upon Lisbon to purchase them, swelling the imperial purse with precious gold and silver currency.[17]

Because it would undermine the economic logic that brought the Dutch to Asia in the first place, Macedo thought his plan would also prove an "infallible" way to promote the "ruin of the Dutch" and thereby deliver control of Indian Ocean trade back to Portugal. And all of this would come without "the cost of blood ... or shipwrecks, or navigation from India."[18] Both personnel and seaworthy ships were not just expensive but now – after decades of war and the deforestation of significant stretches of metropolitan Portugal and the Konkan and Brazilian coasts – scarce

---

[16] This, as I argued in Chapter 4, was precisely what Orta had seen as the promise of the empire.

[17] BNP Res. Cod. 11377, ff. 65, 67.   [18] BNP Res. Cod. 11377, ff. 67v, 83.

resources to be closely guarded and carefully conserved.[19] Even references
to the mines of Potosí and "Sofala" did important strategic work. In both
Spain and Portugal, the actual Andean mines had come to stand instead
for a notional "Potosí" – a source of sudden and fabulous wealth whose
seductions could corrupt, mislead, or both.[20] The point played to nation-
alist sympathies in two ways. It was a subtle commentary on Spanish
mishandling of its own vast riches, reassuring Macedo's readers where his
sympathies lay despite his long absence and difficulties. It also spoke to
Portuguese troubles in Brazil and East Africa. Claims that similar mines of
silver or gold lay just beyond the limits of the Brazilian captaincies had
become a common way for would-be prospectors to swindle benefices
from the Crown before disappearing into the South American interior.[21]
Meanwhile, successive attempts to locate and capture the mines of the
Zambezi highlands upriver from the East African port of Sofala had
proven costly failures. Precisely why was an ongoing matter of debate in
Lisbon – one that chroniclers, missionaries, and other visitors were wont
to resolve.[22] Turning away from Asia was a way to regain control of it;
and plant wealth, unlike mineral wealth, would bring imperial riches
without the corruption and expense of distant mines.

   Those assertions, Macedo assured his readers, "needed no proof."[23]
Others did. What had until the late fifteenth century constituted the
prevailing set of claims about the region of the globe that straddled the
equator – that its proximity to the sun rendered it devoid of vegetation
and human inhabitants, that passage through it was impossible – had
been challenged and then upended by early voyages into the Atlantic.
Macedo's peers – educated at university, perhaps with a degree from one
the higher faculties of theology, law, or medicine – would have learned of
those claims of classical geography in lectures, perhaps at Coimbra or
Evora. The raft of hagiographic literature that had circulated in Portugal
ever since would have reminded them, however, that those claims were
amiss and that it was the Henrican voyages of the fifteenth century that

---

[19] Van Veen, *Decay or Defeat*.
[20] Studnicki-Gizbert, *Nation*; Elvira Vilches, *New World Gold: Cultural Anxiety and Monetary Disorder in Early Modern Spain* (Chicago: University of Chicago Press, 2010).
[21] Schwartz, ed., *A Governor and His Image*.
[22] The ill-fated Barreto-Homen expedition can be traced through the sources published
together as João C. Reis, *A empresa da conquista do senhorio do Monomotapa* (Lisobn:
Heuris, 1984).
[23] BNP Res. Cod. 11377, f. 67v.

had proven them so.[24] In their various overseas travels, Cadamosto, Pereira, Barros, and many others had not found the earthly paradise (although rumors persisted among the Spanish that it lay somewhere in South America[25]), and the kingdom of Prester John had not quite been what they had expected. But beyond the Senegal – as they crossed below the Tropic of Cancer – they had indeed encountered a world that was verdant and fecund, and heavily populated.

Yet even though the mythical torrid zone had proven thickly vegetated, densely populated, and imminently passable (once the wind and ocean currents had been charted), it did not follow that nature behaved everywhere equally throughout that immense region – it did not mean that the climatic symmetry that had characterized the geography inherited from the ancients should still hold true, and that one totalizing vision should replace another. But Macedo, pointing to accounts of India and Brazil, now said that, yes, in fact it did. To substantiate that claim, Macedo turned to a combination of reason and experience. Macedo tended first to reason, hyperbolically announcing his knowledge of "all of the principles of Natural Philosophy," which he assured his readers, "demonstrate that all nature which grows between the equinoctial line and the Tropic of Cancer grow as well between that same line and the Tropic of Capricorn." Highlighting the syllogism as the instrument proper to natural philosophy, he launched into two logical proofs to support his case – one "larger" the other, "smaller."[26] The first and "larger" (by which he meant more general) syllogism concerned climate and environment. "The natural causes that produce plants were heat and the humidity of the land. These two qualities – heat and humidity – were the same in the regions that comprehend the tropics, north and south. For that reason, all of the plants that are produced between the equinoctial line and one tropic to the north must also be produced between that same line and the other to the south." To that he added a "smaller" syllogism that dealt with the matter of seasonal variation: "For when the sun

[24] Wey Gómez, *Tropics of Empire*, 71–79; and on the antagonistic attitude of many Portuguese *letrados* to the classicist bent of their Renaissance peers, see the essays in Maria Berbara and Karl A. E. Enenkel, eds., *Portuguese Humanism and the Republic of Letters* (Leiden: Brill, 2012).

[25] Cañizares-Esguerra, *Nature, Empire, and Nation*, 116–121.

[26] BNP Res. Cod. 11377, f. 68v. On the importance of the syllogism to both natural philosophy and natural history among those concerned with collecting and the overseas world in the sixteenth and seventeenth centuries, see Cook, *Matters of Exchange*, 15–16; and Daston and Park, *Wonders*, 115.

crosses the line toward the Tropic of Cancer it is winter in the Tropic of Capricorn; and to the contrary, when the sun crosses the other way it happens in reverse."[27]

Those two forays into formal logic were the extent of this naturalist's philosophy. But to Macedo they provided sufficient basis for his explanations of what he, his countrymen, and his contemporaries had long observed to happen as plants moved back and forth across the globe. Those arguments were the substance of Macedo's "Observações." He needed to find a way – some technique, tool, or device – by which to demonstrate the coherence of the region of the tropics. In keeping with his botanical ambitions, Macedo turned to the humble coconut palm. By his own account, the coconut palm was one of the most ubiquitous and unremarkable plants to inhabit Portugal's empire. The obscure palm noted in Malacca by Tomé Pires, sketched by the pilot Francisco Rodriguez in the East Indies, and described by Garcia de Orta in Goa had – in ways not entirely unknown to Macedo – made its way to Brazil. In both Asia and Brazil, this plant for which "men have found numerous and diverse uses" thrived. That very combination of banality and ubiquity was what made the coconut "more than any other plant" the one by which "nature demonstrates its fecundity." Macedo turned it into an instrument that measured the internal coherence of the global tropics. As he explained in the "Observacões," the coconut was "cultivated in the East in all lands that run from the [equinoctial] line to the Tropic of Cancer but it does not grow, nor is it cultivated, in any place beyond that Tropic." "And in the same way, with the same virtues and effects, it is grown and is cultivated in Brazil and the lands that run from the line to the Tropic of Capricorn such that the land of Rio, which is at 22 degrees, produces them but they do not grow, nor are they cultivated, in the lands of São Paulo, which is one degree beyond the Tropic of Capricorn."[28]

Macedo thought that the most convincing part of his entire plan and the best evidence of the soundness of his thinking was that, in fact, those global transplantations had already taken place. In the "Observações," Macedo offered detailed instructions on how his scheme was to unfold. In practice, these were rather beside the point. His correspondent in Rome was the Jesuit António Vieira. As a missionary in Brazil, Vieira had made a reputation first as an orator and then as a field missionary. Contemporaries credited him with conversion of the indomitable native inhabitants of

---

[27] BNP Res. Cod. 11377, ff. 68v–69v.   [28] BNP Res. Cod. 11377, ff. 69v–70v.

Marajó Island. His successes in the mission field and his way with words helped him gain an appointment to the court of D. João IV in the wake of the Restoration. While Macedo was in France planning botanical conquest, Vieira had been dispatched to Rome.

When Macedo wrote to Vieira about his proposal, Vieira responded that, in fact, many Asian plants had already taken root in Brazil.[29] What in the 1560s Clusius had assembled together on the page in his *Aromatum et simplicium* had now – by way of the networks of Portuguese empire – already come to pass. Indeed, so rapid, dense, and confused were these global exchanges that Linschoten, and Orta before him, believed cashews and pineapples to be of South Asian rather than South American provenance (Figure 8.1).

Successful or not, Macedo's policy proposals were influential. The same year that Macedo penned his thoughts on the tropics was the year that his friend and confidant Luís de Meneses, the Count of Ericeira, was appointed Lord of the Treasury in Portugal. The diplomat in Paris and the Count of Ericeira in Lisbon kept a steady correspondence. When the Count began what turned out to be the successful but short-lived development of domestic Portuguese industry, he borrowed heavily from Macedo's writings. The diplomat had argued for the importance of domestic wool consumption; the Count of Ericeira made it a centerpiece of his industrial program. Macedo had drawn attention to the portability of the mulberry tree that allowed the production of silk; the Count undertook extensive mulberry cultivation. What Macedo wrote, the Count of Ericeira read and often carried out.

And Macedo was a prolific write – which at first glance makes the fate of his "Observações" and the influence it might have had into something of a mystery. His policy proposals formed part of a considerable body of opinion on matters ranging from natural philosophy and politics to history and jurisprudence. He witnessed the publication of some of his work before his death in 1680.[30] Much of it remained in print long afterward. Volumes of his collected work came off of Lisbon's presses

---

[29] Vieira, *Cartas*, 210–212.

[30] This was true mainly for his writings on politics, jurisprudence, and history. See, for example, Duarte Ribeiro de Macedo, *Discurso Politico que o Conde de Soure, Embaxador extraordinario de Sua Magestade a el Rey Christianissimo, deu ao Cardeal Mazarine em São João da Luz* (Lisbon: Henrique Valente, 1661 [Paris, 1659]); Macedo, *Juizo Historico, Juridico, Politico sobre a paz celebrada entre as coroas de França e Castella, no anno de 1660* (Lisbon: João da Costa, 1666); and Macedo, *Vida da Emperatriz Theodora* (Lisbon: João da Costa, 1677).

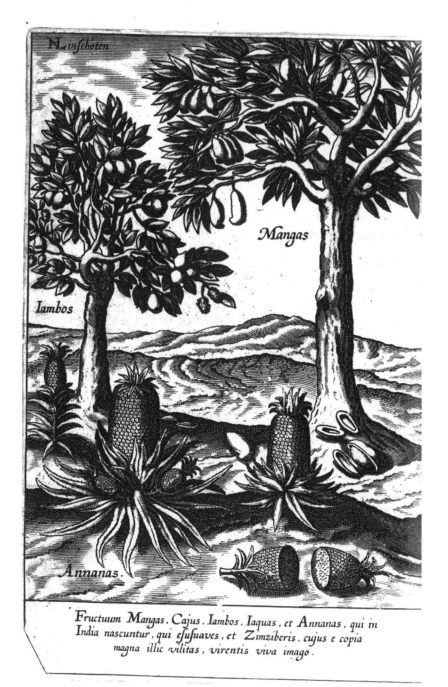

FIGURE 8.1 Assembling Intertropical Nature. Cashews ("Cajus") and pineapples ("Annanas") native to South America mingle with the mangoes ("Mangas") and jackfruit ("Iaquas") of South Asia in an engraving from Jan Huygen van Linschoten, *Histoire de la navigatione de Jan Huygen van Linschoten aux Indes Orientales* (Amsterdam: Evert Cloppenburgh, 1638).
Courtesy of the John Carter Brown Library at Brown University.

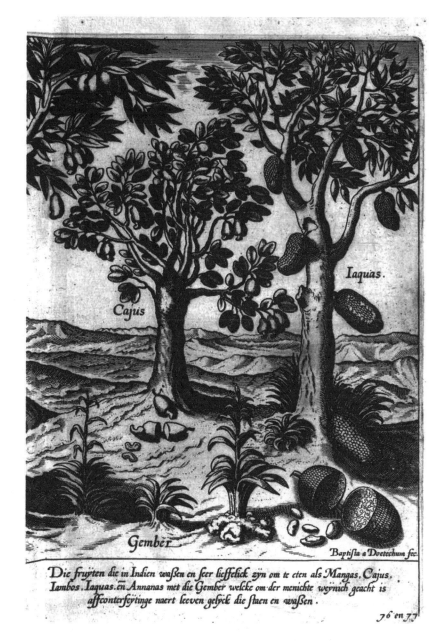

FIGURE 8.1 (*cont.*)

three times from the early eighteenth to the early nineteenth century: first in 1743, then later in 1767 and 1817.[31] Among his numerous works, the essay he penned on the tropics was nearly lost. The "Observações" appeared only in the last of them, tucked anonymously (the edition had no table of contents) into a section blandly titled "Political Works" (*Obras politicas*).[32] The "Observações" had come out once before – separately, bound on its own – in 1782.[33] But for an essay that articulated and defended a novel view of one of the most hotly debated and mythical region of the globe – the very region across which Portuguese policymakers attempted to prop up an ailing empire – it had a notably dubious publication record. By that measure alone (circulation in print), the brief would appear to have been of little consequence. Macedo's proposals for domestic manufacturing received a wide and influential readership but his account of the tropics, nature, and the promise of transplantation received little notice. Macedo the councilor and diplomat became an object of esteem but his writings on natural philosophy seemed to disappear.

Manuscripts tell a different story. Especially for early modern Portugal, where a lively and widespread manuscript culture persisted amid the proliferation of print.[34] Publication was not the only way that Macedo's work stayed in circulation. Nor did it determine what aspects of his work proved most influential to naturalists in metropolitan Portugal in the late seventeenth and eighteenth centuries.[35]

---

[31] Manuel Pinheiro Chagas, ed., *Diccionario Popular: Historico, Geographico, Mythologico, Biographico, Artistico, Bibliographico e Litterario*, 16 vols. (Lisbon: Joaquim Germano de Sousa Neves, 1881), vol. 9, 288.

[32] Duarte Ribeiro de Macedo, *Obras ineditas de Duarte Ribeiro de Macedo*, ed. António Lourenço Caminha (Lisbon, Impressão Regia, 1817), pt. 2, ch. 8: 103. It is the first in a section called "Observações."

[33] Chagas, ed., *Diccionario Popular*, 288.

[34] Fernando Bouza-Álvarez, "Cultura escrita e história do livro: A circulação manuscrita nos séculos XVI e XVII," in *O livro antigo em Portugal e Espanha, séculos XVI–XVIII*, a special issue of *Leituras. Revista da Biblioteca Nacional* 9/10 (2002), 63–98; and José Manuel Herrero Massari, *Libros de viajes de los siglos XVI-XVII en España y Portugal: Lecturas y lectores* (Madrid: Fundación Universitaria Española, 1999), 189–190.

[35] Here I build on the work of Adrian Johns, *The Nature of the Book: Print and Knowledge in the Making* (Chicago: University of Chicago Press, 1998); and for Portugal in particular the essays collected in Palmira Fontes da Costa and Adelino Cardoso, eds., *Percursos na História do Livro Médico (1450–1800)* (Lisbon: Edições Colibri, 2011). Faria, *Duarte Ribeiro de Macedo*, 353, has already inferred this was the case for Macedo based on her extensive review of numerous manuscript copies of his work. The comment I have here found in the publication of the Academia Real confirms that conjecture.

In 1779, metropolitan Portugal became home to its first learned society committed to the study of nature, the *Academia Real das Sciencias de Lisboa*. When in 1789, the Academia published a memorial on the economic applications of accumulated natural knowledge, its members looked not to the writings of Macedo the jurist, ambassador, and political economist but to Macedo the naturalist. Among members of the metropolitan Academia, Macedo's "Observacões" was so well known that it could be cited easily and with little introduction: "On the transplantation of [cinnamon] trees, Duarte Ribeiro de Macedo has already written."[36] Macedo was mentioned several times. He was "a writer who has done great honour to us [his countrymen] by his published writing," but who had done "perhaps more still" by virtue of a treatise (*discurso*) that "circulates in manuscript" (*que anda manuscrito*) and that discusses the "transplantation of Asian spices to Brazil."[37] In fact, there was not one but a number of treatises that Macedo wrote in an effort to recruit natural knowledge to the task of imperial economic improvement.[38]

In the intervening century – and through networks spread from Lisbon and Évora to Porto, London, and beyond – manuscript copies of Macedo's work had proliferated.[39] Not only physicians but a perhaps wideranging community of late-seventeenth- and eighteenth-century naturalists owned, read, or heard talk of it. Apothecaries and shop owners like one José da Fonseca on Rua do Arsenal, just behind the Paço da Ribeira in Lisbon, had copies of the "Observações."[40] A focal point of this activity was almost certainly the library of the Count of Ericeira. When Macedo's friend Luís de Meneses, the third Count of Ericeira, died in

---

[36] Academia Real das Ciências [Academia Real das Sciencias de Lisboa], *Memorias economicas da Academia Real das Sciencias de Lisboa* (Lisbon: Office of the Academia Real das Sciencias, 1789), vol. 1, 197.

[37] Academia Real das Ciências, *Memorias*, v. 1, 324.

[38] In addition to BNP Res. Cod. 11377, and other copies of the "Observações sobre a transplantação dos fructose da Índia ao Brasil" cited here and below, as well as the "Discurso sobre a introdução das artes," discussed above, essays in this vein that were written by Macedo and which circulated in manuscript include ANTT, PT, TT, MSBR, 39, ff. 19–26, "Discurso sobre os generos para o Comercio que há no Maranhão e Pará"; BNP Res. Cod. 3542, ff. 91–105, "Trinta e sete géneros que se tem descoberto no Estado do Maranhão e Pará." Copies of the Obervações arrived in Brazil: BN, CL, I-29, 14, 3-4, doc. 3. In Portugal they underwrote more detailed plans for bioprospecting: BNP Res. Cod. 6941/4, ff. 1–11; and BNP Res. Cod. 11463, ff. 57–60.

[39] In addition to those copies that I have consulted and which I reference here, readers should consult what appears to be an almost exhaustive list of copies of the "Discurso" and related texts in Faria, *Um Diplomata Moderno*, 803–835.

[40] ANTT, MSL, no. 1013.

1690, his son inherited the title and the estate – including the library. Francisco Xavier de Meneses, the fourth Count of Ericeira had a keen interest in natural history, medicine, and philosophy. Medical students regularly gathered in his library.[41] Friends from throughout the empire wrote asking for copies of published work from the Royal Academy of History – a precursor of the Academia Real das Sciencias.[42] Inspired by what he had heard of high society in London and Paris, the fourth Count of Ericeira hosted gatherings of like-minded peers.[43]

Extant manuscript copies of the "Discurso" bear the scars of transcription. Their titles differ slightly. Particular passages in some copies received greater elaboration. They even carried conflicting dates: Was Macedo dispatched to France in 1668 or 1686?[44] Another copyist could not be sure of the date at all at left behind a title page that read "sent from France while on an embassy in [. . .]."[45] Some of these transformations managed to skirt the divide between manuscript and published copy. When the "Discurso" was readied for the 1817 compilation of Macedo's work, it was printed with 1775 rather than 1675 as the date of authorship.[46] Through successive transcriptions and final publication, Macedo's essays changed slightly.[47] His argument for a coherent intertropical region remained the same.

FEVER, PRINT CULTURE, AND REFORM

Macedo had said nothing about disease. Others would. In fact, they already had – and their reasons for doing so may help explain why Macedo's forays into natural philosophy were so frequently copied. Participants in the younger Count of Ericeira's salons began to agitate

---

[41] Costigan, *Through Cracks in the Wall*, 166.   [42] Boxer, *Golden Age*, 362.

[43] José Sebastião da Silva Dias, "Portugal e a cultura Europeia (séculos XVI a XVIII)," *Biblos* 28 (1952): 203–498.

[44] The original was titled "Observações" but most of the copies referenced here, as well as others uncoverd by Faria, *Um Diplomata Moderno*, are titled "Discurso."

[45] ANTT, PT, TT, MSBR 39, f. 1.

[46] This was not the fault of mislaid finger; keyboards did not accelerate the printing process until much later. It is, however, an entirely comprehensible mistake. The ink, for example, in the date at the end of ANTT, PT, TT, MSBR 39, f. 14v. has been smudged in such a way that 1675 might easily be mistaken for 1775. This was the same manuscript with the elliptical title page and the uncertainty caused by that smudge may have been the source of its compiler's befuddlement.

[47] One copy of Macedo's essay on the commercially viable plants of Grão Pará and the Maranhão clearly bears the date 1633, when Macedo would have been fifteen years old. See ANTT, PT, TT, MSBR 39, ff. 19 and 26.

for, among other things, the reform of medicine in metropolitan Portugal.[48] Theirs were an extension of efforts that had begun even before Macedo set out for Paris. The physicians who had taken up these debates would see in Macedo's handwritten briefs a view of intertropical coherence that would support what they increasingly claimed were the exceptional epidemiological perils of that very region. If university-trained physicians gained ascendency in Portugal over the middle of the eighteenth century as a consequence of their alliance with Inquisitors to root out the varied forms of magical healing peddled by quacks and charlatans,[49] those conflicts had roots in these more limited, less concerted but (I will argue) still influential medical contests of the middle and late seventeenth century. The growing authority of university trained physicians in metropolitan Portugal in this period would entail the consolidation of a view of global intertropical coherence in both environmental and epidemiological terms. Fever would be central both to the pursuit of greater influence for physicians and to the consequent vision of the intertropical world. These developments were linked in important ways to midcentury administrative reforms. They are reflective of what Diogo Curto and others have argued was an expanding print culture in early seventeenth-century Lisbon and the state's deepening reliance on men with formal university schooling in the political and economic affairs of Portugal and its empire.[50]

The newly installed House of Bragança derived at least a few administrative lessons from the Habsburgs whom it replaced in 1640.[51] Before the union of the Crowns, the Portuguese House of Aviz had never created an administrative infrastructure as large and centralized as that of the neighboring Habsburg state.[52] In 1642, as part of an effort to strengthen

---

[48] Antótnio Lameira, *Do Informalismo ao Formalismo na Ciência Setecentista em Portugal. Do Conde da Ericeira à Academia Real das Ciências de Lisboa*, MA thesis, Faculdade de Ciências e Tecnologia da Universidade Nova de Lisboa, 2000. See also Walker, *Doctors, Folk Medicine, and the Inquisition*, 96–99; and Dias, "Portugal e a cultura Europeia."

[49] This is the principal argument of Walker, *Doctors*; and Braga, *Assistência, Saúde Pública e Prática Médica em Portugal*, ch. 5. See also Paiva, *Bruxaria e superstição*.

[50] I have in mind Diogo Ramada Curto, *O discurso político em Portugal (1600–1650)* (Lisbon: Universidade Aberta, 1988), chs 2 and 3. See also the essays by Fernando Bouza-Álvarez, Diogo Ramada Curto, Manuela D. Domingos, and Maria Valentina C. A. Sul Mendes in *O livro antigo em Portugal e Espanha, séculos XVI–XVIII*; and Hanson, *Economy and Society*, 42–44.

[51] A. R. Disney, *A History of Portugal and the Portuguese Empire*. 2 vols. (New York: Cambridge University Press, 2009), vol. 1, ch. 11.

[52] Ferreira, *The Crown, the Court, and the Casa da Índia*; and Disney, *History of Portugal*, vol. 1, chs 8–10.

royal control and improve imperial administration, D. João IV created the *Conselho Ultramarino* (the Overseas Council). Overseas service was all but a formal requirement of would-be councillors, and for the next half-century, the Conselho would be dominated by a combination of *letrados* (attorneys) and officials returned from the colonies.[53] Although the Portuguese imperial state had not yet begun to systematically compile the natural knowledge contained in colonial reportage, the Overseas Council would function as something of an institutional surrogate in that area. Through a succession of imperial itineraries that took Crown-appointed officials out to the colonies and back to Lisbon, the Overseas Council amassed not colonial reportage on nature *per se*; rather, it acquired expertise on its colonies by collecting the people who served there. Quite apart from the philosophizing of Macedo, those itineraries gave reason enough to see the Atlantic and Indian Ocean theaters of the empire as uniformly plagued by debilitating illness. Administrators would return with accounts of deadly fevers from West Central Africa, South Asia, and South America alike.

Francisco de Távora, the Conde de Alvor, was just such an official. He had served as the governor of Angola for some eight years, from 1668 to 1676, in the wake of the Dutch occupation and the treaty with Spain. Between 1681 and 1686, Távora was in Goa as viceroy of the Éstado da India.[54] I have already shown that concern with the fevers of sub-Saharan Africa dated at least to the late fifteenth century and continued to figure prominently in the later work of Brito, Abreu, and Brandão. It may have been in Angola that Távora, too, began to appreciate the impact of febrile disease on the empire. If so, Távora's tenure in Goa only sharpened that perception. Ideologically charged reports of Goa's decline dated, as I and others have shown, to the late sixteenth century.[55] When Távora

---

[53] On the growing number and importance of *letrados* in political affairs see Curto, *Discurso político*, 137–138; Hanson, *Economy and Society*, 42–44; and on shifting membership of the *Concelho Ultramarino*, see Erik Lars Myrup, "To Rule from Afar: The Overseas Council and the Making of the Brazilian West, 1642–1807," PhD diss., Yale University, 2006, 99–100.

[54] Távora was also a member of the Council of State from 1688 to 1705. [Luíz de Menezes, the third Count of Ericeira], *Relação do felice successo que conseguiram as armas so Serenissimo principe D. Pedro, nosso senhor, governadas por Francisco de Tavora, governador e capitão general do reino de Angola, contra a rebellião de D. João, re das Pedras e Dongo, no mez de dezembro de 1671* (N.p.: N.p., n.d.); Myrup, "To Rule," 201, 447; Pearson, *Portuguese in India*, xiv. Such itineraries were common; see Russell-Wood, *Portuguese Empire*, 64–71.

[55] See my discussion in Chapter 3 and the sources cited therein.

arrived in Goa in 1681, he found the city already partially abandoned. It was so dilapidated and in such ill-health that renewal seemed impossible. Távora began to advocate for its relocation toward the coast further west, to the windswept and more elevated area of Panjim. It was a years-long effort that he vigorously continued to support as first a member (1693–1702) and then later as president (1702–1705) of the Overseas Council.[56]

Távora would not live to see the fruits of those efforts (Goa was only relocated at the end of the eighteenth century) but as president of the Overseas Council he also addressed the ill-health of the Portuguese Atlantic. While Luanda had been under Dutch occupation, the port of Benguela (on the coast to the south of Luanda) emerged as an important slave trading port. Until Luanda was recaptured, most of the enslaved Africans carried to Brazil departed from Benguela. Fevers associated with the surrounding marshlands had proven so deadly that one of its first Portuguese Governors, Rodrigo de Miranda Rodrigues, died in 1653 in the short time between his arrival and the ceremony by which he was to have been formally installed. As head of the Overseas Council in 1703, Távora addressed the problem by dispatching a university-trained physician not to care for the governor or supervise the hospital (which had been the standard arrangement) but to provide formal medical instruction in Portugal's African enclaves. Távora, with the Overseas Council as his instrument, sought to create a medical school in Portugal's most important slaving port[57] (though ultimately the project came to naught).[58]

What is most important about the failed medical school in Luanda is that it signaled a changed relationship between imperial administration and medical expertise. University-trained physicians and the medical knowledge they proffered were not only increasingly seen by imperial administrators like Távora as critical to imperial fortunes but as superior to the diverse forms of curative knowledge that had long proven critical to colonial survival – so much so that members of the Overseas Council now

---

[56] José Nicolau da Fonseca, *An Historical and Archaeological Sketch of the City of Goa* (Bombay: Thacker and Company Ltd., 1878), 173–179.

[57] Luiz de Pina, *História da Medicina Imperial Portuguesa (Angola)* (Lisbon: Agência Geral das Colónias, 1943), 55.

[58] Of three attempts, in 1703, 1791, and 1844, only the 1791 effort led to formal instruction and had but an "ephemeral existence" according to Augusto de Esaguy, *A abertura da Escola Médica de São Paulo da Assunção de Luanda, 1791* (Lisbon: Editorial Império, 1951), 9.

saw fit to more directly manage colonial medical affairs.[59] The ill-fated attempt to found a medical school in Luanda was itself the first of three such efforts.[60]

State attempts to more directly manage colonial health by deploying the expertise of learned medicine was a second consequence of the administrative changes brought by João IV. Unlike Habsburg Spain, Portugal did not have the institution of the *protomedicato* that brought together physicians for the regulation of medicine.[61] João IV did not create one either but, in the wake of the events of 1640, the new king did insist that physicians compose medical work not in Latin but in vernacular Portuguese.[62] In effect, the royal appeal instigated in print a vigorous and at times heated debate over the state of medicine in the kingdom, about the pernicious influence of lay healers, and about what should be done about it. Amid the better-known pamphleteering campaigns that gave voice to disputes over the political and economic affairs of the kingdom,[63] it seems that physicians used the printed page as vehicle of medical reform.[64] They capitalized on the growing appetite among a small but widening and eager reading public in the capital for information about the empire overseas. While Macedo had articulated and defended the coherence of the intertropical region in environmental terms, the epidemiological coherence of that same region – signalled especially by the apparent ubiquity of tertian fevers – became central to attempts by metropolitan physicians to demonstrate the superiority of learned medicine and to consolidate their influence over metropolitan medical practice.

---

[59] In addition to the discussion later in this chapter, see also the record of the administrative changes to military and maritime health in Henry C. Burdett, *Hospitals and Asylums of the World: Their Origin, History, Construction, Administration, Management, and Legislation* (London: J. and A. Churchill, 1893), 610.

[60] Esaguy, *A abertura da Escola Médica*, 9.

[61] Abreu, "A organização e regulação," 117–120. Nominally, the *físico-mor* (physician-general) handled this, although enforcement was highly irregular.

[62] Maximiano Lemos, *História da medicina em Portugal: doutrinas e instituições* 2 vols. (Lisbon: n.p., 1899), vol. 2, 113–114; José Pedro Sousa Dias, *Droguistas, Boticários e Segredistas: Ciência e Sociedade na Produção de Medicamentos na Lisboa Setecentos* (Lisbon: Fundação Calouste Gulbenkian and the Fundação para a Ciência e a Tecnologia, 2007), 199. See also Abreu, "A organização e regulação."

[63] Curto, *Discurso político*, 102, 108–109.

[64] Pre-Philippine efforts at medical reform had already begun to take advantage of the growth in literacy and print culture and were every bit as rancorous as those later. Afonso de Miranda, the *contador* of D. Sebastião before his disastrous invasion of Morocco, had written a critique of learned medicine but withheld it from publication for fear of recrimination. His son had it published in 1562. See BL vol. 1, 81, 45.

The empire overseas helped set the stage for the ensuing debate in a number of ways – not least by fostering the development of Lisbon's book trade. Seaborne commerce in general and the spice trade in particular helped expand pockets of literacy in Lisbon and financed speculative publishing.[65] Although few in the sixteenth century and always small in proportion to the total number of publications,[66] medical authors and printed medical texts multiplied in seventeenth-century Portugal. Surgeons, apothecaries, physicians and many others wrote books that covered everything from diet and regimen to women's medicine and reproductive health.[67] Among those who could afford them, private libraries became fashionable.[68] The close relationship between the empire overseas and print culture in Lisbon was made manifest even on the city's streets. Printers shops clustered alongside those of apothecaries, confectioners, silk merchants, and others that lined Lisbon's main commercial thoroughfare, the Rua Nova dos Mercadores. And in many of those same shops, medical books were bought and sold.[69]

Empire set the stage for late seventeenth-century medical contests in other ways too. Much as in Goa or along the Brazilian coast, so too in metropolitan Lisbon: the empire contributed to the proliferation of disparate medical knowledges, the diversification of medical practice, and the expansion of readily available *materia medica*. Persons of West and Central African descent in particular became common fixtures of the clinical landscape of Portugal from at least the beginning of the sixteenth

---

[65] Valentim Fernandes made a fortune as the royal publisher printing law codes (*Ordenações*) for João III, and was paid at one point in nutmeg and pepper. See Artur Anselmo, *Estudos de história do livro* (Lisbon: Guimarães Editores, 1997), 77–78; and Curto, *Discurso político*, 104–105. Literacy expanded more slowly in Portugal and England than in other parts of Europe according to Vivan Nutton, "Books Erudition and Medicine, 1450–1700," in Costa and Cardoso, eds., *Percursos*, 36.

[66] Jorge Borges de Macedo, *Livros impressos em Portugal no século XVI: Interesse e formas de mantalidade* (Paris: Fundação Calouste Gulbenkian, 1975), 203–210.

[67] The speculation about a persistent Galenism in so many treatises on dietary regimen in Ian MacLean, "'Lusitani Periti': Portuguese Medical Authors, National Identity, and Bibliography in the Late Renaissance," in *Learning and the Market Place: Essays in the History of the Early Modern Book* (Boston: Brill, 2009), ch. 13, is borne out by Inês de Ornellos e Castro, "Prática médica e alimentação nos textos portugueses seiscentistas," in Costa and Cardoso, eds., *Percursos*, 73–91.

[68] That was so much the case that at least one author at the end of the sixteenth century saw fit to publish a guide explaining "why one ought to form a library" and how to go about doing so. See Curto, *Discurso político*, 11–114; and José Manuel Herrero Massari, *Libros de viajes de los siglos XVI-XVII en España y Portugal: lecturas y lectores* (Madrid: Fundación Universitaria Española, 1999), 188–195.

[69] Curto, *O discurso político*, 104.

century. While by 1504 in the Hospital de Todos-os-Santos in the middle of Lisbon, four African slaves (probably from the Guinea Coast) worked among the sick and handled the dead, others served in the households of Lisbon's physicians. Some tended the gardens and distilled water for medicines near the popular healing springs of Caldas da Rainha, along the coast to the north of the capital.[70] In the eighteenth century, among the carpenters, caulkers, and coopers, and alongside the stevedores, fish-mongers, and prostitutes who crowded Lisbon's waterfront were healers like António. A slave from Benin, António's ambiguous gender (he donned women's dress and referred to himself as Vitória) was part of a carefully cultivated persona whose transgressive capacity implied the profound curative power by which António (as Vitória) earned both a reputation and a daily (and nightly) wage. By the beginning of the seventeenth century, men and women like António spanned the Portu-guese Atlantic, trafficking in forms of healing that Inquisition officials were keen to prosecute.[71] Countless such lay healers made their way into the Portuguese countryside, where they worked as *saludadores* and *cur-andeiros*, *sangradores* and *barbeiros*, *feitiçeiros* and *bençadeiros* – all of whom tended in various ways to the health of subjects of the Portuguese Crown. They, too, increasingly fell under the suspicion of physicians and – especially in the case of *feitiçeiros* and *bençadeiros* – of Inquisition officials.[72]

Meanwhile over the seventeenth century, metropolitan apothecaries multiplied. Bezoar stones from India and Peru, tobacco from the Amer-icas, tamarind from West Africa, and cloves from the Banda Islands were but a fraction of the drugs and spices from the intertropical world that filled pantries, market stalls, and the drug shops that lined the streets and side shops of central Lisbon. Recipes curative, alchemical, and culinary circulated in print and manuscript alike. Recipe collections grew larger and were themselves items of exchange in Lisbon. They changed hands

---

[70] A. C. de C. M. Saunders, *A Social History of Black Slaves and Freedmen in Portugal, 1441–1555* (New York: Cambridge University Press, 1982), 65, 67, 97, 171.

[71] António was tried for sodomy. See James H. Sweet, "Mutual Misunderstandings: Ges-ture, Gender and Healing in the African Portuguese World," *Past and Present* (2009), Supplement 4, 128–143; and a similar case treated at greater length in Sweet, *Domingos Álvares*.

[72] Walker, *Doctors*, 212–217, discusses the distinctions between these different designa-tions. Vocational categories generally failed to account fully for the kinds of curative work that any one practitioner regularly undertook. See Fissell, Introduction 1–17.

literally and metaphorically, as even individual recipe books accumulated the varied languages and penmanship of generations of owners.[73]

It was the tumultuous medical world of seventeenth-century Portugal that physicians claimed was a threat to the city, the kingdom, and the empire. Beginning in the middle of the seventeenth century, a coterie of assertive and well-placed physicians took to the presses. Their attacks on medical practice were not just against lay healers but against what they saw as the corrupt and deficient state of medical training and practice more broadly. That they turned to the printed page amid what appears to have been a lasting and dynamic manuscript culture was hardly surprising. Literacy, debate, and commentary had long been the stock in trade of physicians. Their schooling, access to and ownership of books (especially, but not exclusively, key medical texts), and their ability to engage in theoretical debates about the causes of disease were, so they claimed, precisely what made them superior clinicians. That, at least, was what generations of physicians had argued, and it was on the basis of their command of a textual corpus that physicians advocated for systems of examination and licensure over which they could claim authority.[74] In Lisbon by the middle of the seventeenth century, there was probably no better place to put on full display for an influential public readership the skills that defined their profession than on the printed page.[75]

Empire would give their reformist project a geographical and topical focus. The rise of Benguela as a slaving port and the febrile death of the governor in 1653 were indicative of the ramifying connections between Portuguese Africa and Portuguese America that had made the southern Atlantic into an integrated regional system and the focus of imperial

---

[73] WC Mss. 363; BNF, FP, Cod. 59, ff. 1–334; Braga, *Assistência, Saúde Pública e Prática Médica em Portugal*; Castro, "Prática médica e alimentação"; and Maximiano Lemos, *Farmacopoeia Portuguesa dos séculos XVI à XVIII* (Porto: Tipografia da Emprêsa Guedes, 1922).

[74] Their efforts were not always successful in an institutional sense (lay healers found it easy enough to attract clients without formal licensure). But in Portugal as elsewhere, physicians did manage to reorganize the medical landscape to varying degrees in much of late medieval Europe. In Lisbon in particular, the increasing influence of the physician-general came also as a consequence of the removal of its university to Coimbra in 1537. See Abreu, "Organização e regulação." On Portugal in particular, see Iona McCleery, "Medical Licensing in Late Medieval Portugal," in *Medicine and the Law in the Middle Ages*, eds. W. J. Turner and S. M. Butler (Leiden: Brill, 2014), 196–219; and Dutra, "Practice of Medicine." On the wider pattern for early modern Europe, I have relied on Green, *Making Women's Medicine Masculine*, 1–28.

[75] Curto, *Discurso político*, 106–108.

policy well before Távora was seated at the head of the Concelho Ultramarino.[76] The Concelho had already begun to oversee the movement of people across the South Atlantic in both directions.[77] Enslaved African persons were forced westward to labor on Brazilian plantations. The settlement of Benguela and the continuation of the slave trade there depended on *degredados* (Portuguese exiles, often convicts) from Luanda, as well as on the merchants, soldiers, and convicts who sailed in the opposite direction from Brazil. Motley crews of "Brazilians" were instrumental, too, in the recapture of Angola from the Dutch in 1648. "Without Angola, there is no Brazil," one observer insisted. But it was also true that without Brazil, there would be no Angola.[78]

By tackling the foremost illnesses of what was by now the most important theatre of Portugal's empire – by some accounts, the only one still worthwhile[79] – physicians could showcase their therapeutic acumen and enhance both their clinical authority and political influence. In this context Abreu's *Tratado de las siete enfermedades* took on particular importance. In it, Abreu had identified a single disease, tertian fever, as the most common plague of the Atlantic. Abreu had provided both a theoretical discussion of its causes and an extensive discussion of what he believed to be the most effective treatments. The whole text amounted to an assertion that Abreu's having been overseas had given him superior knowledge about the body; such an imperial itinerary made his claims about tertian fever more credible, his text more authoritative. Metropolitan physicians followed Abreu's lead – and in more ways than one.

Abreu's *Tratado* was not just an examination of debilitating fevers and their associated afflictions, and it not only made malignant fevers in general and tertian fever in particular a focus of learned medical commentary and debate, but it also strengthened the weight of an appeal to experience in the empire as a foundation of medical authority.[80] Two decades after Abreu's text was published, as metropolitan administrative attention focused increasingly on the South Atlantic, and as controversy

---

[76] Alencastro, *Trato dos viventes*.   [77] Pina, *História da Medicina*, 44.

[78] Mariana P. Cândido, "South Atlantic Exchanges: The Role of Brazilian-Born Agents in Benguela, 1650–1850," *Luso-Brazilian Review* 50 (2013): 57–58 and 77, n. 23. See also AHU Angola, cx. 5, doc. 108.

[79] In contrast to Macedo, a coterie of royal advisors counseled leaving Asia altogether. See Subrahmanyam, *Portuguese Empire*, ch. 6.

[80] In addition to what follows, see the examples of the surgeon António de Viana and the physician Francisco Correia de Amaral Castello Branco in *BL* vol. 1, 415; and *BL* vol. 2, 135–136.

over the state of medical practice swelled, no category of disease more quickly became central to practical and theoretical debates than fever, and especially tertian fever. Empire had become a professional, clinical, and epistemic resource.

As a group, the physicians who took up these debates in print – among them: Duarte Madeira Arrais, Francisco Morato Roma, Simão Pinheiro Mourão, João Ferreira da Rosa, Manuel de Azevedo, João Curvo Semedo, and Francisco da Fonseca Henriques – had a number of things in common.[81] They abided by the royal instruction to write in the vernacular (Spanish or Portuguese, depending on when they wrote and where their careers took them). They were well placed (socially) and well connected (politically). They all spent their careers in Portugal or (in the case of Abreu, Mourão, and Rosa) Portugal's empire. They were also well published and probably well known, at least by name. Indeed, as I discuss below, Mourão was notorious. Their publications often went through multiple editions, and as authors they tended to reference one another's work.[82] They shared a concern with correcting both what they saw as professional malpractice as well as the errors of popular healers. They all took an interest in illnesses that were either new at home or common overseas. Arrais was the author of what was probably the best selling treatise on *morbo gallico* (the "French disease") in seventeenth-century Portugal but, increasingly over the latter half of the century, he and other physicians concentrated their efforts on a catalog of afflictions that included mal de Luanda, dysentery, pox, and especially malignant and tertian fevers.[83] The concern with fevers was so pronounced, their coverage so obligatory, that treatises addressing them often sat somewhat incongruously within books otherwise devoted to different topics altogether. Henriques's compendious *Medicina lusitana* may be the best example. It was divided into three sections; the last one addressed the diagnosis and treatment of fever but the first two were given over,

---

[81] A detailed prosopography and a comprehensive account of their shifting medical work is comfortably beyond the scope the present chapter. I have culled these details from their medical writings, which are listed in the bibliography, as well as from their entries in *BL*. These are, respectively, *BL* vol. 1, 734–735; *BL* vol. 2, 148, 210–211, 643, 658; and *BL* vol. 3, 184–185, 720. These were not the only physicians whose medical publications reflect an increasing preoccupation with diseases common to colonial settings. See also *BL* vol. 2, 241; and *BL* vol. 3, 451, and 585.

[82] This was an increasingly common tactic among Portuguese authors broadly. On which see Diogo Ramada Curto, "A história do livro em Portugal."

[83] For example, *BL* vol. 2, 241; and *BL* vol. 3, 451, and 585.

respectively, to a discussion of the health of the fetus in utero and to the health of the young child.[84] In their medical recipes, these physicians tended to embrace exotic *materia medica*. Arrais, like many of his contemporaries, favored guaiacum for morbo gallico. He, Semedo, and others advocated the use of china root (*raiz da china*), sarsaparilla, cinchona (*quinaquina*), chocolate, and a cornucopia of other therapeutics.[85] Tobacco was also common, though it had prominent and outspoken detractors in Lisbon.[86]

The work of Francisco Morato Roma and Manuel de Azevedo provide both a portrait of these shifting midcentury medical debates and an indication of the place of fever within them. Roma was Abreu's junior by some two decades and as the aging Abreu was in Lisbon composing the *Tratado*, the young Roma was in Coimbra finishing his medical degree. As Abreu's book made its way through the lengthy process of review and licensure for publication in May of 1623, Roma took up a post in the Braganza household. With the ascent of João IV in 1640, he became physician of the royal chamber and hence the physician general for the kingdom. Roma's *Luz da medicina* was published for the first time in 1664.[87] Meant as a guide to "practical, rational, and methodical" medicine, it covered diseases of the body in its entirety – not simply from head to toe but, as Roma put it, "from the head to the very soles of the feet." It was to be of use "not only for professors in the arts of medicine and surgery" but to anyone caring for the sick (*enfermeiros*) and to "the father of every family."[88] The physician of the royal body became physician to the body politic.

The *Luz da medicina* fared well on the Portuguese book market. Although its author died in 1668, printers in Lisbon and Coimbra produced new editions in 1672, 1686, 1700, 1726, and again in 1753.[89] The first three editions of the *Luz da medicina* carried a title page that detailed at some length its contents and made clear that the treatise on fever was

---

[84] Francisco da Fonseca Henriques, *Medicina Lusitana, Socorro Delphico aos clamores da natureza humana para total profligacão de seus males dividio em tres partes* (Amsterdam: Miguel Dias, 1710).

[85] *BL* vol. 1, 734–735; *BL* vol. 3, 595; and *BL* vol. 4, 34. On Semedo, see below.

[86] *BL* vol. 2, 241.

[87] Francisco Morato Roma, *Luz da medicina, pratica racional, e methodica, guia de enfermeyros* (Lisbon: Henrique Valente de Oliveira, 1664).

[88] These promises appear on the title page of Roma, *Luz*.

[89] *BL* vol. 2, 210–211. The 1686 edition is not listed by Barbosa Machado in the *BL*, but a copy is held in the Biblioteca Nacional de Portugal: BNP, Res., Cod. 6316 P.

the one part of the book in Latin. As in Abreu's *Tratado* the theoretical discussion of the causes of fever stood apart and remained under the purview of those with university training. Otherwise, the text was given over largely to the vernacular and focused on treatment. By 1726, someone – perhaps the printer who hoped to profit from republication – changed both of those features of the text. The title was shortened and Roma's treatise on fevers now appeared in the vernacular,[90] alongside the extensive and already very popular guide to *materia medica* by the surgeon Gonçalo Rodrigues de Cabreira (by 1671 it had already gone through some five separate editions).[91]

Roma never referenced Abreu directly, though he referred often and obliquely to the diverse opinions of "many authors." He shared Abreu's concern with fevers in general and tertian fevers in particular. "Intermittent tertian fevers," he noted, were "popularly called *maleitas*."[92] Roma also shared Abreu's reservation about the potential to effectively treat afflictions like fever. "Not all illnesses," he cautioned his readers, "can be cured" (*as doenças nem todas são curaveis*).[93]

Whereas Roma divided his original treatise on fever between four classes (those he described as simple, putrid, malignant, and contagious), the newly appended, vernacular text focused more narrowly on one kind: tertian fever. And it did so in considerable detail. The "single treatise on pernicious and malignant tertian fevers" divided the affliction into six distinct kinds of tertian fever, cautioning that it was possible as well to have a "double tertian fever" – that is: two of them simultaneously. It was largely an exercise in Galenic humoralism. Five of the six fevers were attributed to humors that were either crude or putrid, often but not always this was yellow bile. These fevers were further classed according to the corrupting humor's movement within the body (whether inward toward the heart or outward toward the extremities) and by the particular organ in which it came to rest (those seated in the heart and liver received particular attention).[94] Their prognosis varied and the author noted that "sudden death," though unlikely, was always a possibility.[95] It was the sixth and final fever that was most dangerous and whose victims were unlikely to survive. It was provoked by some unspecified – and, given the nuance with which he discussed the other fevers, probably unknown –

---

[90] *BL* vol. 2, 211.   [91] *BL* vol. 2, 403.   [92] Roma, *Luz*, 2–12, 133–156, 343–367.
[93] Roma, *Luz*, 2.   [94] Roma, *Luz*, 456–458.   [95] Roma, *Luz*, 459.

"pestilential quality." The real danger was that it also appeared to be "contagious."[96] This deadly fever could afflict whole populations simultaneously. When discovered, it demanded immediate attention.

So much nosological hair-splitting notwithstanding, the author proposed courses of treatments that were generally similar for all of these fevers.[97] They included bathing, ginseng, and bezoar-based elixirs, and, more commonly, bloodletting.[98] Careful attention had to be given to the intervals between bloodletting, eating, and sleeping, lest the fever or its location shift. The most important treatments were cinchona (*chyna chyna*) and "agua da Inglaterra," a cinchona-containing "water." But even that, he cautioned, may not work.[99]

Subtle, complex, arcane – the level of technical complexity was a measure of just how vigorous the debates about tertian had become.[100] By the early eighteenth century, debates over fever in general and tertian fever in particular seem to have spilled beyond the community of physicians and were now, like Macedo's vision of intertropical coherence, part of a wider discussions among metropolitan naturalists.

The final 1753 edition of the *Luz da medicina* retained Cabreira's guide but included a treatise on fever that was altogether different from Roma's original.[101] The title page made the dubious assertion that the surgeon Cabreira was its author. But nothing about Cabreira's publication record suggested even to the contemporary eighteenth-century bibliographer Diogo Barbosa Machado that Cabreira had written, let alone published, a treatise on fevers. What is more likely is that a third, unknown author, wrote the piece. It may have been of quite recent vintage, perhaps already circulating in manuscript. If so, it was one among numerous other, similar pieces of writing. According to the bibliographer Machado, manuscript treatises on tertian fever now circulated commonly and had begun to collect in royal and private libraries alike.[102]

Not everyone concerned with fever had ventured out into the empire. Roma, for one, had not. But the physician Manuel de Azevedo, author of

---

[96] Roma, *Luz*, 458–459.   [97] Roma, *Luz*, 477–479.   [98] Roma, *Luz*, 460–463.

[99] Roma, *Luz*, 480.

[100] Pace Latour: "when controversies flare up the literature becomes technical," in *Science in Action*, 30–44.

[101] Francisco Morato Roma, *Luz da medicina, pratica racional, e methodica, guia de enfermeyros* (Coimbra: Francisco de Oliveira, 1753).

[102] *BL* vol. 1, 734–735; *BL* vol. 2, 99, 135–136, *BL* vol. 3, 437; and *BL* vol. 4, 52, 101, and 185–186. Several of such manuscripts ended up in the library of one Paulo Pinto Coelho, see *BL* vol. 4, 260.

the *Correcção de abusos*, had – and he was the first since Abreu to return to Portugal to publish a book about the diseases he had found there.[103] In 1631, during the union of the Crowns, he was appointed the chief physician (*protomedico*) of the Spanish armada dispatched to Brazil as part of the effort to reverse Dutch advances there. Over the course of the next seven years, Azevedo crossed the Atlantic, journeyed between Bahia and "the Indies," twice battled Dutch fleets, and then sailed to Catalonia in 1638, where a revolt against Castilian rule was underway. It was the Catalan revolt that helped embolden Portuguese dissidents and made victory more likely in 1640. Because Azevedo had put his expertise in the service of Spain, and in light of the vigorous anti-Spanish sentiment at court, Azevedo excused himself in his introduction for not detailing his work for the Spanish Crown in Catalonia.[104]

For Azevedo, the omission was immaterial. It was not his work in the Mediterranean but his years in the Atlantic – and in particular the region below what he referred to as "the latitude of Cape Verde" – that underwrote his claims about nature and disease. In those years, he treated mal de Luanda, which was "unknown to physicians as it is the result of long sea voyages." He tended to seamen suffering from bloody dysenteries, which he came to believe were "especially deadly at the latitude of Cape Verde." But in Bahia, further into the intertropical region, it was a host of malignant fevers that were most pervasive (he claimed to have treated some seven hundred cases of it), and which thereby found its way into his *Correcção de abusos*, where – as was the case in Roma's *Luz da medicina* – it was given an entire treatise.[105]

Azevedo, believed that his experience in the empire distinguished his work from that of his peers. Doubting readers, he cautioned, should "consider well the diverse kingdoms and climates that I faced, the diversity of perilous diseases that I have confronted, and the countless number of sick patients whom I have cured." That range of experience – not just in the kingdom but beyond "the latitude of Cape Verde" and amid hundreds of cases of debilitating fever – was sufficient to give him a "confidence that is not excessive in what I have written, [and in] what you will read."[106]

---

[103] Manuel de Azevedo, *Correcção de abusos introduzidos contra o verdadeiro method da medicina* (Lisbon: Officina de Diogo Soares de Bulhões, 1668).

[104] Azevedo, *Correcção*, v–xiv.   [105] Azevedo, *Correcção*, xiii, xvi–xix.

[106] Azevedo, *Correcção*, viii.

Azevedo's introduction was as unflinchingly critical as the title of his treatise – the "correction of bad practices (*abusos*)" – was direct. He warned readers no to be fooled by the fact that his book was "so slim" and then launched into a criticism of metropolitan medical practice, beginning first with his colleagues. Anyone with a medical degree – and indeed many without one – could and did write guides to medicine. But even a medical degree was insufficient to ensure practical know-how. Surveying the landscape of medical publications, Azevedo concluded that it was their lack of experience that led his younger colleagues to focus so heavily on theory at the expense of useful, practical information that would promote health. Azevedo's *Correcção* much more overtly targeted what he saw as the bad medicine proffered by lay healers. The situation in the capital was so bad that "ancient and modern authors alike would find the city riddled with noxious sects of medicine." Azevedo thought it necessary to "eradicate" from all of Portugal "the noxious abuses that are prejudicial to health and life." He would not rest content until the "entire kingdom is without the abominable and misguided ways that some medics of this city have introduced into medicine."[107]

Seclusion probably enabled Azevedo's candor. Having returned to the kingdom in 1638, Azevedo practiced medicine for another decade. In 1648, piety, he claimed, compelled him to choose a more cloistered life. Azevedo entered the Carmelite novitiate and ten months later earned the simple cloth scapular that adorned the shoulders of Carmelite monks. For the next two decades, Azevedo cared for his professed brothers and composed the *Correcção de abusos*. In an age when royal favor determined careers, courtly discourse was suffused with calculated diffidence.[108] Such public attacks upon the physicians in whom the king and his courtiers placed not only their confidence but their lives could be counterproductive. Azevedo would hardly have been able to attack the "medicine practiced at this court" if he were still a part of it.[109]

Published in 1668, copies of Azevedo's *Correcção* circulated in Lisbon just as Macedo was settling into life at the French court. Among physicians in metropolitan Portugal there was as yet no hard and fast medical distinction that paralleled the environmental one soon drawn so sharply by Macedo. But Azevedo articulated just such a distinction. He referred repeatedly to "diverse climates" and relegated the most pervasive and

---

[107] Azevedo, *Correcção*, xxi.
[108] These themes are explored at length in Mario Biagioli, *Galileo, Courtier*.
[109] Azevedo, *Correcção*, xix–xxv.

deadliest fevers to the region below "the latitude of Cape Verde." Perhaps nowhere in the *Correcção* was the connection between the empire, inter-tropical locations, and debilitating tertian fevers more apparent than in the book's opening illustration (Figure 8.2). A humble friar – surely this was Azevedo – kneels before the heavens to receive the Carmelite order's characteristic rough-hewn scapular from the mythical Virgin of Carmo – all in the midst of a figure wielding a fiery blade. Here again was the flaming sword of the Cherubim – that image used in the thirteenth century to reconcile contradictory claims about the nature and climate of the torrid zone, the same "flaming sword of deadly fevers" invoked by Barros in the sixteenth century to explain the cause of death of so many Portuguese who ventured into the intertropical region.[110]

Now it was Azevedo, the pious physician, who confronted the deadlier fevers peculiar to the intertropical world.

Azevedo's experience with fevers in Brazil suggests the final dissolution even of the edenic myth that had surrounded Portugal's South American colonies. Indeed, just as the *Correcção de abusos* was coming to print, Brazil was in the throes of an epidemiological catastrophe. This time, colonial epidemics would be embraced as a bodily phenomenon. Health and disease in Portuguese America would increasingly be interpreted in light of its intertropical (as opposed to its regional, Atlantic) location. As that happened, epidemiological coherence became not just a possibility but a philosophically defensible position – one taken up by another ambitious physician. The tropics loomed.

INTERTROPICAL CONTAGION

Simão Pinheiro Mourão crossed the Atlantic to escape a sordid past. Before his eyes ever fell across the long, verdant arch of coastal Pernambuco, this son of an attorney had attended two of the oldest and most prestigious universities in Iberia. He held a degree in medicine from

---

[110] For the association references, see Chapter 1 and the references there. The scriptorium of the Lisbon convent housed a collection of the chronicles of the early West African voyages, including that of Zurara. By the early eighteenth century, the institution was not only associated with healing but had acquired a reputation for saving supplicants from deadly fevers. See Joseph Pereira de Santa Anna, *Chronica dos Carmelitas da antiga, e regular observancia nestes Reynos de Portugal, Algarves, e seus Dominios* (Lisbon: António Pedroso Galrão, 1745), 195, 486, 508–528, and 547–551; see also 283 for a wonderful engraving of the façade of the convent, now largely destroyed.

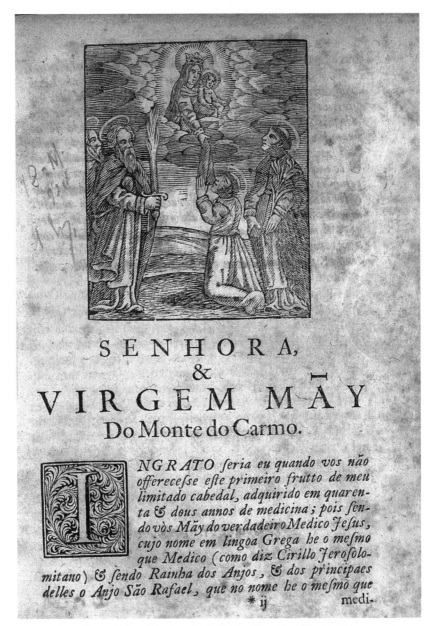

SENHORA,
&
VIRGEM MĀY
Do Monte do Carmo.

NGRATO *feria eu quando vos não
offerecefse efte primeiro frutto de meu
limitado cabedal, adquirido em quaren-
ta & dous annos de medicina; pois fendo vos Māy do verdadeiro Medico Jefus,
cujo nome em lingoa Grega he o mefmo
que Medico (como diz Cirillo Jerofolo-
mitano*) & *fendo Rainha dos Anjos, & dos principaes
delles o Anjo São Rafael, que no nome he o mefmo que*
* ij   medi-

FIGURE 8.2 Inventing an Intertropical Illness. The flaming sword becomes a
symbol of intertropical fevers in this image from Manuel de Azevedo, *Correcção
de abusos introduzidos contra o verdadeiro methodo da medicina* (Lisbon: Diogo
Soares de Bulhões, 1668).
Courtesy of the Biblioteca Nacional de Portugal.

Coimbra, had received a license to practice medicine anywhere in the empire, and – at least for a few years in the early 1660s – could boast of connections to the royal household, a thriving practice in Almada, a medical reputation on the make, the prospect of an honorable marriage, and a prosperous future perhaps in the imperial capital of Lisbon. But by the time Mourão sailed for Brazil in 1672, he had also already been imprisoned not once but four times – on one occasion for trafficking in stolen goods, on another for breaking his promise of marriage after having consummated the relationship. He had been sentenced to one of Portugal's African colonies but was allowed to serve instead in Alenquer after the Portuguese queen decided his expertise could be put to better use in the kingdom. After a few years, the townspeople of Alenquer decided otherwise. Mourão was forced to flee. He appeared twice before the Inquisition, was compelled to attend the *auto-da-fé* of his father, and was himself finally reconciled to the Church on the condition that he clothe himself in a *sambenito* – that rough-hewn vestment an unmistakable mark of dishonor – for the rest his life.[111]

That sartorial discipline could have ended his career. Physicians donning the *sambenito* were forbidden to practice in the kingdom. But not in the empire: Mourão sailed for Brazil.[112] In a colony in which university-education in general and degreed physicians in particular were scarce, a medical diploma from Coimbra endowed graduates with particular privilege.[113] In slightly different circumstances, Mourão would have had every reason to think his fortunes should improve. But in Brazil too it would have been impossible to catch sight of Mourão and not immediately understand the gravity of the accusations against him. With the *sambenito*, Mourão was instead derogated to the colonial category of the suspect, the morally degenerate.[114]

---

[111] *MRP*, 430–433; On the symbolism of the sambenito, see Alejandro Cañeque, "Theater of Power: Writing and Representing the Auto de Fe in Colonial Mexico," *The Americas* 52 (1996): 321–343.

[112] *MRP*, 433–434.

[113] The absence of the university forced those seeking education to return to Europe, usually to Coimbra – a shared experience that Schwartz has argued was formative of a unified Brazilian identity. See Stuart B. Schwartz, "The Formation of a Colonial Identity in Brazil," in *Colonial Identity in the Atlantic World, 1500–1800* eds. Nicholas Canny and Anthony Pagden (Princeton, NJ: Princeton University Press), 15–50.

[114] Vainfas, *Trópico dos pecados*.

Yet in the colonies, family histories could be revised or invented, personal failures hidden and fortunes reversed.[115] Men who in metropolitan Portugal would have been constrained by distinctions of family, trade, or religious heritage, might in the colonies improve their lot – sometimes considerably. It was true that by the end of the sixteenth century access to land, credit, and labor all grew more expensive and credit was less readily available.[116] But some boundaries could still be crossed – even erased – and others drawn in their place. By 1676, Mourão had begun to do just that. A petition to prince regent D. Pedro, with the support of Pernambuco's governor João de Souza, won approval and for the first time in four years – and forever thereafter – Mourão could leave his residence, pass along the streets, and tend to clients in Pernambuco without the shame of his *sambenito*.[117]

Just as he reinvented himself, so too did Mourão try to refashion medical practice in Portuguese America. There, Mourão became a medical author. Of the two texts that survive, Mourão's *Queixas repetidas* was by far the more caustic. The *Queixas* was an indictment of the colony's lay practitioners and amounted to an extended critique of colonial medicine. At the heart of it was the problem of tertian fever.[118] It was tertian fever, Mourão argued, that was "the most common illness in this climate," and the proliferation of lay medical practices that had sustained Portugal's American colonies for nearly two centuries were simply ill suited to handle the interpretive challenges and bodily dangers it posed.[119] Mourão divided the *Queixas* into two books. The first began with a list of the problems with medicine, which Mourão tried to rectify with chapters explaining the operations and transformations of the humors, rules for medical treatment, and three chapters on fever. The second book moved from diseases acute and deadly to cover ailments

---

[115] This is a long-running theme. See, for example, Júnia Ferreira Furtado, *Chica da Silva: A Brazilian Slave of the Eighteenth Century* (New York: Cambridge University Press, 2009); Herson, *Cristãos*; Studnicki-Gizbert, *Nation*; Wadsworth, *Agents*.

[116] Alexander Marchant, *From Barter to Slavery: The Economic Relations of Portuguese and Indians in the Settlement of Brazil, 1500–1580* (Gloucester, MA: P. Smith, 1966); and Schwartz, "Commonwealth."

[117] *MRP*, 433–434.

[118] The text remained in manuscript for nearly three centuries before it was published as Simão Pinheiro Mourão, *Queixas repetidas em ecos dos arrecifes de Pernambuco contra os abusos medicos que nas suas capitanias se observam tanto em dano das vidas de seus habitantes*, ed. Jamie Walter (Lisbon: Junta de Investigações do Ultramar, 1965 [1677]).

[119] Mourão, *Queixas*, 17.

chronic and debilitating – apoplexy, paralysis, spasms and convulsions, epilepsy, mania, and delirium.[120]

Mourão's critique of colonial lay healers may have been well received but his preoccupation with fever of any kind was rather beside the point – at least as far as Governor D. João de Souza, among Mourão's most influential and politically powerful patrons, was concerned. Mourão had arrived in Brazil in the wake of a succession of pox epidemics – one in 1664 and another in 1666 – and would practice medicine in the midst of another in 1683. It was to the problem of pox that the governor asked Mourão to turn his attention. In both practical and professional terms, it was a smart shift of emphasis for Mourão. He would surely not be able to transform medical practice in Pernambuco but he believed (and the governor, it seems, agreed) that his philosophical training gave him an advantage over his often unlettered and largely unlicensed counterparts in the colonies. Mourão's *Tratado único das béxigas e sarampo* was a much more theoretical treatise than his *Queixas*. In eight chapters, the *Tratado único* dealt at much greater length with explanations for the multiple causes of, and subtle distinctions between, the varied kinds of pox that swept the colonies; he dwelt much more on questions of pathogenesis and prognosis than on questions of treatment, prevention, or regimen.[121]

Tedious epistemic and ontological distinctions drawn at the request of no less an authority than the colonial governor were an opportunity to burnish his own reputation and enhance his standing among the well-to-do of the Brazilian northeast. Mourão welcomed it. His *Tratado único do sarampo e bexigas*, printed in Lisbon in 1683, was the first published medical treatise written entirely about Brazil. It was one of the few to discuss diseases in the colony at any length since Abreu's *Tratado* a half-century earlier. With his *Tratado único do sarampo e bexigas*, Mourão expanded the range of illnesses available for learned inquiry and debate. His book moved beyond Abreu's overarching concern for fevers and introduced discussion of the causes of what he argued were not only two but a number of different kinds of pox.

What began as the kind of exercise by which learned physicians secured their reputations and, crucially, some of their best-paying clients ensnared Mourão in the thorny issue of colonial epidemiology and the problematic combination of prodigious nature and debilitating febrile

---

[120] Mourão, *Queixas*, 5–62, 63–98.
[121] Romão Mosia Reinhipo [Simão Pinheiro Mourão], *Tratado unico das bexigas e sarampo* (Lisbon João Galrão, 1683).

illness. At stake in the *Tratado único das bexigas e sarampo* were a number of important issues. The first was the identity of the pox that had repeatedly swept the colonies during the preceding decade. Pox was well known in the corpus of medical literature but it seemed to erupt with peculiar ferocity in Brazil.[122] Mourão would ultimately have to explain why that was so and whether it was indeed the same pox that was so familiar to writers of earlier ages. The second and related question was the relationship between pox and fever. The two occurred together and, at least among the writers most influential for Mourão, the pox was often understood to be a consequence of fever. Properly identifying and treating the fever therefor also implied a treatment for the pox, too. Mourão would have to decide whether to continue to argue for that position or come up with an alternative. The third question concerned the fundamental character of the climate and environment of Brazil and whether it was indeed as healthy as generations of his countrymen had claimed it was. If Brazil were both verdant and deadly – and both conditions seemed increasingly undeniable – then Mourão would be compelled to explain how that could be so. The first question was not only easy but was in fact rather common; the second allowed Mourão to demonstrate his skillful reasoning. It was in response to the third question that Mourão articulated a philosophical explanation that resolved the very issue thrust to the fore by the earliest West African encounters: how could it be that at place could be characterized simultaneously by prodigious nature and debilitating illness? To answer that question, Mourão would resort to a minor and generally obscure element of Galenic theory to explain disease in Brazil. In so doing, Mourão rendered the intertropical region not just environmentally coherent but epidemiologically coherent as well.

For Mourão, as any properly trained physician well knew, the first order of business was the identification and explanation of the disease in question. On those questions hung all attempts to stop it, prevent it, and treat those afflicted with it. Pox was commonplace. By the seventeenth-century pox was already a longstanding object of medical inquiry and a host of physicians had addressed it. To this most common question – What was pox? – Mourão gave a commonplace answer. Susceptibility to

---

[122] Indeed, many questions about the virulence of what many have claimed was smallpox beginning in the late fifteenth century remain unsettled. A probing discussion is found in Ann G. Carmichael and Arthur Silverstein, "Smallpox in Europe before the Seventeenth Century: Virulent Killer or Benign Disease?," *Journal of the History of Medicine and Allied Sciences* 42 (1987): 147–168.

pox was inherent in human generation itself, communicated to the fetus *in utero* by the menstrual blood that sustained it until birth. Indeed, menstrual blood communicated to the fetus an array of potentially pernicious qualities that, if given the proper configuration of circumstances, would manifest themselves as varied kinds of pox. Mourão was quite specific about the relationship between menstrual blood and pox. The thinner blood (*mais delgado*) contributed the bad qualities that could produce a kind of pox that Mourão termed "sarampo"; the thicker blood (*mais crasso*) produced the pox he called "bexigas."[123]

His explanation for the universality of pox – that susceptibility lay in the vagaries of human generation – had a prestigious pedigree and was one around which there were centuries of scholarly consensus. Of the many ancient and contemporary authors Mourão might have chosen as a source for this account, he cited the German physician Daniel Sennert. On the question of the causes of pox, Mourão referenced Sennert repeatedly. But to demonstrate his own intellectual prowess and to thereby secure his own theoretical and clinical authority on the disease as it manifested itself in Brazil, Mourão had to distinguish his account from that of the well-regarded Sennert on whom he relied so heavily. Mourão turned to the resource most readily to hand: his own experience. That he had actually witnessed pox sweep through northeastern Brazil with unimaginable ferocity was an experience that he believed distinguished his work from that of his metropolitan peers. Those observations formed the basis of his own attempt to draw finer distinctions between what he argued were in fact an array of five different kinds of pox. The effort was as important clinically as it was professionally. Once finer distinctions were known, surer treatment and more certain prognosis were possible.[124]

It was in distinguishing his own work from that of his chief reference that Mourão also addressed the question of fever. Mourão had not only multiplied the kinds of pox available for diagnosis, but that work entailed a second important claim as well. Pox – in all their diversity – occurred almost simultaneously with fevers. And yet, although pox and fevers occurred together and were a consequence of common causes, they were nevertheless ontologically distinct afflictions. For Mourão, the question was which of these illnesses to treat first. Sennert had followed many others before him in affording clinical primacy to fever. Indeed, Sennert's work on pox comprised a single section in a much larger commentary

---

[123] Mourão, *Tratado*, 22–26.
[124] Mourão, *Tratado*, 77–82, identified five difference kinds of pox.

focused on the problem of fevers. His *De febre maligna cum variolis et morbiliis* circulated in Latin and a number of European vernaculars,[125] and it was likely from that text that Mourão knew of Sennert's work. For the German physician, pox was important not by itself but for what it revealed about the nature of the fever that it accompanied. Details about pox were indicators of which humors had been most corrupted by the fever. They were, in short, a guide to treating the fever that was, in turn, the real threat to the patient's life. Hence, for example, Sennert's explanation that "on the third or fourth day, the fever brings about spots which become either bexigas or sarampo. The color of the pox material indicates the humor affected and their location suggests which internal parts had been affected."[126] In this way, Sennert viewed pox in all of their varied manifestations as products of particular fevers. The fevers themselves had curative priority and were the object of treatment. Taken together, bleeding, the use of medicines, and diet helped the body "resist [the] malignancy" of fevers.[127]

Mourão, too, linked fevers with humors and the particular organs that synthesized them.[128] But rather than take the pox as a guide to the treatment of fever, Mourão reversed their clinical priority. He used the fever as an indication of what humors constituted the different pox.[129] For Mourão, treating pox first would resolve the fever as well. By first elaborating novel explanations for the causes and types of pox and redefining their relationship to fever, Mourão leveraged his own personal observations in Brazil to establish a place for himself in theoretical debates over both fevers and pox. Intellectually and professionally, Mourão managed to straddle the divide that separated metropolitan medical debates (that afforded primacy to fevers) and colonial medical imperatives (of which pox seemed to be the most pressing).

The more fundamental problem remained. Mourão still had to account for why pox of any sort seemed to erupt with an epidemic ferocity the likes of which, according to Mourão, were unknown in the corpus of Latin and Islamic medical writing to which he was privy. Perhaps the easiest thing to do was what Mourão had already done with tertian fever:

---

[125] *MRP*, 78.   [126] *MRP*, 299.   [127] *MRP*, 300.

[128] This was by no means novel. Distinct fevers were always linked to individual humors, themselves associated with individual organs. Notions of fever and contagion as understood by early modern German physicians and mapped onto the body are examined in Luke Demaitre, *Leprosy in Premodern Medicine: A Malady of the Whole Body* (Baltimore, MD: Johns Hopkins University Press, 2007), 184–189.

[129] Mourão, *Tratado*, 97–99.

blame the inadequate medicine of Brazil's varied practitioners. But he did not. Mourão might have followed Abreu and claimed that so much disease was simply characteristic of the South Atlantic – that the colonies of Portuguese America were unhealthy just like those of Portuguese Africa, and that the Atlantic was a single coherent epidemiological field. But he did not do that either. Instead, Mourão adopted the more global perspective that was then up for debate among his colleagues in metropolitan Portugal. He defined disease in Brazil in terms of its latitude. Mourão, however, was much more precise than his colleagues in Lisbon had been. Attuned to the epidemiological challenges facing every major theatre of Portugal's intertropical empire, and schooled in the Hippocratic-Galenic corpus, Mourão would claim that certain diseases were characteristic of the entire intertropical world. He would identify this global region as an epidemiological unity and explain how that could be so.

To recapitulate: I argued in Chapter 2 that West African encounters presented an enigmatic contradiction for seafarers who were even vaguely familiar with the Hippocratic-Galenic medical corpus that by the late fifteenth century was not only foundational for the learned medicine of the universities but influenced lay assessments of health in unfamiliar places. Bountiful nature was supposed to signal a healthy environment propitious for human settlement. But on verdant shores beyond the Senegal, European travelers fell ill and died. According to the Hippocratic-Galenic corpus, such a combination should have been a product of local factors like heat and humidity that accentuated the processes of growth, decay, rot, and putrefaction and thereby generated illnesses. Those, as I have shown, were precisely the parameters within which generations of sailors, merchants, chroniclers, missionaries, plantation owners and physicians from sub-Saharan Africa to South Asia and South America explained illness. And yet, despite centuries of colonial settlement, there was still no explanation for why the most globally verdant region seemed so often to be so deadly, and why the cause of that death was so often fever.

Brazil had been the exception that proved the rule. Now colonial epidemics of pox and fever, combined with a metropolitan preoccupation especially with intertropical fever, compelled Mourão to explain the still-confounding coincidence of verdant nature and debilitating febrile illness – and not just in Brazil but throughout the intertropical world. Here again, Mourão turned to the work of the German physician and the intellectual tradition of which he was a part. Senert's pathology, his approach to epidemic disease in general, no less than his approach to pox and to pestilential fevers in particular, was derived from the work of the French physician Jean Fernel. When Mourão turned to Sennert on questions such as this, he was in fact reading Sennert's reiteration of Fernel's work. Over the early and middle sixteenth century, Fernel was among a number of physicians who had tried to explain plague and the great pox of the turn of the sixteenth century – the two diseases that had so recently swept through Europe and which had been of greatest concern to the emergent, transnational community of physicians and naturalists.[130] Fernel had observed that none of the standard causes of disease – repletion, inanition, obstruction, or putrefaction – could account for the variety of symptoms that diseases like plague and pox presented or for their violent and pervasive effects on the body. Nor did standard explanations account for the particularity with which acute diseases seemed to strike. As the author of one recent study of Fernel's work posed the dilemma, the cause of diseases like these could not "simply [be] a corruption of the air," as was so often claimed, because "'healthy air' contains a spirit which sustains and protects all living things; made putrid or corrupt, it endangers all life in equal measure." As Fernel saw it, pestilence like plague and pox could not really be explained in this way, for those afflictions attacked only one kind of organism. Those diseases therefore demanded a distinct explanation.[131]

To resolve this problem Fernel took a cue from Galen, who had explained that while most medicines ameliorate an illness through its action on one or more of the body's constituent humors, the actions of a few medicines were not susceptible to humoral explanation but seemed instead to act by what Fernel referred to as the "total substance" (*tota substantia*) of the body. Fernel inverted Galen's logic. He argued that not only did some medicines act on the total substance of the body but that some diseases, rather than corrupt any individual humor or upset the balance among them, acted on the body's "total substance" – that is it afflicted a particular kind organism in its entirety. Among the diseases

---

[130] Ann G. Carmichael. *Plague and the Poor in Renaissance Florence* (New York: Cambridge University Press, 1986); Kathryn Park, *Doctors and Medicine in Early Renaissance Florence* (Princeton, NJ: Princeton University Press, 1985); Arrizabalaga, Henderson, and French, *The Great Pox*; and French, *Medicine before Science*, 157–184.

[131] Linda Deer Richardson, "The Generation of Diseases: Occult Causes and Diseases of the Total Substance," in *The Medical Renaissance of the Sixteenth Century*, eds. A. Wear, R. K. French, and I. M. Lonie (New York: Cambridge University Press, 1985), 184.

that could act on the body in this way were those whose causes Fernel described as "occult" or "hidden." According to the French physician, there were three kinds of occult illness, each defined by its mode of transmission: pestilential illnesses were communicated by air, contagious illnesses were transmitted by direct external contact with a poisonous substance, and poisonous diseases were produced within the body or taken in (consumed with food or drink, or produced within the body itself).[132]

Fernel found this explanation more satisfying than the conventional Hippocratic-Galenic one because it seemed to account for the observable precision of epidemic disease – it affected only human life but not that of plants and animals. True pestilence, in other words, attacked only one kind. Mourão agreed. It was to that first category of occult diseases that Mourão turned in order to explain the pronounced effects of pox and fever. Pestilential epidemics like these were, Mourão argued, partly a consequence of "poisonous impurities" – but impurities produced not only by putrid waters, rotting bodies, and hot and balmy airs but also by a causal configuration of heavenly bodies. Earthly sources of rot and contamination were important for when the peculiar alignment of particular stars, comets, and planets produced their own dangerous airborne impurities, those local factors gave epidemics their precise contours. They determined the precise effects of disease in a certain place and at a certain time of year. But they were especially characteristic of the intertropical world, argued Mourão, because the intertropical region itself was much more susceptible to heavenly influences.[133]

Hence, with an explanatory apparatus developed by Fernel to account for disease in sixteenth-century Europe, Mourão managed to explain how it was that the intertropical region could be at once verdant and healthy and yet everywhere also (potentially) diseased. In effect, Mourão had claimed that what made Brazil so healthy – a warm, humid climate and

---

[132] For this analysis, I rely on Richardson, "Generation of Diseases"; Iain M. Lonie, "Fever Pathology in the Sixteenth Century: Tradition and Innovation," *Medical History* 1 (1981): 19–44; Vivian Nutton, "The Seeds of Disease: An Explanation of Contagion and Infection from the Greeks to the Renaissance," *Medical History* 27 (1983): 1–34; Vivian Nutton, "The Reception of Fracastoro's Theory of Contagion: The Seed That Fell among Thorns?," *Osiris*, 2nd ser., 6 (1990): 196–234; J. Coomans and G. Geltner, "On the Street and in the Bathhouse: Medieval Galenism in Action?" *Anuario de Estudios Medievales* 43 (2013): 53–82; and the discussion of debates over fever and contagion in Arrizabalaga, Henderson, and French, *The Great Pox*; and Hamlin, *More Than Hot*.

[133] Mourão, *Tratado*, 105–109.

prodigious nature – was also the very quality that made it so liable to febrile illness, since those factors amounted to the preconditions that enabled epidemic diseases whose causes lay in the heavens. This was how Mourão accounted for the simultaneous occurrence of prodigious nature and debilitating illness. The entire verdant, intertropical world was uniformly more deadly – more prone throughout to such things as debilitating fevers – and that fact of nature had a causal explanation grounded in the authoritative intellectual lineage that tied Mourão directly to Galen.

ASSEMBLING THE TROPICS

In his *Tratado único das bexigas e sarampo*, Mourão provided a philosophical justification for the simultaneous occurrence of prodigious nature and debilitating febrile illness and identified that peculiar combination as the distinctive condition of the intertropical world. He derived that perspective from the work of Daniel Sennert and, through Sennert, from a marginal strain of Galenic medical theory elaborated by the French physician Jean Fernel that posited seeds as the cause of creature-specific contagion. In so doing, Mourão managed to side-step a fundamental contradiction inherent in the medical epistemology that had variously underwritten epidemiological speculation in Portuguese colonies for centuries. Even within the intellectual world of the Portuguese Atlantic, his work was not unprecedented. Brandão had speculated that seeds caused the principal diseases of the South Atlantic at the turn of the seventeenth century. Mourão's midcentury metropolitan predecessors had already begun to insist variously upon the environmental (pace Macedo) and epidemiological (pace Azevedo and others) coherence not of the Atlantic but of the intertropical world more generally. Mourão, however, produced a philosophical justification for that coincidence.

The printed work of João Curvo Semedo concretized in clinical and therapeutic terms the vision of intertropical coherence that took shape across metropolitan diplomatic, administrative, and medical circles. Between the cosmographic lines of Macedo (that linked celestial lines of latitude with earthly landscapes) and the lines of pathology charted by the physicians (which delimited a space of subtle, unseen seeds of febrile contagion), Semedo conjured a sensorially rich, densely diseased, and therapeutically diverse world. One of the best known and most prolific physicians in Portugal at the turn of the eighteenth century, Semedo had come to Lisbon in 1662, with a medical degree from Coimbra and just as debates about fever, medicine, and the empire were picking up. Over time, and much like Abreu, Roma, and Azevedo, he won the patronage of some of the most influential officials in imperial Portugal. He became a physician of the royal household, member of the prestigious Order of Christ, familiar of the Inquisition, and personal physician to members of both the Council of State and the Overseas Council.[134]

The combination of the sheer volume of his published work and its evident commercial success – tens of thousands of printed pages – suggest, if not his influence,[135] then at least the degree to which his work spoke to and reflected metropolitan medical concerns and perspectives. In fluid Portuguese prose (he had a knack for economy and precision) Semedo addressed wide-ranging questions of medicine and health. He was best known for a guide to household medicine published under the title *Polyanthea medicinal*.[136] Printed in small type and nearing a thousand pages per copy, the *Polyanthea* was dense, massive, and compendious. It was also a best seller. First printed in 1697, Semedo published new editions of it in 1704 and 1716.[137] Each volume was thicker than the last.[138] The first edition ran to 1,060 copies. The second, at 2,150 copies, was more than twice as large (and Semedo readily conceded that it took over twice as long, twelve years rather than five, to sell all of them). Though sprawling, Semedo constructed the *Polyanthea* to be as thoroughly accessible as possible. Each of the three treatises and the nearly 150 chapters that comprised the *Polyanthea* were neatly surveyed in an expansive table of contents. An alluringly titled "Index of the most notable things contained within this book" (*Indice das cousas mais notaveis, que se contèm neste Livro*), which ran to about 150 pages, located individual diseases and particular remedies with even greater precision.

---

[134] José Pedro Sousa Dias, "Terapéutica Química y polifarmacia en Portugal: La contribución de João Curvo Semedo (1635–1719)," in *Construyendo las ciencias químicas y biológicas* (Mexico City: Universidad Autónoma Metropolitana, 1998), 67–88.

[135] This is the argument of Dias, "Terapéutica," 177.

[136] Here I work from João Curvo Semedo, *Polyanthea Medicinal. Noticias Galenicas e Chemicas* (Lisbon: António Pedroso Galrão, 1716).

[137] After Semedo's death in 1719, it was also published twice more, once in 1727 again in 1741. As Adrian Johns, *Nature of the Book*, demonstrates, the fact of publication did little to stabilize a text. Although the various editions of the *Polyanthea* are generally discussed collectively, as in the otherwise superb discussion in Dias, "Therapéutica," these editions are far from identical. There is some divergence between the findings of Dias, the claims of the bibliographer Barbosa Machado, and the holdings of Lisbon's Biblioteca Nacional. To my knowledge there is yet no study of the successive transformations of this medical text or a definitive count of new editions.

[138] Semedo, *Polyanthea*, *3, finally apologized to his readers for what he judged the undeniable "corpulence" of the 1716 edition.

The *Polyanthea* was one work among many. Before his death in 1719, as he busily shuffled between royal bedsides, printers, apothecary shops, and the city's wharves, Semedo also managed to publish a raft of other titles. By comparison to the swollen *Polyanthea*, most of these were anemic. But they were legion. They included:

Atalaia da vida contra as hostildades da morte;
Manifesto em que se mostra com autoridades de gravissimos doutores que se podem dar purgas estando os humores crus;
Manifeso que o Doutor João Curvo Semedo ... faz aos amantes da Saúde;
Memorial de vários simplices;
Observações médicas doutrinais;
Proposta que o Doutor João Curvo Semedo, Médico, morador em Lisboa, faz aos amantes da saude, e attentos às suas consciencias;
Tratado do ouro diaforético.

All were medical. Some, like the *Proposta*, were leaflets of between ten and eleven pages. The *Memorial* was a pamphlet of slightly more than thirty pages. Exactly how many copies of any one of these were printed is an open question. What is clear is that they were printed in multiple runs, sometimes separated by several years. Differing versions of the *Manifesto*, the *Proposta*, and the *Memorial* remain. They are distinguishable by differences both subtle (such as paragraph organization) and obvious (like title changes: the *Proposta* and one of the two pamphlets titled *Manifesto* are virtually identical).

The *Polyanthea* was surely meant for the curated shelves of his patron's personal libraries, the chambers of practicing physicians, or the busy shops of prosperous apothecaries. Semedo's pamphlets – slimmer, cheaper – were probably meant for wider and less exclusive circulation. Although Semedo's published works might be considered in isolation, a more careful reading reveals a much closer relationship between them.[139] Not only do all of the smaller pamphlets reference the *Polyanthea* but different versions of each pamphlet reference particular editions of that

---

[139] Readers may have had difficulty keeping track of Semedo's work. For that complaint, as for ills more serious and bodily, Semedo offered a remedy. Tucked into the front matter of the third edition of the *Polyanthea* was a list of Semedo's various printed works: those "already in print" as well as those "in preparation." See Semedo, *Polyanthea*, unnumbered first page.

larger text – and they do so with specific chapter, page, and paragraph citations. Later editions of the *Polyanthea* incorporated some of the pamphlets, and also advertised current and forthcoming versions of them. Semedo did not simply write and publish ancillary material. He frequently rewrote and republished it.

Semedo's printed work is best conceived as a massive, mutually-reinforcing corpus of therapeutic understanding. Of course, given the litany of cross-references, that was exactly what Semedo had intended. In the ever-widening expanse that separated the covers of each subsequent edition of the *Polyanthea* yawned an immense catalog of what Semedo described in the *Memorial* (itself appended to the 1716 edition) as "various simples from the East Indies, America, and other parts of the world."[140]

The self-referential world of paper that Semedo repeatedly set in motion within Lisbon drew on the books, letters, and material objects that Portugal's empire had mobilized globally. Semedo noted the provenance of his drugs but he said little about their regionally-specific significance. He nodded at the curative expertise of unnamed "Moors [in Africa], Gentios [of Brazil], and Iogues [in Asia]" on whom his own work ostensibly depended.[141] But not even the most basic techniques of that vaguely-referenced cast of specialists were ever spelled out in any detail. The diverse range of medical expertise and the therapeutic techniques that populated the intertropical world – and which were inextricably a part of the colonial cultures of natural inquiry and medical practice that I have explored here – were left out of the *Polyanthea*. In their place were what Semedo claimed to be his own, proprietary, and (by implication) superior formulas. Semedo encouraged his readers to acquire them at any one of a number of apothecary shops spread from the Chiado neighborhood in central Lisbon to the outskirts of the city. These shops peddled the pills, pastes, and other medicaments that he claimed to make with his very own hands. Semedo left aside details about their preparation but put on display the exotic plant and mineral matter from which he concocted them.

In the *Polyanthea*, Semedo staged the promiscuous intermingling of widely-scattered therapeutics drawn from disparate approaches to healing. When readers consulted the text, they waded into a cacophony

[140] Semedo, *Polyanthea*, 226. [141] Semedo, *Polyanthea*, 226.

of nature, color, taste, smell, and disease. The book (and especially the smaller and ultimately appended pamphlet, the *Memorial*) was an eclectic assortment that included sapphires, the ear of a snow leopard, seahorse genitals, ginger, and Peruvian spiders. Of some seventy-nine simples, a dozen were common to the area from Portugal to France; a number of others were from locations as disparate as Kandahar and the Spanish Indies.

But there was more to Semedo's seemingly haphazard juxtapositions. Contemporary claims of intertropical coherence provided an underlying spatial logic to Semedo's vertiginous arrangements. Most of these *materia medica* – no fewer than forty-three – were from the intertropical world, and often but not always from Portuguese dominions: from Bahia to Benguela, and from Melindi to the Maldives, Malacca, and beyond. Most of these were, according to Semedo, medical panaceas. The afflictions they treated, much like their origins, ranged widely. Yet among the most sought after drugs, those that got the most elaboration, and those to which Semedo returned most frequently were *materia medica* for fevers. From the Canara Coast to the south of Goa came a root so valuable in treating malignant tertian or quartan fevers that "out of devotion" it was popularly referred to as the "root of Our Lady of Fevers." It was best if taken in the morning, or when a fever begins to decline, or when over the course of an infirmity, the tongue seemed black or yellow.[142] The "Cannanore stone," made its way to Semedo's attention in two brilliant colors, yellow and green. The green ones were better. But either one, if finely ground and given with water were excellent for fevers – and even better, especially for intermittent fevers, if the water was first boiled with pure gold.[143] The "Manica root" grew among the gold deposits of the Manica highlands in the interior of Mozambique. Semedo cautioned readers that it must not be taken with any kind of oil, lest the root turn to poison.[144] In Brazil, unicorn horns were finally found – on the crown of an Amazonian bird that, according to Semedo, the natives called the "ave inhuma" – and they too were put to effective use against fevers.[145] Much else from the intertropical world could also treat fevers: elephant tusks (especially when prepared with rose water and coconut from the Maldives), Colombo root (when ground and soaked with juice of lime), and even a mermaid's rib.[146] The drugs to which individual names were irrevocably bound were

---

[142] Semedo, *Polyanthea*, 186.   [143] Semedo, *Polyanthea*, 217.
[144] Semedo, *Polyanthea*, 335–336.   [145] Semedo, *Polyanthea*, 254–257.
[146] Semedo, *Polyanthea*, 377.

invariably those for fever. One was the "root of João Pires."[147] The other was the "root of João Lopes Pinheiro," which was a particularly "admirable remedy for tertian and quartan fevers."[148]

In the pages of the *Polyanthea*, Semedo assimilated exotic therapeutics to one another through their common efficacy against fever. Through reference to the disparate intertropical origins of these drugs, he conjured a vision of distant but seamlessly fecund intertropical landscapes. By insisting on their use in the treatment of fevers locally throughout the vast equinoctial region, he located those afflictions, too, across the same global space. Between the covers of the thickening *Polyanthea*, a vast and variegated intertropical world had been neatly assembled into an internally consistent, globally coherent one.

Seeds of plants and seeds of contagion commingled. The relationship between the world that Semedo conjured and the one variously elaborated by Macedo and by Portuguese physicians in the middle and late seventeenth century was neither incidental nor implicit. As he took care to point out at the opening of the *Polyanthea*, Semedo's survey of the diseases and treatments therein was predicated on the work of the very succession physicians whose writings stressed intertropical epidemiological coherence: Duarte Madeira Arrais, Amborios Nunes, Aleixo de Abreu, Francisco Morato Roma, Simão Pinheiro Mourão, João Ferreira da Rosa, Manuel de Azevedo, and Semedo's contemporary Francisco da Fonseca Henriques.

As a new vision of the intertropical world was summoned into being, so old language was given new meaning in the attempt to reference it. What to call this single vast region, the intermingling constituents of which were now inventoried in such stunning, lurid detail in the multiplying pages of the *Polyanthea*? One answer came in the form of a poem. Pascoal Ribeyro Coutinho's lyrical tribute to Semedo was one of several meant to celebrate the *Polyanthea*.[149] The untitled poem was modeled on the sixteenth-century *Os Lusiadas* by the sixteenth-century humanist Luís de Camões. That Homeric epic by Portugal's best-known bard celebrated the Portuguese voyages of exploration.[150] Camões's original cast Vasco

---

[147] Semedo, *Polyanthea*, 409.

[148] Discussions of these appear in varying degrees of detail throughout the *Polyanthea*. The basic references here are to the *Memorial* included in the 1716 edition, the pagination of which is not continuous with the rest of the volume in which it was included. See the discussion of these in Semedo, *Polyanthea*, 111.

[149] The poem first appeared in the second, 1704, edition.

[150] It was (and remains) seen not only as a major literary accomplishment but foundational in the development of the Portuguese language itself.

da Gama in the lead role and culminated in that explorer's epochal
1498 passage to Calicut.[151] In the poem by Camões, the glorious *fidalgo*
was richly rewarded for his oceanic conquests by his lover Tethys (the
Greek Titaness of the ocean), who not only revealed to da Gama the
glories that were to follow in his wake but who led him to the top of a
heavenly summit from which da Gama was allowed to gaze upon the vast
máquina do mundo – the machinery of the Ptolemaic universe – in its
entirety.[152]

With a global empire, mortal eyes achieved godly perspective: that
extended metaphor neatly suited Coutinho's purpose. In his poem meant
to celebrate Semedo's accomplishments, Coutinho simply replaced the
explorer with the physician. Semedo had attained global vision, but as a
man of medicine in Lisbon rather than a gentleman seafarer in Asia.
Instead of complete knowledge of the inner-workings of the universe,
Semedo's labors won him unequaled knowledge of bodily ills and worldly
medicine – of things "anatomical, chymical, herbal."[153] Just as da Gama
had surveyed the oceans and brought new peoples and new lands under
the control of the Crown, so Semedo had examined exotic vegetable and
mineral objects and delivered their curative powers to metropolitan
subjects.

When Coutinho referenced the vast intertropical world from which
Semedo assembled his career and reputation, he invoked merely "the
ardent tropic."[154] It was a subtle but significant shift. What had once
been a single line of latitude now referenced an entire region. The "tropic"
had become a place. To be sure, this language was not yet widely used.
The Portuguese lexicographer, Rafael Bluteau, who also contributed
words of praise for Semedo to the opening of the *Polyanthea*, would still
distinguish between the tropic (a "term of astronomy") and the torrid
zone (a "cosmographical term"). Yet neither was this the torrid zone of
old. Writing at the turn of the eighteenth century and capturing the spatial
transformation that had unfolded in the last two centuries, Bluteau's
definition merits quotation at length. The "torrid zone" he wrote,

---

[151] Although just how epochal it really was remains a point of contention. Compare K. N.
Chaudhuri, *Trade and Civilization in the Indian Ocean World: An Economic History
from the Rise of Islam to 1750* (New York: Cambridge University Press, 1985); and
Subrahmanyam, *Political Economy of Commerce*.

[152] This was not the first time that maritime exploits inspired Portuguese poets to reference
this particular goddess. See Subrahmanyam, *The Career and Legend of Vasco da Gama*,
76–77, and n. 2.

[153] Semedo, *Polyanthea*.   [154] Semedo, *Polyanthea*, xxix.

lies immediately beneath the path of the sun, between the Tropics of Cancer and Capricorn [where it] receives the rays of the Sun perpendicularly, and so direct and constant, and abundant that the Ancients believed it to be totally uninhabitable. And there is no doubt that across this swath of land there are many places that are indeed dry, sterile, and scorched ... and yet there are many parts, principally in America where frequent rains and large, extensive rivers temper the heat. One finds the same to be true in Asia ... particularly in Golconda and the City of Goa ... [where] the rains irrigate the lands and render them fertile.[155]

Much like the Humboldtian tropics later, a new vision of the intertropical world as unified and coherent despite evident internal variation had become an imperial matter of fact. And a repurposed language was available to refer to it. Lines of latitude now stood in for the landscapes of empire.

---

[155] Rafael Bluteau, *Vocabulario portugues e latino*, 10 vols. (Lisbon: Oficina da Música, 1712–1728), vol. 8, 310 and 647.

9

Epilogue

Somewhere between the theoretical mapping that inscribes cosmographic lines around the imagined globe to produce "the tropics," the empirical geography of lands, seas, and airs that characterize these parts of the globe, and the environments and peoples that make places in the equinoctial regions of the globe, epistemology and ontology constantly rework one another.

Dennis Cosgrove[1]

ALCHEMY, TRANSPLANTATIONS, AND THE LANGUAGE OF EMPIRE

In a world in which vocational skills and hence livelihoods ran in families, João Curvo Semedo was something of an interloper. His father was not a physician, attorney, or theologian. He enjoyed no official appointment and held no title. He was a blacksmith. Perhaps for that reason, Semedo the successful physician placed so much emphasis on the value of craftsmanship. True to his upbringing, Semedo made his living by personally "fabricating" the medicines he sold.[2] He was a "mechanic" among philosophers. Semedo's colleagues assured readers that even Galen would have approved.[3] It was a prestigious if perhaps increasingly outdated warrant for Semedo's professional practice.

[1] Cosgrove, "Tropic and Tropicality," 215.
[2] Semedo, *Polyanthea*, [unnumbered p. 19].
[3] Semedo, *Polyanthea*, [unnumbered p. 23].

Portugal's empire endowed the mechanical arts with new value. In Semedo's hands, it also wrenched learned medicine in Portugal from its more conventional Galenic orientation. Solving the problem of intertropical fevers – diseases brought about by imperceptible seeds – meant making medicines that acted in the same way. Like the diseases they were meant to treat, the requisite drugs acted upon the entire human organism all at once – on the so-called *tota substantia* – rather than upon individual humors.[4]

For Semedo, the drugs in question were not simply combinations of exotic ingredients. They were the products of chemical medicine, and it was, above all, chemical medicine that most interested Semedo in the *Polyanthea*. Instead of the more conventional Galenic therapeutics (plant-derived medicinal simples whose properties could be plotted along the twin axes of hot/cold and moist/dry), Semedo touted the superiority of an expanded range of *materia medica* centered on minerals, stones, and metals – things that were not so easily classed. His preferred ingredient was "antimony" (*antimonio*).[5] The whole of Book Two in the *Polyanthea* was given over to a survey of the ways in which the obdurate metallic substance could be prepared to treat a host of diseases – tertian fever first among them – that "were incurable in the times of Hippocrates and Galen."[6] Through the practice of chemical medicine, the sage physician would use his "secret knowledge" (*segredos*) to unleash the occult forces, the "specific, volatile spirits," of the sublunary in order to enact "marvelous" cures upon the body.[7] Chemical medicine was to the imperial physician as "arms to a soldier, rudders to a pilot, and oils to a painter."[8] Antimony enabled medicine's "perfection."[9]

Semedo was not alone in his belief that antimony had hidden and profound transformative powers.[10] Rather, antimony was widely thought to be the precursor of the so-called philosopher's stone – the material

---

[4] Semedo, *Polyanthea*, 59 offered readers an explanation of the concept "toda a substancia." See also Richardson, "The Generation of Disease"; and Andrew Wear, "Explorations in Renaissance Writings on the Practice of Medicine," in *The Medical Renaissance of the Sixteenth Century*, eds. A. Wear, R. K. French, and I. M. Lonie (New York: Cambridge University Press, 1985), 118–145.

[5] Semedo also used the popular names "estíbio" (stibnite) and "pòs [*sic*] de Quintilio" (Quintilian's powders). According to Principe, *Secrets of Alchemy*, 138–141, early modern "antimony" was not pure antimony but antimony sulfide ("sulfur of antimony").

[6] Semedo, *Polyanthea*, [unnumbered p. 21], 703.

[7] Semedo, *Polyanthea*, 696, but see the discussion on 693–724.

[8] Semedo, *Polyanthea*, 693.   [9] Semedo, *Polyanthea*, [unnumbered p. 20].

[10] These were quite apart from its Galenic properties, which Semedo *Polyanthea*, 17, listed as cold in the first degree and dry in the second.

agent by which the alchemist "transmuted" metals of one kind into another (most famously base metals into gold).[11]

By the turn of the eighteenth century, the creation of a global intertropical empire and the promiscuous intermingling of once-disparate plants, animals, and seeds of contagion made the language of alchemy useful to areas quite apart from imperial health. Its metaphors of transformation, and its emphasis on occult powers and arcane knowledge made alchemical language into a lexicon for speaking across domains of imperial expertise. From medicine and geography to political economy, the language of contemporary alchemy prevailed. Abreu conceived of the hidden transformations of febrile diseases within the body as a succession of "transmutations."[12] Even before Semedo wrote of the "transplantation" of fever-inducing seeds, Macedo planned to transform South American landscapes through the "transplantation" of South Asian drugs and spices.[13] So seductive, uncertain, and (possibly) transformative was Macedo's plan to reverse to imperial fortunes that he compared it to the elusive "philosopher's stone" itself.[14] Of course, the transplantation of drugs and spices from South Asia to South America would not turn lead into gold but it just might reverse the fortunes of an embattled, impoverished intertropical empire.[15]

The uncertainties that compelled this language were a long time in the making. It took two centuries to assemble the tropics. It also took an intertropical empire, the mobilization of plants, animals, and objects, and the potent but also contingent combination of administrative reform, economic turmoil, seeds of contagion, and professional self-interest. "The tropics" was a consequence of countless human entanglements with both intertropical objects and disease agents. These began in the middle of the fifteenth century. They culminated in the late seventeenth century. Epidemiological encounters along the Upper Guinea Coast gave the lie to long-standing and contradictory claims about the health of intertropical

---

[11] Principe, *The Secrets of Alchemy*, 25–26, 112–127.

[12] See, for example, Abreu, *Tratado*, 24v, 61v, 63, and 117v.

[13] Semedo, *Polyanthea*, 74, 79; Macedo's comment can be found in BNP Res. Cod. 11377 ff. 68, 71v, 75–75v, 82v. On "transplantation" in the thinking of contemporary alchemists, see Principe, *The Secrets of Alchemy*, 114 and 235, n. 11.

[14] BNP Res. Cod. 11377 f. 67.

[15] The language of alchemy persisted. Marshall Hodgson would critically refer to the stunning, destructive achievement of Western imperial primacy "the great Western transmutation." See Hodgson, *Rethinking World History: Essays on Europe, Islam, and World History*, ed. Edmund Burke III (New York: Cambridge University Press, 1993), ch. 4.

Africa. Aristotle insisted the whole intertropical region was scorched and barren. Seafarers found that, at least in the Gulf of Guinea, that was not so. Theologians, philosophers, and seafarers alike variously located the earthly paradise and the mythical kingdom of Prester John in intertropical Africa only to find that that was not quite true either. They did find a bountiful natural world. Yet contrary to the claims of the Hippocratic framework, natural abundance did not necessarily mean the region was propitious for colonial settlement. All along the West African coast, prodigious nature was accompanied by debilitating illness. Fevers, in particular, proved pervasive.

Those encounters had consequences. First, in the African Atlantic, Iberian and other European travelers turned to indigenous therapeutics and then to indigenous medical specialists. That move, I have repeatedly suggested, was not a hard one for travelers to make. Clinical plurality characterized the plague-stricken kingdoms from which European travelers had come. From the outset, febrifuges were central to cross-cultural medical exchanges and they remained so to colonial cultures of natural inquiry as they emerged across Portugal's empire. If exotic *materia medica* had long been a prized component of long-distance trade, the creation of a global intertropical empire would ultimately mean not only a more globalized drugs trade but one in which treatments for enigmatic tertian fevers were increasingly prominent.

Second, those encounters posed other questions. One was whether or not the West African situation was a generalized condition of the entire intertropical world. Were all intertropical regions characterized by abundant nature and febrile disease? The other was how illness could be widespread and so utterly pervasive in a place that appeared profoundly healthy. This was an epidemiological situation that the Hippocratic epistemology could not accommodate. If the culprit were bad air or some other environmental cause, the offending element should have had similarly deleterious effects on all living creatures. But in the intertropical world, it was only human life that seemed imperilled. Nature continued to thrive. How could a place be at once verdant and deadly?

Much as happened with plague and the great pox in Mediterranean Europe, so, too, with fevers among European seafarers in the African Atlantic: the unexpected prevalence and inexplicable virulence of fevers along the West African coast challenged European ideas about the causes of disease. Speculation about causes began aboard the first ships to sail beyond the Senegal. For university-trained Portuguese physicians at the end of the seventeenth century, the solution to the question of causes would lay in what, according to Vivian Nutton, was a minor and largely forgotten bit of Galenic medical theory.[16] Rather than an individual, humoral imbalance within the body, some afflictions were caused by seeds acting upon it from the outside.

In the late seventeenth century, claims of intertropical coherence –both environmental and epidemiological – became foundational to contests for the imperial authority of learned medicine. With its insistence on intertropical fever as a signal clinical concern, its proffering of intertropical nature as the principal source of effective therapeutics, and its assertions of medicinal improvement through metropolitan chemical-medical modifications, João Curvo Semedo's *Polyanthea medicinal* appears as a culminating statement of this metropolitan perspective.

RELOCATING EXPERTISE IN THE EARLY MODERN WORLD

If the deadliest fevers were located in the tropics, expertise about them no longer could be. Semedo's *Polyanthea* also appears symptomatic of a will to dominate, displace, or to outright erase the multiple ways of knowing and healing that, I have argued, inhabited the Portuguese colonial world and which I have tried to highlight in the preceding chapters. Domination and displacement may often have been central to the imperial programs of conversion, cultural tutelage, and colonial improvement variously hatched in Lisbon, Madrid, London, Paris, and elsewhere beginning in the sixteenth century.[17]

But on the ground, across empires, what actually happened was more complex and necessarily entailed a good bit more borrowing and collaboration than postcolonial studies are often willing to concede. Improvised arrangements – commercial and curative alike – hinged on transgressing the very lines of race, ethnicity, culture, and religion meant to demarcate boundaries between colonized and colonizer.[18] Generations of scholarship have shown the early modern colonial world to be violent and stringently hierarchical. Portuguese colonies both in South Asia and the South Atlantic were no different. But imperial rhetorics of strict cultural

---

[16] Nutton, "Seeds of Disease"; and Nutton, "Reception of Fracastoro."

[17] On cultural exclusivism as a hallmark of European empires, see Jane Burbank and Frederic Cooper, *Empires in World History: Power and the Politics of Difference* (Princeton, NJ: Princeton University Press, 2010).

[18] Here I point to a common theme in much writing on European empires both early modern and modern. See, for example, Gruzinski, *Mestizo Mind*; Xavier and Županov, *Catholic Orientalism*; Jasanoff, *Edge of Empire*; Tilley, *Africa as a Living Laboratory*.

conformity masked quotidian colonial realities of tolerance and collaboration.[19] Following Serge Gruzinski (on the colonial Americas) and Sanjay Subrahmanyam (on Portuguese Asia), I have tried to recognize the brutality of this world but without overlooking the pervasive uncertainty that came with the experience of early modern colonialism and which made Portugal's colonies places simultaneously ripe with curiosity, doubt, and innovation.[20] Goa, Luanda, and Pernambuco were home to cultures of inquiry characterized by investigative and therapeutic collaboration that defy easier postcolonial formulations.[21]

Whether Iberian contemporaries could boast of institutions that centralized global reconnaissance, institutionalized empirical practices, and mounted experimental programs has become central to debates over when and where a scientific revolution took place. By focusing on Goa, on Jesuit missions along the coast of Brazil, and on the Atlantic itineraries of a physician and a sugar planter in the seventeenth century, I have attempted to reorient and pluralize the history of early modern science, and to decouple it from Eurocentric, modernist narratives of scientific revolution that orient so many studies of early modern – especially Iberian – science. I have argued that the creation of Portugal's empire entailed the convergence of diverse epistemic practices and that these helped constitute distinct (although by no means entirely divergent) colonial cultures of natural inquiry in each theater of colonial engagement.

By moving between scales – the institutional infrastructure of Portugal's global empire, the unstable milieu of south Asian commercial networks, the shifting arrangements of material within early modern books, and a colonial household in Goa, I have tendered an argument about natural inquiry as it was practiced by the best-known physician in Portuguese Asia. Rather than an extension of either the prevailing metropolitan fascination with exotica or the humanist pursuit of unadulterated ancient knowledge, I argued that Garcia de Orta's work of accumulating, comparing, and identifying Asian nature spoke first and foremost to the intertwined commercial and epidemiological concerns of disadvantaged colonial traders. Orta's epistemology was highly functional and shuttled between texts and experience, and is not reducible to teleological narratives of empiricism and

---

[19] See Schwartz, *All Can Be Saved*; Studnicki-Gizbert, *Nation*.

[20] Gruzinski, *Mestizo Mind*, 45–51; Subrahmanyam, *Explorations in Connected History: From the Tagus to the Ganges*, ch. 1.

[21] See also the discussion in Jasanoff, *Edge of Empire*, 10–13; and in William Dalrymple, *White Mughals: Love and Betrayal in Eighteenth Century India* (New York: Penguin, 2004), 7–43.

experimentalism. Fevers were among the most frequently cited illnesses in Orta's book. But the study of medicine for Orta meant primarily the identification of tradable medicinal plants. It did not entail arguments about the intertropical situation of Portuguese Asia. It did mean grappling artfully with the antagonisms of Portuguese colonial society.

Natural inquiry in Portuguese America had a distinct chronology. I have countered the frequent claim that Jesuit missionaries advocated the disciplined study of natural phenomena. I show instead that debates within the Jesuit order over the allocation of their own personnel and expertise led Jesuits to encourage a learned ignorance of Brazil's unfamiliar flora and fauna, and to dismiss epidemic disease as a medical concern. By insisting that Brazilian nature was unworthy of study, Jesuits helped deflect contemporary interest in Brazilian nature and thereby also helped delay efforts to catalog it. Their dismissal of the curative attributes of Brazilian flora helped foreclose the possibility that Brazilian *materia medica* would become part of an expanding imperial pharmacopoeia. With this interpretation, I have insisted that an understanding of the culture of inquiry that characterized the Company demands not only a hard look at the spiritual and philosophical aspects of Jesuit life but also attention to the material constraints, competing priorities, and personal outlooks that polarized debates among Company members.

With questions about disease in particular shunted to the margins of colonial inquiry, claims that Brazil was both verdant and healthy would continue to circulate for over a century. The culture of natural inquiry that came to characterize the Portuguese Atlantic in the early seventeenth century challenged such sanguine assertions of colonial epidemiology, and expanded the catalog of Brazilian nature. That culture of inquiry, I have suggested, enabled distinctive geographical imaginings and entailed the emergence of a new investigative persona. Abreu had argued that the most pernicious and theoretically challenging illnesses of the empire were found throughout the Atlantic and were common equally in Lisbon, Luanda, and along the coast of Brazil. His *Tratado* would prove formative for metropolitan medical debates of the mid- to late seventeenth century. Signally, it gave intellectual authority to a view of the Atlantic – not the tropics – as a single, coherent, epidemiological region. Brandão's work moved from a pan-Atlantic perspective to a colonial Brazilian one. His *Diálogos das grandezas do Brasil* reveals some of the ways by which Brazilian nature entered the imaginations, pipes, and apothecary stalls of turn-of-the-century Portugal. The history of the *Diálogos* is the story of the economic and cultural shifts not just in the Atlantic but across

Portugal's empire that finally compelled the study of Brazilian nature. The *Diálogos* reveals the ways in which sorting the unfamiliar flora and fauna of Portuguese America demanded as well the creation of new epistemic tools and the new investigative persona of the planter naturalist. The case of Brandão challenges longstanding portrayals of colonial sugar planters as intellectually unimaginative and as focused single-mindedly on finance and social status.

Early modern empires enabled colonial convergences of humans, objects, and disease-causing entities. They scattered but did not necessarily disrupt knowledges. They inspired regional and global geographical frameworks and the crafting of novel epistemologies – and that was true in Goa and the Portuguese Atlantic no less than in London, Lisbon, Paris, or Madrid.

Bibliography

ARCHIVES AND COLLECTIONS

Brazil

Biblioteca Nacional (BN)
    Coleção Linhares (CL)

France

Bibliothèque Nationale de France (BNF)
    Fonds Portugais (FP)

India

Historical Archives of Goa (HAG)
    Cristandade (CR)
        Leis a favor da Cristandade, 1562–1843
    Monções do Reino (MR)
    Provisões, alvarás e regimentos (PAR)
        Provisões a favor da Cristandade, 1515–1840
        Catalogo dos Vice-Reis, 1604–1837

Portugal

Arquivo Histórico Ultramarino (AHU)
    Administração Central (ACL)
        Conselho Ultramarino (CU)

Arquivo Nacional da Torre do Tombo (ANTT)
    Cartório Jesuítico (CJ)
    Chancelarias (CH)
    Colecção de Cartas (COL)
    Corpo Chronológico (CC)
    Manuscritos da Livraria (MSL)
    Manuscritos do Brasil (MSBR)
    Tribunal do Santo Ofício (TSO)
      Inquisição de Lisboa (IL)
Biblioteca Nacional de Portugal (BNP)
    Colecção Geral (CG)
    Reservados (RES)
      Codices (Cod.)
      Manuscritos (Mss.)

United Kingdom

British Library
    Additional Manuscripts (Add. Mss.)
Wellcome Collection (WC)
    Manuscripts (Mss.)

PRINTED CONTEMPORARY SOURCES (INCLUDING EARLY
MODERN BOOKS OF MEDICINE AND NATURAL HISTORY)

Abreu, Aleixo de. *Tratado de las siete enfermedades. De la inflammacion universal del higado, zirbo, pyloron, y riñones, y de la obstrucion de la satiriasi, de la terciana y febre maligna, y passion hipocondriaca: Lleva otros tres tratados, del mal de Loanda, del guzano, y de las fuentes y sedales.* Lisbon: Pedro Craesbeeck, 1623.

Abreu, João Capistrano de, ed. *Primeira visitação do Santo Ofício às partes do Brasil pelo Licenciado Heitor Furtado de Mendonça: Confissões da Bahia, 1591–1592.* Rio de Janeiro, F. Briguiet, 1935.

    ed. *Primeira visitação do Santo Ofício às partes do Brasil pelo Licenciado Heitor Furtado de Mendonça: Denunciações da Bahia, 1591–1593.* São Paulo: Paulo Prado, 1925.

Academia Real das Ciências [Academia Real das Sciencias de Lisboa]. *Memorias economicas da Academia Real das Sciencias de Lisboa.* 1st series. Lisbon: Office of the Academia Real das Sciencias, 1789–1815.

"Breve relação das escrituras dos gentios da India Oriental e dos seus costumes." In *Collecção de Notícias para a Historia e Geografia das Nações Ultramarinas, que vivem nos domínios portuguezes, ou lhes são vizinhas.* Lisbon: Typografia da Academia, 1812.

Memorias economicas da Academia Real das Sciencias de Lisboa. Para o adiantamento da agricultura das artes e da industria em Portugal e suas conquistas. 2nd edn. 5 vols. Lisbon: Typographia da Academia, 1885 [1789–1815].

Afzel, Adam. *Plantarum Guineensium*. Uppsala: Typis Edmannianis, 1804.

Albuquerque, Afonso de. *Comentários do grande Afonso de Albuquerque, Capitão Geral que foi das Indias Orientais em tempo do muito poderoso Rey D. Manuel, o primeiro deste nome*. 2 parts. 4th edn. Revised and with an introduction by António Baião. Coimbra: Imprensa da Universidade, 1922.

Albuquerque, Viriato A. C. R. de, ed. "Postura dos Fizicos, Cirurgiões, Sangradores e Boticários." In *O Senado de Goa: Memória Histórico-Arqueológico*, ed. Albuquerque, 423–425. Nova Goa: Imprensa Nacional, 1909.

Alvares, Simão. "Emformação que me dey symão alluẽz buticayro mor delRey noso sõr do naçymento de todelas droguas que vão pera o Reyno o quoal ha xxxix Anos q̃ serue nestas partes da Imdia seu o ficio homẽ gramdemente curyoso destas cousas." Reprinted in Jaime Walter, "Simão Alvares e o seu rol das drogas da Índia." *Studia* 10 (1962): 136–149.

Antonil, Andre João. *Cultura e opulência do Brasil por suas drogas e minas*. Lisbon: Officina Real Deslandesiana, 1711.

Arrães, Duarte Madeira [Madeyra]. *Methodo de conhecer e curar o morbo gallico. Primeira parte: Propoem-se definitivamentte a essencia, especies, causas, sinaes, pronosticos, e cura do morbo gallico, e todos seus effeitos, e se trata do azougue, sarsaparilha, Guaiação, pao Santo, raiz da China, e de todos os mais remedios desta enfermidad*. Lisbon: Lourenço de Anvers, 1642.

Methodo de conhecer e curar o morbo gallico. Primeira parte. Propoem-se definitivamentte a essencia, especies, causas, sinaes, pronosticos, e cura do morbo gallico, e todos seus effeitos, e se trata do azougue, sarsaparilha, Guaiação, pao Santo, raiz da China, e de todos os mais remedios desta enfermidad: Segunda parte. Disputação-se largamente por questoens em forma todas as duvidas que se podem mover sobre a essencia, especies, causas, sinaes, e pronosticou da cura do morbo gallico, e as que pode haver sobre o azougue &c. Lisbon: Antonio Crasbeek de Mello, 1683.

Methodo de conhecer e curar o morbo gallico. Primeira parte. Propoem-se definitivamentte a essencia, especies, causas, sinaes, pronosticos, e cura do morbo gallico, e todos seus effeitos, e se trata do azougue, sarsaparilha, Guaiação, pao Santo, raiz da China, e de todos os mais remedios desta enfermidad: Segunda parte. Disputação-se largamente por questoens em forma todas as duvidas que se podem mover sobre a essencia, especies, causas, sinaes, e pronosticou da cura do morbo gallico, e as que pode haver sobre o azougue &c. Illustrated and with annotations by D. Francisco da Fonseca Henriquez Mirandella. Lisbon: Antonio Pedrozo Galrão, 1715.

Arte Palmarica escrita por um Padre da Companhia de Jesus. Nova Goa: Imprensa Nacional, 1918.

Azevedo, Manuel [Manoel] de. *Correcção de abusos introduzidos contra o verdadeiro method da medicina*. Lisbon: Officina de Diogo Soares de Bulhões, 1668.

Baião, António, ed. *A Inquisição de Goa: Correspondência dos inquisidores da Índia*. 2 vols. Coimbra: Imprensa da Universidade, 1930

Barbosa, Duarte. *O Livro de Duarte Barbosa (edição crítica e anotada)*. 2 vols, edited by Maria Augusta da Veiga e Sousa. Lisbon: Ministério da Ciência e da Technologia, the Instituto de Investigação Científica Tropical, and the Centro de Estudos de História e Cartografia Antiga, 1996.

Barros, João de. *Da Ásia de João de Barros e de Diogo de Couto*. New edn. Lisbon: Regia Officina Typografica, 1778.

Diálogo em louvor da nossa linguagem. Lisbon, 1540.

Bluteau, Rafael. *Vocabulario portugues e latino*. 10 vols. Lisbon: Oficina da Música, 1712–1728.

Bocarro, António. *O livro das plantas de todas as fortalezas, cidades, e povoações do Estado da Índia oriental*. 2 vols, edited by Isabel Cid. Lisbon: Casa da Moeda, 1992 [1635].

Bontius, Jacobus. *An Account of the Diseases, Natural History, and Medicines of the East Indies*. London: T. Noteman, 1769.

De medicina Indorum. Leiden: Franciscus Hackius, 1642.

Brandão, Ambrósio Fernandes. *Diálogos das grandezas do Brasil*, edited by José Antonio Gonsalves de Mello. 2nd edn. Recife: Imprensa Universitária, 1966.

Brandão, João. *Tratado da majestade, grandeza e abastança da cidade de Lisboa na segunda metade do século XVI*, edited by Anselmo Braamcamp Freire and Gomes de Brito. Lisbon: Livraria Ferin, 1923 [1552].

Brásio, António, ed. *Monumenta Missionaria Africana. África Ocidental (1471–1531)* 1st series. 15 vols. Lisbon Agência Geral do Ultramar, 1952–1988.

Brásio, António, ed. *Monumenta Missionaria Africana. África Ocidental (1342–1499)*. 2nd series. 5 vols. Lisbon: Agência Geral do Ultramar, 1958–1985.

Brito, Domingos Abreu e. *Inquerito à vida administrative e economica de Angola e do Brasil*. Coimbra: Imprensa da Universidade, 1933 [1592].

Cadamosto, Alvise. "The voyages of Cadamosto and Pedro de Sintra." In *The Voyages of Cadamosto and Other Documents on Western Africa in the Second Half of the Fifteenth Century*. Translated and edited by G. R. Crone. London: Hakluyt Society, 1937 [1507], 1–84.

Cardim, Fernão. *Tratados da terra e gente do Brasil*, edited by Baptista Caetano, Capistrano de Abreu, and Rodolpho Garcia. Rio de Janeiro: Editores J. Leite, 1925 [ca. 1580].

Castanheda, Fernão Lopes de. *História do descobrimento e conquista da Índia pelos portugueses*. 2 vols. Porto: Lello and Irmão, 1979.

Chagas, Manoel Pinheiro, ed. *Diccionario Popular: Historico, Geographico, Mythologico, Biographico, Artistico, Bibliographico e Litterario*. 16 vols. Lisbon: Joaquim Germano de Sousa Neves, 1842–1895.

Clusius, Carolus. *Aromatum et simplicium aliquot medicamentorum apud indos nascentium historia*. Facsimile edn. with an introduction by M. de Jong and D. A. Wittop Koning. Delft and The Hague: B. de Graaf, 1963 [Frankfurt: Christopher Plantin, 1567].

Comissão Executiva das Comemorações do V Centenário da Morte do Infante D. Henrique, ed. *Monumenta Henricina*. 14 vols. Coimbra: Atlântida, 1960–1973.

Cordeiro, Luciano, ed. *Memorias do ultramar: Viagens, explorações e conquistas dos Portuguezes. Producções, commercio e governo do Congo e de Angola segundo Manuel Vogado Sotomaior, Antonio Diniz, Bento Banha Cardoso, e Antonio Beserra Fajarado, 1620–1629.* Lisbon: Imprensa Nacional, 1881.

Correia, Gaspar. *Lendas da Índia.* 4 vols, edited and with an introduction by M. Lopes de Almeida. Porto: Lello and Irmão, 1975 [ca. 1556].

Costa, Cristovão da [Acosta, Cristobal]. *Tractado Delas Drogas, y medicinas de las Indias Orientales, con sus Plantas debuxadas al biuo por Christoual Acosta medico y cirujano que las vio ocularmente.* Burgos: Martin de Victoria, 1578.

Tratado en loor de las mvgeres. Y dela Castidad, Onestidad, Constancia, Silencio, y Iusticia. Con otras muchas particularidades, y varias Historias. Venice: Giacomo Cornetti, 1592.

Cunha Rivara, J. H., da., ed. *Archivo Portuguez-Oriental.* 6 vols. Nova Goa: Imprensa Nacional, 1857–1876.

Diretoria do Arquivo, divulgação e estadística da Prefeitura do Salvador, ed. *Documentos históricos do Arquivo Municipal. Atas da Câmara.* 10 vols. Salvador: Perfeitura Municipal do Salvador, 1944–[n.d.].

Dobzhansky, Theodosius. "Evolution in the Tropics." *American Scientist* 38 (1950): 209–221.

Documentos sobre os Portugueses em Moçambique e na África Central, 1497–1840. 9 vols. Lisbon: National Archives of Rhodesia and Nyasaland, and the Centro de Estudos Históricos Ultramarinos, 1962–1969.

França, Eduardo d'Oliveira, and Sônia Siqueira, eds. "Segunda visitação do Santo Ofício às partes do Brasil. Livro das Confissões e Ratificações da Bahia, 1618–1620." *Anais do Museu Paulista* 17 (1963): 123–547.

Fryer, John. *A New Account of East India and Persia. Being Nine Years Travels, 1672–1681.* 3 vols, edited with notes and an Introduction by William Crooke. London: Hakluyt Society, 1909–1915.

Gallardo, Bartolome Jose. *Ensayo de una Biblioteca Española de libros raros y curiosos.* Expanded by M. R. Zarco del Valle and J. Sancho Rayón. 4 vols. Madrid: M. Rivadaneyra, 1863–1889.

Galvão, Antonio. *Tratado dos descobrimentos antigos, e modernos.* 2nd edn. Lisbon: Officina Ferreiriana, 1731 [1563].

Gama, Vasco da. *Em Nome de Deus: The Journal of the First Voyage of Vasco da Gama to Índia.* Translated and edited by Glenn J. Ames. Leiden: Brill, 2009.

Gândavo, Pedro de Magalhães. *História da provincia de Santa Cruz a que vulgarmente chamamos Brasil.* Lisbon: António Gonçalves, 1576.

Regras que ensinam a maneira de screver a ortographia da líingua Portuguesa, com um Diálogo que adiante se segue em defenão da mesma língua. Lisbon, 1574.

Garcia, Rodolfo, ed. *Primeira visitação do Santo Ofício às partes do Brasil. Denunciações de Pernambuco, 1593–1595.* São Paulo: Paulo Prado, 1929.

Garcia, Rodolfo, ed. *Diálogos das grandezas do Brasil.* Rio de Janeiro: Tecnoprint Gráfica, 1968.

Góis, Damião de. *Chronica do felicissimo rei Dom Emanuel.* 4 parts. Lisbon: Francisco Correia, 1566–1567.

Urbis Oilisiponis descriptio. Évora, 1554.

Gonçalves, Sebastiam. *Primeira Parte da Historia dos Religiosos da Companhia de Jesus e do que fizeram com a divina graça na conversão dos infieis a nossa sancta fee catholica nos reynos e provincias da India Oriental.* 3 vols, edited by Joseph Wicki. Coimbra: Atlântida, 1957–1962 [ca. 1619].

Hall, Frederick Holden, William F. Harrison, and Dorothy Winters Welker, trans. and eds. *Diálogos das grandezas do Brasil.* Albuquerque, NM: University of New Mexico Press, 1987.

Henriques, Francisco da Fonseca. *Medicina Lusitana, Socorro Delphico aos clamores da natureza humana para total profligacão de seus males dividio em tres partes.* Amsterdam: Miguel Dias, 1710.

Hooker, William Jackson, ed. *Niger Flora; or, An Enumeration of the Plants of Western Tropical Africa, Collected by the Late Dr. Theodore Vogel, Botanist to the Voyage of the Expedition Sent by Her Britannic Majesty to the River Niger in 1841, under the Command of Capt. H. D. Trotter, R. N., &c.* London: Hippolyte Bailliere, 1849.

Humboldt, Alexander von. *Personal Narrative of Travels to the Equinoctial Regions of the New Continent, during the Years 1799–1804.* 3 vols. Translated by Helen Maria Williams. London: Longman, Hurst, Rees, Orme, and Brown, 1814–1822.

Leite, Serafim, ed. *Monumenta brasiliae,* 5 vols. Rome: Monumenta Historica Societatis Iesu, 1956–1968.

"Livro das Cidades, e Fortalezas, que a Coroa de Portugal tem nas Partes da Índia, e das Capitanias, e mais Cargos que Nelas ha e da Importancia Delles." *Studia* 6 (1960): 15–16.

Macedo, Duarte Ribeiro de. *Obras ineditas de Duarte Ribeiro de Macedo,* edited by Antonio Lourenço Caminha. Lisbon: Impressão Regia, 1817.

Discurso Politico que o Conde de Soure, Embaxador extraordinario de Sua Magestade a el Rey Christianissimo, deu ao Cardeal Mazarine em São João da Luz (Lisbon: Henrique Valente, 1661 [Paris, 1659].

Juizo Historico, Juridico, Politico sobre a paz celebrada entre as coroas de França e Castella, no anno de 1660 (Lisbon: João da Costa, 1666).

Vida da Emperatriz Theodora (Lisbon: João da Costa, 1677).

Libro del conosçimiento de todos los reinos y tierras y señoríos que son por el mundo y de las señales y armas que han cada tierra y señorío por si y de los reyes y señores que los poseen. Madrid: Alejandro Pueyo, 1920.

Machado, Diogo Barbosa. *Bibliotheca Lusitana: Historica, Critica, e Cronologica.* 4 vols. Lisbon: Antonio Isidoro da Fonseca, 1741–1759.

Maler, Bertil, ed. *Orto do esposo.* Rio de Janeiro: Ministério da Educação e Cultura and the Instituto Nacional do Livro, 1956.

Malfante, Antoine. "The Letter of Antoine Malfante from Tuat, 1447." In *The Voyages of Cadamosto and Other Documents on Western Africa in the Second Half of the Fifteenth Century,* edited by G. R. Crone, 85–90. London: Hakluyt Society, 1937.

Matos, Artur Teoodoro de, ed. *Documentos Remetidos da Índia ou Livros das Monções (1625–1736).* 2 vols. Lisbon: Academia das Ciências, 1999–2001.

Mello, José Antonio Gonsalves de, ed. *Diálogos das grandezas do Brasil*. 2nd edn. Recife: Imprensa Universitária, 1966.

ed. *Primeira visitação do Santo Ofício às partes do Brasil. Confissões de Pernambuco, 1594–1595*. Recife: Universidade Federal de Pernambuco, 1970.

[Menezes, Luíz de.] *Relação do felice successo que conseguiram as armas do Serenissimo principe D. Pedro, nosso senhor, governadas por Francisco de Tavora, governador e capitão general do reino de Angola, contra a rebellião de D. João, re das Pedras e Dongo, no mez de dezembro de 1671*. N.p., n.d.

Montemayor, Jorge de. *Los siete livros de Diana*. Granada: Rene Rabut, 1564 [1559].

Mourão [Morão], Simão Pinheiro. *Queixas repetidas em ecos dos arrecifes de Pernambuco contra os abusos medicos que nas suas capitanias se observam tanto em dano das vidas de seus habitantes*, edited by Jaime Walter. Lisbon: Junta de Investigações do Ultramar, 1965 [1677].

[Romão Mosia Reinhipo]. *Tratado unico das bexigas e sarampo*. In *Morão, Rosa e Pimenta. Notícias dos três primeiros livros em vernáculo sôbre a medicina no Brasil*. Edited by Gilberto Osório de Andrade and Eustáquio Duarte, 73–125. Recife: Arquivo Público Estadual de Pernambuco1956 [Lisbon: João Galrão, 1683].

Roma, Francisco Morato. *Luz da medicina, pratica racional, e methodica, guia de enfermeyros*. Coimbra: Francisco de Oliveira, 1753.

Luz da medicina, pratica racional, e methodica, guia de enfermeyros. Lisbon: Henrique Valente de Oliveira, 1664.

Nichols, Rose Standish. *Spanish and Portuguese Gardens*. London: Constable and Company, 1922.

Orta, Garcia de [Orta, Garcia da]. *Colóquios dos simples e drogas da Índia*. 2 vols, edited by Conde de Ficalho. Lisbon: Imprensa Nacional, 1895.

[Orta, Garcia d']. *Coloquios dos simples, e drogas e cousas medicinais da India, e assi dalg̃uas frutas achadas nella onde se tratam alg̃uas cousas tocantes amediçina, pratica, e outras cousas boas, pera saber cõpostos pello Doutor garcia dorta: fisico del Rey nosso senhor, vistos pello muyto Reverendo senhor, ho liçenciado Alexos diaz: falcam desenbargador da casa da supricacçã inquisidor nestas partes*. Goa: Joannes de Endem, 1563.

Paré, Ambroise. *The Apologie and Treatise of Ambroise Paré, Containing the Voyages made into Divers Places with Many of His Writings upon Surgery*, edited by Geoffrey Keynes. London: Falcon Educational Books, 1951 [ca. 1564].

Pato, Bulhão. *Cartas de Afonso de Albuquerque seguidas de documentos que as elucidam*. 6 vols. Lisbon: Acadêmia Real das Ciências, 1884–1903.

Pereira, Duarte Pacheco. *Esmeraldo de situ orbis*, edited by Augusto Epiphanio da Silva Dias. Lisbon: Typographia Universal, 1905 [ca. 1506].

Pimentel, Luis Serrão. *Arte pratica de navegar e regimento de pilotos*. Lisbon: Antonio Craesbeeck de Mello, 1681.

Pina, Rui de. "Chronica d'Elrey D. João II." In *Crónicas de Rui de Pina*, ed. M. Lopes de Almeida. Porto: Lello and Irmão Editores. 1977.

Piso, Willem and Georg Marcgraff. *Historia naturalis Brasiliae.* Leiden: Franciscum Hackium and Lud. Elzevirium, 1648.

Pissurlencar, Panduronga S. S. *Regimentos das Fortalezas da Índia: Estudo e Notas.* Bastorá: Tipografia Rangel, 1951.

Pliny the Elder. *The Natural History of Pliny.* 6 vols. Translated by John Bostock and H. T. Riley. London: George Gell and Sons, 1855–1857.

República Portuguesa, Ministério das Colónias, ed. *Os sete único documentos de 1500, conservados em Lisboa, referents à vaigem de Pedro Álvares Cabral.* Lisbon: Agência Geral das Colónias, 1940.

Ruel, Jean [Ruello, Ioanne]. *Pedanii Dioscoridis Anazarbei. De Medica Materia Libri Sex.* Basel: n.p., 1542.

Santa Anna, Joseph Pereira de. *Chronica dos Carmelitas da antiga, e regular observancia nestes Reynos de Portugal, Algarves, e seus Dominios.* Lisbon: Antonio Pedrozo Galram, 1745.

Santa Maria, Agostinho de. *Historia da fundação do Real Convento de Santa Monica.* Lisbon: Antonio Pedrozo Galram, 1699.

São Boaventura, Fortunato de. *Collecção de ineditos Portuguezes dos seculos XIV e XV.* 3 vols. Coimbra: Real Imprensa da Universidade, 1829.

Semedo, João Curvo. *Polyanthea Medicinal. Noticias Galenicas e Chemicas.* Lisbon: Antonio Pedrozo Galram, 1716.

Sen, Surendranath, ed. *Indian Travels of Thevenot and Careri: Being the Third Part of the Travels of M. de Thevenot into the Levant and the Third Part of a Voyage Round the World by Dr. John Francis Gemelli Careri.* New Delhi: National Archives of India, 1949.

Sousa, Francisco de. *Oriente Conquistado a Jesus Cristo pelos Padres da Companhia de Jesus da Província de Goa.* Revised with an introduction by M. Lopes de Almeida. Porto: Lello and Irmão, 1978.

Sousa, Gabriel Soares de. *Tratado Descriptivo do Brazil,* edited by Francisco Adolpho de Varnhagen (Rio de Janeiro: Typographia Universal de Laemmert, 1851 [1587]).

Sprat, Thomas. *The History of the Royal Society of London for the Improvement of Natural Knowledge.* London: n.p., 1734 [1667].

Strobaeus, Bilibaldus, trans. *Tertia pars Indiae Orientalis.* Frankfurt: Matthaeus Beckerus, 1601.

Reede, Henricus van, tot Drakenstein. *Hortus indicus Malabaricus.* 12 vols. Amsterdam: Joannis van Someren and Joannis van Dyck, 1678–1703.

Tavernier, Jean Baptiste. *Travels in India of Jean Baptiste-Tavernier, Baron of Aubonne.* 2nd edn. 2 vols. Edited by William Crooke and translated by V. Ball. London: Macmillan, 1925 [1676].

Teixera, Pedro. *Relaciones del origen, descendencia y sucesion de los reyes de Persia, y de Hormuz, y de un viage hecho por el mismo autor desde la India Oriental hasta Italia por tierra.* Amberes: n.p., 1660 [1610].

Thevet, Andre. *Singularitez de la France Antarctique, autrement nommee Amerique, & de plusieurs terres & isles decouvertes de nostre temps.* Paris: Christopher Plantin, 1558.

Trancoso, Gonçalo Fernandes. *Tratado do Padre Gonçalo Fernandes Trancoso sobre o Hinduísmo,* edited by José Wicki. Lisbon: Centro de Estudos Históricos Ultramarinos, 1973 [Maduré, 1616].

Vasconcelos, Simão de [Vasconellos, Simam de]. *Vida do veneravel Padre Ioseph de Anchieta, da Companhia de Iesu, taumaturgo do Novo Mundo, na Provincia do Brasil.* Lisbon: João da Costa, 1672.

Vieira, António. *Cartas do Padre Antonio Vieyra da Companhia de Jesus a Duarte Ribeiro de Macedo.* Lisbon: Eugenio August, 1827.

Wicki, Jospeh, ed. *Documenta Indica.* 18 vols. Rome: Monumenta Historica Societatis Iesu, 1948–1988.

Zurara [Azurara], Gomes Eannes de. *Chronica do descobrimento e conquista de Guiné* Paris: J. P. Aillaud, 1841.

Reis, João C. *A empresa da conquista do senhorio do Monomotapa.* Lisbon: Heuris, 1984.

MODERN SOURCES

Abreu, Laurinda. "A organização e regulação das *profissões médicas* no Portugal Moderno: entre as orientações da Coroa e os interesses privados." In *Arte Médica e Imagem do Corpo: de Hipócrates ao final do século XVIII,* edited by Adelino Cardoso, António Braz de Oliveira, and Manuel Silvério Marques, 97–122. Lisbon: Biblioteca Nacional de Portugal, 2010.

Abulafia, David. *The Discovery of Mankind: Atlantic Encounters in the Age of Columbus.* New Haven, CT: Yale University Press, 2008.

Achim, Miruna. *Lagartijas medicinales: Remedios americanos y debates científicos en la ilustración.* Mexico City: Consejo Nacional para la Cultura y las Artes, 2008.

Adas, Michael. *Dominance by Design: Technological Imperatives and America's Civilizing Mission.* Cambridge, MA: Belknap Press, 2006.

Machines as the Measure of Men: Science, Technology, and Ideologies of Western Dominance. Ithaca: Cornell University Press, 1989.

Adas, Michael and Hugh Glenn Cagle. "Age of Settlement and Colonisation." In *The Ashgate Research Companion to Modern Imperial Histories,* edited by Philippa Levine and John Marriott, 41–74. Burlington, VT: Ashgate, 2012.

Adelman, Jeremy, ed. *Colonial Legacies: The Problem of Persistence in Latin American History.* New York: Routledge, 1999.

Adorno, Rolena. "The Negotiation of Fear in Cabeza de Vaca's *Naufragios.*" *Representations* 33 (1991): 163–199.

Agnolin, Adone. *Jesuítas e Selvagens: A Negociação da Fé no Encontro Catequético-Ritual Americano-Tupi (séc. XVI-XVII).* São Paulo: Humanitas Editorial, 2007.

Alavi, Seema. *Islam and Healing: Loss and Recovery of an Indo-Muslim Medical Tradition, 1600–1800.* New York: Palgrave, 2008.

Albuquerque, Luis de. "A 'aula da esfera' do Colégio de Santo Antão no século XVII." *Anais da Academia Portuguesa de História* 21 (1972): 337–391.

Alden, Dauril. *The Making of an Enterprise: The Society of Jesus in Portugal, Its Empire, and Beyond, 1540–1750.* Stanford, CA: Stanford University Press, 1995.

Alden, Dauril and Joseph C. Miller. "Out of Africa: The Slave Trade and the Transmission of Smallpox to Brazil, 1560–1831." *The Journal of Interdisciplinary History* 18 (1987): 195–224.

Alegria, Maria Fernanda, Suzanne Daveau, João Carlos Garcia, and Francesc Relaño. "Portuguese Cartography in the Renaissance." In *The History of Cartography, Volume 3: Cartography in the European Renaissance,* 975–1068. Chicago: University of Chicago Press, 2007.

Alencastro, Luis Felipe de. *O Trato dos Viventes: Formação do Brasil no Atlântico Sul, séculos XVI e XVII.* São Paulo: Companhia das Letras, 2000.

Almeida, Onésimo T. "Portugal and the Dawn of Modern Science." In *Portugal, the Pathfinder: Journeys from the Medieval toward the Modern World, 1300-ca. 1600,* edited by George Winius, 341–361. Madison, WI: A Special Publication of the *Luso-Brazilian Review,* 1995.

"Sobre a revolução da experiência no Portugal do século XVI: Na pista do conceito de 'Experiência a Madre das Cousas.'" In *Actas do Quinto Congresso da Associação Internacional de Lusitanistas,* 3 vols., edited by T. F. Earle, 1617–1627. Coimbra: Associação Internacional de Lusitanistas, 1998.

Alpers, Svetlana. *The Art of Describing: Dutch Art in the Seventeenth Century.* Chicago: University of Chicago Press, 1983.

Alves, Ana Maria. *Iconologia do Poder Real no Período Manuelino.* Lisbon: Imprensa Nacional, 1985.

Andaya, Leonard Y. "The Portuguese Tribe in the Malay-Indonesian Archipelago in the Seventeenth and Eighteenth Centuries." In *The Portuguese Tribe and the Pacific,* edited by Francis A. Dutra and João Camilo dos Santos, 129–148. Santa Barbara, CA: Center for Portuguese Studies at the University of California at Santa Barbara, 1995.

Anderson, Warwick. *Colonial Pathologies: American Tropical Medicine, Race, and Hygiene in the Philippines.* Durham, NC: Duke University Press, 2006.

"Climates of Opinion: Acclimatization in Nineteenth-Century France and England." *Victorian Studies* 35 (1992): 135–157.

Anselmo, Artur. *Estudos de história do livro.* Lisbon: Guimarães Editores, 1997.

Amos, Thomas L. *The Fundo Alcobaça of the Biblioteca Nacional, Lisbon.* 3 vols. Collegeville, MD: Hill Monastic Manuscripts Library, 1988.

Araújo, Ana Cristina. *A Cultura das Luzes em Portugal: Temas e problemas.* Lisbon: Livros Horizonte, 2003.

Arnold, David. *Colonizing the Body: State Medicine and epidemic Disease in Nineteenth-Century India.* Berkeley, CA: University of California Press, 1993.

"Envisioning the Tropics: Joseph Hooker in India and the Himalayas, 1848–1850." In *Tropical Visions in an Age of Empire,* edited by Felix Driver and Luciana Martins, 137–155. Chicago: University of Chicago Press, 2005.

"India's Place in the Tropical World, 1770–1930." *Journal of Imperial and Commonwealth History* 26 (1998): 1–21.

The Problem of Nature: Environment, Culture, and European Expansion. Cambridge, MA: Blackwell, 1996.

The Tropics and the Travelling Gaze: India, Landscape, and Science, 1800–1856. Seattle, WA: University of Washington Press, 2006.

"'Illusory Riches': Representations of the Tropical World, 1840–1950." *Singapore Journal of Tropical Geography* 21 (2000): 6–18.

Arnold, David ed. *Warm Climates and Western Medicine: The Emergence of Tropical Medicine, 1500–1900.* Atlanta, GA: Rodopi, 1996.

Arrizabalaga, Jon, "Garcia de Orta in the Context of the Sephardic Diaspora." In *Medicine, Trade and Empire: Garcia de Orta's Colloquies on the Simples and Drugs of India (1563) in Context,* edited by Palmira Fontes da Costa, 11–32. Burlington, VT: Ashgate, 2015.

"Problematizing Retrospective Diagnosis in the History of Disease." *Asclepio* 54 (2002): 51–70.

Arrizabalaga, Jon, John Henderson, and Roger French. *The Great Pox: The French Disease in Renaissance Europe.* New Haven, CT: Yale University Press, 1997.

Askari, S. Hasan. "Medicine and Hospitals in Muslim India." *The Journal of the Bihar Research Society* 43 (1957): 7–21.

Asúa, Miguel de, and Roger French. *A New World of Animals: Early Modern Europeans on the Creatures of Iberian America.* Burlington, VT: Ashgate, 2005.

"Los jesuítas y el conocimiento de la naturaleza Americana." *Stromata* 59 (2003): 1–20.

Attewell, Guy. *Refiguring Unani Tibb: Plural Healing in Late Colonial India.* Delhi: Orient Longman, 2007.

Axelrod, Paul and Michelle A. Fuerch. "Flight of the Deities: Hindu Resistance in Portuguese Goa." *Modern Asian Studies* 30 (1996): 387–421.

Azevedo, Pedro de. "António de Gouveia, alchimista do século XVI." *Archivo Histórico Portuguez* 3 (1905): 179–208 and 274–286.

Azman, Andrew S., Kara E. Rudolph, Derek A. T. Cummings, and Justin Lessler. "The incubation period of cholera: A systematic review." *Journal of Infection* 66 (2013): 432–438.

Baldini, Ugo. "The Academy of Mathematics of the Collegio Romano from 1553 to 1612." In *Jesuit Science and the Republic of Letters,* ed. Mordechai Feingold, 47–98. Cambridge, MA: MIT Press, 2003.

Baldini, Ugo, and Bernardino Fernandes. "As Assistências ibéricas da Companhia de Jesus e a actividade científica nas missões asiáticas (1578–1650)." *Revista Portuguesa de Filosofia* 54 (1998): 195–246.

Ballong-Wen-Mewuda, Joseph Bato'ora. *São Jorge da Mina: 1482–1637.* Lisbon: Fundação Calaouste Gulbenkian, 1993.

Barrera-Osorio, Antonio. *Experiencing Nature: The Spanish American Empire and the Early Scientific Revolution.* Austin, TX: University of Texas Press, 2006.

Barreto, Luís Filipe. *Descobrimentos e renascimento: Formas de ser e pensar nos séculos XV e XVI.* Lisbon: Imprensa Nacional-Casa da Moeda, 1983.

"Garcia da Orta e o dialogo civilizacional." *Actas do seminário internacional de história Indo-Portuguesa.* Lisbon: Centro de Estudos de História e Cartografia Antiga, 1985.

Basham, A. L. "The Practice of Medicine in Ancient and Medieval India." 18–43. In Charles Leslie, ed. *Asian Medical Systems: A Comparative Study.* Berkeley, CA: University of California Press, 1977.

Bauer, Ralph. "A New World of Secrets: Occult Philosophy and Local Knowledge in the Sixteenth-Century Atlantic." In *Science and Empire in the Atlantic*

World, edited by James Delbourgo and Nicholas Dew, 99–126. New York, Routledge, 2008.

Bedini, Silvo A. *The Pope's Elephant*. Nashville, TN: J.S. Sanders and Company, 1998.

Bell, Aubrey F. G. "Damião de Goís, a Portuguese Humanist." *Hispanic Review* 9 (1941): 243–251.

Bennet, Jane *Vibrant Matter: A Political Ecology of Things*. Durham, NC: Duke University Press, 2010.

Bennett, Herman L. "'Sons of Adam': Text, Context, and the Early Modern African Subject." *Representations* 92 (2005): 16–41.

Bennett, Jim. "Early Modern Mathematical Instruments." *Isis* 102 (2011): 697–705.

Benton, Lauren. *A Search for Sovereignty: Law and Geography in European Empires, 1400–1900*. New York: Cambridge University Press, 2010.

Berbara, Maria, and Karl A. E. Enenkel, eds. *Portuguese Humanism and the Republic of Letters*. Leiden: Brill, 2012.

Bewell, Alan. *Romanticism and Colonial Disease*. Baltimore, MD: Johns Hopkins University Press, 2003.

Bhardwaj, Surinder M. "Disease Ecologies of South Asia." In *The Cambridge World History of Human Disease*, edited by Kenneth F. Kiple, 642–649. New York: Cambridge University Press, 1993.

Biagioli, Mario. *Galileo, Courtier: The Practice of Science in the Culture of Absolutism*. Chicago: Chicago University Press, 1993.

Birmingham, David. *Trade and Conflict in Angola: The Mbundu and their Neighbors under the Influence of the Portuguese, 1483–1790*. Oxford: Clarendon Press, 1966.

Blackmore, Josiah. "Imaging the Moor in Medieval Portugal." *Diacritics* 36 (2006): 27–43.

Blair, Ann. *Too Much to Know: Managing Scholarly Information before the Modern Age*. New Haven, CT: Yale University Press, 2010.

   The Theater of Nature: Jean Bodin and Renaissance Science. Princeton, NJ: Princeton University Press, 1997.

Bleichmar, Daniela. *Visible Empire: Botanical Expeditions and Visual Culture in the Hispanic Enlightenment*. Chicago: University of Chicago Press, 2012.

   "Atlantic Competitions: Botany in the Eighteenth-Century Spanish Atlantic." In *Science and Empire in the Atlantic World*, edited by James Delbourgo and Nicholas Dew, 225–252. New York: Routledge, 2008.

   "Books, Bodies, Fields: Sixteenth-Century Transatlantic Encounters with New World *Materia Medica*." In *Colonial Botany: Science Commerce, and Politics in the Early Modern World*, edited by Londa Schiebinger and Claudia Swan, 83–99. Philadelphia: The University of Pennsylvania Press, 2005.

Bleichmar, Daniela, Paula de Vos, Kristin Huffine, and Kevin Sheehan, eds. *Science in the Spanish and Portuguese Empires, 1500–1800*. Stanford, CA: Stanford University Press, 2009.

Bleichmar, Danilea, and Peter C. Mancall, eds. *Collecting Across Cultures: Material Exchanges in the Early Modern Atlantic World*. Philadelphia, PA: University of Pennsylvania Press, 2013.

Blier, Suzanne Preston. "Imaging Otherness in Ivory: African Portrayals of the Portuguese ca. 1492." 75 (1993): 375–396.

Borges, Charles J. "Foreign Jesuits and Native Resistance in Goa, 1542–1759." In *Essays in Goan History*, edited by Teotonio R. de Souza, 69–80. New Delhi: Concept Publishing Company, 1989.

Bouza-Álvarez, Fernando. "Cultura escrita e história do livro: a circulação manuscrita nos séculos XVI e XVII." In *O livro antigo em Portugal e Espanha, séculos XVI-XVIII*, a special issue of *Leituras*. Revista da Biblioteca Nacional 9/10 (2002): 63–98.

Bowd, Gavin, and Daniel Clayton. "Tropicality, Orientalism, and French Colonialism in Indochina: The Work of Pierre Gourou, 1927–1982." *French Historical Studies* 28 (2005): 297–327.

Boxer, Charles. Ralph. *The Golden Age of Brazil, 1695–1750*. Berkeley, CA: University of California Press, 1962.

The Portuguese Seaborne Empire, 1415–1825. New York: Alfred A. Knopf, 1969.

Portuguese Society in the Tropics: The Municipal Councils of Goa, Macao, Bahia, and Luanda, 1510–1800. Madison, WI: University of Wisconsin Press, 1965.

Three Historians of Portuguese Asia: Barros, Couto and Bocarro. Macau: Imprensa Nacional, 1948.

"Some remarks on the Social and Professional Status of Physicians and Surgeons in the Iberian World, Sixteenth-Eighteenth Centuries." *Revista de História* 100 (1974): 197–215.

Braga, Isabel Drumond. *Assistência, saúde pública e prática médica em Portugal (séculos XV-XIX)*. Lisbon: Universitária Editora, 2001.

Braga-Pinto, César. *As Promessas da História: Discursos Proféticos e Assimilação no Brasil Colonial (1500–1700)*. São Paulo: Editorial da Universidade de São Paulo, 2002.

Braudel, Fernand. *The Mediterranean and the Mediterranean World in the Age of Philip II*. 2 vols. Translated by Siân Reynolds. Berkeley, CA: University of California Press, 1995 [1949].

Brockway, Lucile H. *Science and Colonial Expansion: The Role of the British Royal Botanic Gardens*. New Haven, CT: Yale University Press, 1979.

Brody, David. *Visualizing American Empire: Orientalism and Imperialism in the Philippines*. Chicago: University of Chicago Press, 2010.

Brooks, George E. "Kola Trade and State-Building: Upper Guinea Coast and Senegambia, 15th-17th Centuries." Working Paper 38, African Studies Center, Boston University, 1980.

Brown, Vincent. *Reaper's Garden: Death and Power in the World of Atlantic Slavery*. Cambridge, MA: Harvard University Press, 2008.

Buchanan, Iain. "The Collection of Niclaes Jongelinck: II The 'Months' by Pieter Bruegel the Elder." *The Burlington Magazine* 132 (1990): 541–550.

Buono, Amy. "Crafts of Color: Tupi *Tapirage* in Early Colonial Brazil." In *The Materiality of Color: The Production, Circulation, and Application of Dyes and Pigments, 1400–1800*, edited by Andrea Feeser, Maureen Daly Goggin, and Beth Fowkes Tobin, 235–246. New York: Routledge, 2012.

"Interpretive ingredients: formulating art and natural history in early modern Brazil." *Journal of Art Historiography* 11 (2014): 1–21.

Burbank, Jane and Frederick Cooper. *Empires in World History: Power and the Politics of Difference.* Princeton, NJ: Princeton University Press, 2010.

Burdett, Henry C. *Hospitals and Asylums of the World: Their Origin, History, Construction, Administration, Management, and Legislation.* London: J. and A. Churchill, 1893.

Burnett, D. Graham. *Masters of All They Surveyed: Exploration, Geography, and a British El Dorado.* Chicago: University of Chicago Press, 2001.

Cagle, Hugh. "Cultures of Inquiry, Myths of Empire: Natural History in Colonial Goa." In *Medicine, Trade and Empire: Garcia de Orta's Colloquies on the Simples and Drugs of India (1563) in Context,* edited by Palmira Fontes da Costa, 107–128. Burlington, VT: Ashgate, 2015.

"Beyond the Senegal: Inventing the tropics in the late Middle Ages." *Journal of Medieval Iberian Studies* 7 (2015): 197–217.

Cândido, Mariana P. "South Atlantic Exchanges: The Role of Brazilian-Born Agents in Benguela, 1650–1850." *Luso-Brazilian Review* 50 (2013): 53–82.

Cañeque, Alejandro. "Theater of Power: Writing and Representing the Auto de Fe in Colonial Mexico." *The Americas* 52 (1996): 321–343.

Cañizares-Esguerra, Jorge. *Puritan Conquistadors: Iberianizing the Atlantic, 1550–1700.* Stanford, CA: Stanford University Press, 2006.

"The Colonial Iberian Roots of the Scientific Revolution." In *Nature, Empire, Nation: Explorations of the History of Science in the Iberian World.* Stanford, CA: Stanford University Press, 2006.

"Iberian Science in the Renaissance: Ignored How Much Longer." *Perspectives on Science* 12 (2004): 86–124.

Nature, Empire, and Nation: Explorations of the History of Science in the Iberian World. Stanford, CA: Stanford University Press, 2006.

How to Write the History of the New World: Histories, Epistemologies, and Identities in the Eighteenth-Century Atlantic World. Stanford, CA: Stanford University Press, 2001.

"New World, New Stars: Patriotic Astrology and the Invention of Amerindian and Creole Bodies, 1600–1650." *American Historical Review* 104 (1999): 33–68.

Carita, Heldar. *Palácios de Goa.* 2nd edn. Lisbon: Quetzal Editores, 1996

Carmichael, Ann G. *Plague and the Poor in Renaissance Florence.* New York: Cambridge University Press, 1986.

Carmichael, Ann G., and Arthur Silverstein. "Smallpox in Europe before the Seventeenth Century: Virulent Killer or Benign Disease?" *Journal of the History of Medicine and Allied Sciences* 42 (1987): 147–168.

Carney, Judith, and Nicholas Rosomoff. *In the Shadow of Slavery: Africa's Botanical Legacy in the Atlantic World.* Berkeley, CA: University of California Press, 2009.

Carter, Paul. *The Road to Botany Bay: An Exploration of Landscape and History.* Minneapolis, MN: University of Minnesota Press, 1987.

Carvalho, Augusto da Silva. "Garcia d'Orta. Comemoração do quarto centenário da sua partida para a India em 12 de Março de 1534." *Revista da Universidade de Coimbra,* 12 (1934): 130–133.

A Medicina Portuguesa no século XVII. Lisbon: Academia das Ciências de Lisboa, 1940.

Carvalho, Teresa Nobre de. *Os desafios de Garcia de Orta. Colóqios dos Simples e Drogas da Índia*. Lisbon: Esfera do Caos, 2015.

"A Behind-the-Scenes Glimpse into the Princeps Edition of *Colóquios dos simples* (Goa, 1563)." *Early Science and Medicines* 21 (2016): 232–251.

Casale, Giancarlo. *The Ottoman Age of Exploration*. New York: Oxford University Press, 2010.

Castelnau-L'Estoile, Charlotte de. *Les Ouvriers d'une vigne stérile: Les Jésuites et la conversion des Indiens au Brésil, 1580–1620*. Lisbon: Fundação Calouste Gulbenkian, 2000.

"The Uses of Shamanism: Evangelizing Strategies and Missionary Models in Seventeenth Century Brazil." In *The Jesuits: Cultures, Sciences, and the Arts, 1540–1773*, 2 vols, edited by John W. O'Malley, S. J., Gauvin Alexander Bailey, Steven J. Harris, and T. Frank Kennedy, S. J., vol. 2, 616–637. Toronto: University of Toronto Press, 2006.

Castro, Eduardo Viveiros de. "Cosmological Deixis and Amerindian Perspectivism." *Journal of the Royal Anthropological Institute* 4 (1998): 469–488.

Castro, Inês de Ornellas e. "Prática médica e alimentação nos textos portugueses seiscentistas." In *Percursos na História do Livro Médico (1450–1800)*, edited by Palmira Fontes da Costa and Adelino Cardoso. Lisbon: Edições Colibri, 2011, 73–92.

Caulfield, Sueann. *In Defense of Honor: Sexual Morality, Modernity, and Nation in Early Twentieth-Century Brazil*. Durham, NC: Duke University Press, 2000.

Cell, John W. "Anglo-Indian Medical Theory and the Origins of Segregation in West Africa." *The American Historical Review* 91 (1986): 3017–3335.

Cervantes, Fernando. *The Devil in the New World: The Impact of Diabolism in New Spain* (New Haven, CT: Yale University Press, 1997).

Chakrabarti, Pratik. *Materials and Medicine: Trade, Conquest and Therapeutics in the Eighteenth Century*. Manchester: University of Manchester Press, 2010.

Chaplin, Joyce. "The Atlantic Ocean and Its Contemporary Meanings, 1492–1808." In *Atlantic History: A Critical Appraisal*, edited by Jack P. Greene and Philip D. Morgan, 35–51. New York: Oxford University Press, 2009.

Charles, Loïc, and Paul Cheney. "The Colonial Machine Dismantled: Knowledge and Empire in the French Atlantic." *Past and Present* 219 (2013): 127–163.

Chaudhuri, K. N. *Trade and Civilization in the Indian Ocean World: An Economic History from the Rise of Islam to 1750*. New York: Cambridge University Press, 1985.

Clastres, Hélèn. *The Land-Without-Evil: Tupí-Guaraní Prophetism*. Translated by Jacqueline Grenez Brovender. Urbana, IL: University of Illinois Press, 1995 [1975].

Clendinnen, Inga. *Ambivalent Conquests: Maya and Spaniard in Yucatan*. New York: Cambridge University Press, 1987.

Clossey, Luke. *Salvation and Globalization in the Early Jesuit Missions*. New York: Cambridge University Press, 2011.

Coates, Timothy J. *Convicts and Orphans: Forced and State-Sponsored Colonizers in the Portuguese Empire, 1550–1755.* Stanford, CA: Stanford University Press, 2001.

Cohen, Thomas M. *The Fire of Tongues: António Vieira and the Missionary Church in Brazil and Portugal.* Stanford, CA: Stanford University Press, 1998.

Conklin, Alice L. *In the Museum of Man: Race, Anthropology, and Empire in France, 1850–1950.* Ithaca, NY: Cornell University Press, 2013.

Conrad, Lawrence I, Michael Neve, Vivian Nutton, Roy Porter, and Andrew Wear. *The Western Medical Tradition, 800 BC to AD 1800.* New York: Cambridge University Press, 1995.

Cook, David Noble. *Born to Die: Disease and New World Conquest, 1492–1650.* New York: Cambridge University Press, 1998.

Cook, Harold J. *The Decline of the Old Medical Regime in Stuart London.* Ithaca, NY: Cornell University Press, 1986.

"Global Economies and Local Knowledge in the East Indies: Jacobus Bontius Learns the Facts of Nature." In Londa Schiebinger and Claudia Swan, eds., *Colonial Botany: Science, Commerce, and Politics in the Early Modern World,* 100–118. Philadelphia, PA: University of Pennsylvania Press, 2005.

Matters of Exchange: Commerce, Medicine, and Science in the Dutch Golden Age. New Haven, CT: Yale University Press, 2007.

"The new philosophy and medicine in seventeenth-century England." In *Reappraisals of the Scientific Revolution,* edited by David C. Lindberg and Robert S. Westman, 365–397. New York: Cambridge University Press, 1990.

Coomans, J., and G. Geltner. "On the Street and in the Bathhousel: Medieval Galenism in Action?" *Anuario de Estudios Medievales* 43 (2013): 53–82.

Cooper, Alix. *Inventing the Indigenous: Local Knowledge and Natural History in Early Modern Europe.* New York: Cambridge University Press, 2007.

Cooper, Donald B., and Kenneth F. Kiple. "Yellow Fever." In *The Cambridge World History of Human Disease,* edited by Kenneth Kiple, 1100–1107. New York: Cambridge University Press, 1993.

Corkill, David, and José Carlos Pina Almeida. "Commemoration and Propaganda in Salazar's Portugal: The *Mundo Português* Exposition of 1940." *Journal of Contemporary History* 44 (2009): 381–399.

Correia, Alberto C. Germano da Silva. *La Vieille-Goa.* Bastorá: Tipografia Rangel, 1931.

Cortesão, Armando. *Cartografia e cartógrafos Portugueses dos séculos XVI e XVII.* Lisbon: Imprensa Nacional, 1935.

Cortesão, Armando, ed. *The Suma Oriental of Tomé Pires and the Book of Francisco Rodrigues.* 2 vols. London: Hakluyt Society, 1944.

Cosgrove, Denis. "Tropic and Tropicality." In *Tropical Visions in an Age of Empire,* edited by Felix Driver and Luciana Martins, 197–216. Chicago: University of Chicago Press, 2005.

Costa, Palmira Fontes da. "Geographical expansion and the reconfiguration of medical authority: Garcia de Orta's *Colloquios on the Simples and Drugs of India* (1563)." *Studies in History and Philosophy of Science* 43 (2012): 74–81.

"Secrecy, Ostentation, and the Illustration of Exotic Animals in Sixteenth Century Portugal." *Annals of Science* 66 (2009): 59–82.

ed. *Medicine, Trade and Empire: Garcia de Orta's* Colloquies on the Simples and Drugs of India *(1563) in Context*. Burlington, VT: Ashgate, 2015.

Costa, Palmira Fontes da, and Adelino Cardoso, eds. *Percursos na História do Livro Médico (1450–1800)*. Lisbon: Edições Colibri, 2011.

Costa, Palmira Fontes da, and Henrique Leitão. "Portuguese Imperial Science, 1450–1800: An Historiographical Review." In *Science in the Spanish and Portuguese Empires, 1400–1800*, edited by Daniela Bleichmar, Paula de Vos, Kristin Huffine, and Kevin Sheehan, 35–53. Stanford, CA: Stanford University Press, 2009.

Costigan, Lúcia Helena. *Through Cracks in the Wall: Modern Inquisitions and New Christian Letrados in the Iberian Atlantic World*. Boston, MA: Brill, 2010.

Cox, Virginia. *The Renaissance Dialogue: Literary Dialogue in its Social and Political Contexts, Castiglione to Galileo*. New York: Cambridge University Press, 2008.

Crawford, Matthew James. *The Andean Wonder Drug: Cinchona Bark and Imperial Science in the Spanish Atlantic, 1630–1800*. Pittsburgh, PA: University of Pittsburgh Press, 2016.

Crosby, Alfred W. *Ecological Imperialism: The Biological Expansion of Europe, 900–1900*. New York: Cambridge University Press, 1986.

The Columbian Exchange: Biological and Cultural Consequences of 1492. Westport, CT: Greenwood, 1972.

Cunha, Ana Cannas da. *A Inquisição no Estado da Índia: Origens (1539–1560)*. Lisbon: Arquivo Nacional Torre do Tombo, 1995.

Cunningham, Andrew. "Identifying Disease in the Past: Cutting the Gordian Knot." *Asclepio* 54 (2002): 13–34.

"Getting the Game Right: Some Plain Words on the Identity and Invention of Science." *Studies in History and Philosophy of Science Part A* 19 (1988): 365–389.

Curtin, Philip D. *Disease and Empire: The Health of European Troops in the Conquest of Africa*. New York: Cambridge, 1998.

Death by Migration: Europe's Encounter with the Tropical World in the Nineteenth Century. New York: Cambridge University Press, 1989.

Cross-Cultural Trade in World History. New York: Cambridge, 1984.

The Image of Africa: British Ideas and Action, 1780–1850. 2 vols. Madison, WI: University of Wisconsin Press, 1964.

Curto, Diogo Ramada. "A história do livro em Portugal: uma agenda em aberto." In *O livro antigo em Portugal e Espanha, séculos XVI-XVIII*, a special edition of *Leituras: Revista da Biblioteca Nacional* 9/10 (2002): 13–62.

O Discurso político em Portugal (1600–1650). Lisbon: Universidade Aberta, 1988.

Dalziel, J. M. *The Useful Plants of West Tropical Africa*. London: The Crown Agents for the Colonies, 1937.

Dalgado, Sebastião Rodolfo, ed. *Glossário Luso-Asiático*. 2 vols. Hamburg: Helmut Buske Verlag, 1982 [Coimbra, 1919–1921].

Daston, Lorraine. "The Nature of Nature in Early Modern Europe." *Configurations* 6 (1998): 149–172.

"Curiosity in Early Modern Science." *Word and Image* 11 (1995): 391–404.

Daston, Lorraine, and Katherine Park. *Wonders and the Order of Nature, 1250–1750*. New York: Zone Books, 1998.

Daston, Lorraine, and Peter Galison. "The Image of Objectivity." *Representations* 40 (1992): 81–128.

Davies, Surekha. *Renaissance Ethnography and the Invention of the Human: New Worlds, Maps, and Monsters*. New York: Cambridge University Press, 2016.

Dear, Peter. "What is the History of Science the History Of? Early Modern Roots of the Ideology of Modern Science." *Isis* 96 (2005): 390–406.

The Intelligibility of Nature: How Science Makes Sense of the World. Chicago: University of Chicago Press, 2006.

"Jesuit Mathematical Science and the Reconstitution of Experience in the Early Seventeenth Century." *Studies in History and Philosophy of Science* 18 (1987): 133–175.

Delbourgo, James, and Nicholas Dew. "Introduction." In *Science and Empire in the Atlantic World*, edited by James Delbourgo and Nicholas Dew, 1–6. New York, Routledge, 2008.

Delumeau, Jean. *History of Paradise: The Garden of Eden in Myth and Tradition*. Translated by Matthew O'Connell. Urbana, IL: University of Illinois Press, 2000 [1992].

Demaitre, Luke. *Leprosy in Premodern Medicine: A Malady of the Whole Body*. Baltimore, MD: Johns Hopkins University Press, 2007.

Dettelbach, Michael. "Global physics and aesthetic empire: Humboldt's physical portrait of the tropics." In *Visions of Empire: Voyages, Botany, and Representations of Nature*, edited by David Philip Miller and Peter Hanns Reill, 258–292. New York: Cambridge University Press, 1996.

Dias, José Pedro Sousa. *Droguistas, boticários e segredistas: Ciência e Sociedade na Produção de Medicamentos na Lisboa de Setecentos*. Lisbon: Fundação Calouste Gulbenkian and the Fundação para a Ciência e Tecnologia, 2007.

"Terapéutica Química y polifarmacia en Portugal: La contribución de João Curvo Semedo (1635–1719)." In *Construyendo las ciencias químicas y biológicas*, 67–88. Mexico City: Universidad Autónoma Metropolitana, 1998.

Dias, José Sebastião da Silva. "Potugal e a cultura Europeia (séculos XVI a XVIII)." *Biblos* 28 (1952): 203–498.

Diffey, Bailey W., and George D. Winius. *Foundations of the Portuguese Empire, 1415–1580*. Minneapolis, MN: University of Minnesota Press, 1977.

Disney, Anthony R. *A History of Portugal and the Portuguese Empire*. 2 vols. New York: Cambridge University Press, 2009.

Domingos, Manuela D. ed. *Estudos sobre História do Livro e da Leitura em Portugal, 1995–2000*. Lisbon: Biblioteca Nacional, 2002.

Domingos, Manuela D. "Erudição no tempo joanino: a Livraria de D. Francisco de Almeida." In *O livro antigo em Portugal e Espanha, séculos XVI-XVIII*, a special edition of *Leituras: Revista da Biblioteca Nacional* 9/10 (2002): 191–222.

Domingues, Francisco Contente. "Science and Technology in Portuguese Navigation: The Idea of Experience in the Sixteenth Century." In *Portuguese Oceanic Expansion, 1400–1800*, edited by Francisco Bethencourt and Diogo Ramada Curto, 460–479. New York: Cambridge University Press, 2007.

Domingues, Francisco Contente, and Inácio Guerreiro. *A vida a bordo na carreira da Índia (século XVI)*. Separata of the *Revista da Universidade de Coimbra*. Lisbon: Instituto de Investigação Científica Tropical, 1988.

Drayton, Richard. *Nature's Government: Science, Imperial Britain, and the Improvement of the World*. New Haven, CT: Yale University Press, 2000.

"Knowledge and Empire." In *The Oxford History of the British Empire. Volume II: The Eighteenth Century*, 231–252. New York: Oxford University Press, 1998.

Dunn, Frederick L. "Malaria." In *The Cambridge World History of Human Disease*, edited by Kenneth F. Kiple. New York: Cambridge, 1993.

Durbach, Nadja. *Spectacle of Deformity: Freak Shows and Modern British Culture*. Berkeley, CA: University of California Press, 2010.

Dutra, Francis A. "The Practice of Medicine in Early Modern Portugal: The Role and Social Status of the *Físico-mor* and the *Surgião-mor*." In *Libraries, History, Diplomacy, and the Performing Arts: Essays in Honor of Carleton Sprague Smith*, edited by Israel Katz, 135–169. New York: Pendragon Press, 1991.

"A New Look into Diogo Botelho's Stay in Pernambuco, 1602–1603." *Luso-Brazilian Review* 4 (1967): 27–34.

Dwyer, Doris. *Fact and Legend in the Catalan Atlas of 1375*. Chicago: The Herman Dunlap Smith Center for the History of Cartography and the Newberry Library, 1997.

Earle, Rebecca. *The Body of the Conquistador: Food, Race, and the Colonial Experience in Spanish America, 1492–1700*. New York: Cambridge University Press, 2012.

"'If You Eat Their Food ...': Diets and Bodies in Early Colonial Spanish America." *American Historical Review* 3 (2010): 688–713.

Eaton, Richard M. *A Social History of the Deccan, 1300–1761: Eight Indian Lives*. New York: Cambridge University Press, 2005.

Egmond, Florike. "Figuring Exotic Nature in Sixteenth-Century Europe: Garcia de Orta and Carolus Clusius." In *Medicine, Trade and Empire: Garcia de Orta's Colloquies on the Simples and Drugs of India (1563) in Context*, edited by Palmira Fontes da Costa, 167–193. Burlington, VT: Ashgate, 2012.

Elliott, J. H. *The Old World and the New, 1492–1650*. New York: Cambridge University Press, 1970.

Esaguy [d'Esaguy], Augusto de. *A abertura da Escola Médica de São Paulo da Assunção de Luanda, 1791*. Lisbon: Editorial Império, 1951.

Espinosa, Mariola. *Epidemic Invasions: Yellow Fever and the Limits of Cuban Independence, 1878–1930*. Chicago: University of Chicago Press, 2009.

Fabian, Ann. *The Skull Collectors: Race, Science, and America's Unburied Dead*. Chicago: The University of Chicago Press, 2010.

Fabian, Johannes. *Out of Our Minds: Reason and Madness in the Exploration of Central Africa*. Berkeley, CA: University of California Press, 2000.

Fagg, William. *The Afro-Portuguese Ivories*. London: Batchworth Press, 1959.

Farelo, Mario Sérgio. "On Portuguese Medical Students and Masters Travelling Abroad: An Overview from the Early Modern Period to the Enlightenment." In *Centers of Medical Excellence? Medical Travel and Education in Europe, 1500–1789*, edited by Ole Peter Grell, Andrew Cunningham, and Jon Arrizabalaga, 125–147. New York: Routledge, 2010.

Faria, Alice Cabral Caldeira Santiago. "Understanding Pangim as a Transformed Landscape." In *Histories from the Sea*, edited by Francisco José Gomes Caramelo et al., eds. [n. p.] New Delhi: Jawarharlal Nehru University Center for French and Francophone Studies, 2009.

Faria, Ana Maria Homem Leal de. *Duarte Ribeiro de Macedo: Um Diplomata Moderno (1618–1680)*. Lisbon: Biblioteca Diplomática do Ministério dos Negócios Estrangeiros, 2005.

Fausto, Boris. "Fragmentos de história e cultura Tupinambá: Da etnologia como instrumento crítico de conhecimento etno-histórico." In Manuela Carneiro da Cunha, ed. *História dos Índios no Brasil*. São Paulo: Companhia das Letras 1992.

Feldhay, Rivka. "The Cultural Field of Jesuit Science." In *The Jesuits: Cultures, Sciences, and the Arts, 1540–1773*, 2 vol., edited by John W. O'Malley, S. J. Gauvin, Alexander Bailey, Steven J. Harris, and T. Frank Kennedy, S. J., vol. 1, 107–130. Toronto: University of Toronto Press, 1999.

"Knowledge and Salvation in Jesuit Culture." *Science in Context* 2 (1987): 195–213.

Fernández-Armesto, Felipe. *Before Columbus: Exploration and Colonization from the Mediterranean to the Atlantic, 1229–1492*. Philadelphia: University of Pennsylvania Press, 1987.

Ferreira, Susannah Humble. *The Crown, the Court, and the Casa da Índia: Political Centralization in Portugal, 1479–1521*. Boston: Brill, 2015.

"Inventing the Courtier in Early Sixteenth-Century Portugal." In *Contested Spaces of Nobility in Early Modern Europe*, edited by Matthew P. Romaniello and Charles Lipp, 85–102. Burlington, VT: Ashgate, 2011.

Ficalho, Conde de. *Garcia da Orta e o seu tempo*. Lisbon: Imprensa Nacional, 1886.

Plantas Úteis da África Portuguesa. 2nd edn. Lisbon: Imprensa Nacional, 1947 [1884].

Figueiredo, John M. de. "Ayurvedic Medicine in Goa according to European Sources in the Sixteenth and Seventeenth Centuries." *Bulletin of the History of Medicine* 58 (1984): 228–229.

Figueiredo, Jõao Manuel Pacheco de. "Goa Pré-Portuguesa." *Studia* 12 (1963): 139–259.

"Goa Pré-Portuguesa." *Studia* 13–14 (1964): 139–259.

"The Practice of Indian Medicine in Goa during the Portuguese Rule, 1519–1699." *Luso-Brazilian Review* 4 (1967): 51–60.

Findlen, Paula. "Inventing Nature: Commerce, Art, and Science in the Early Modern Cabinet of Curiosities." In *Merchants and Marvels: Commerce, Science, and Art in Early Modern Europe*, edited by Pamela H. Smith and Paula Findlen, 297–320. New York: Routledge, 2002.

"Natural History." In *The Cambridge History of Science. Volume 3: Early Modern Science*, edited by Katharine Park and Lorraine Daston, 435–468. New York: Cambridge University Press, 2003.

Possessing Nature: Museums, Collecting, and Scientific Culture in Early Modern Italy. Berkeley, CA: University of California Press, 1994.

Fissell, Mary. "Introduction: Women, Health, and Healing in Early Modern Europe." *Bulletin of the History of Medicine* 82 (2008): 1–17.

Flint, Richard W. "American Showmen and European Dealers: Commerce in Wild Animals in Nineteenth Century America." In *New Worlds, New Animals: From Menagerie to Zoological Park in the Nineteenth Century*, edited by R. J. Hoage and William A. Deiss, 97–108. Baltimore, MD: Johns Hopkins University Press, 1996.

Fleck, Eliane Cristina Deckman. *Entre a caridade e a ciência: a prática missionária e a científica da Companhia de Jesus (América platina, séculos XVII e XVIII)*. São Leopoldo: Oikos and Editora Unisinos, 2014.

Foucault, Michel. *The Birth of the Clinic: An Archaeology of Medical Perception*. Translated by A. M. Sheridan. New York: Pantheon Books, 1973 [1963].

Franco, Isabel Maria Madureira. "Les Dynamique familiales et sociales dans un village de pêcheurs des environs do Porto (1449–1497)." In *The Medieval Household in Christian Europe, c. 850–1550: Managing Power, Wealth, and the Body*, edited by Cordelia Beattie, 271–293. Turnhout: Brepols, 2003.

Freedman, Paul. *Out of the East: Spices and the Medieval Imagination*. New Haven, CT: Yale University Press, 2008.

French, Roger. "Astrology in Medical Practice." In *Practical Medicine from Salerno to the Black Death*, edited by Luís García-Ballester, Roger French, Jon Arrizabalaga, and Andrew Cunningham, 30–59. New York: Cambridge, 1994.

Medicine before Science: The Business of Medicine from the Middle Ages to the Enlightenment. New York: Cambridge University Press, 2003.

Friedlein, Roger. "El diálogo renacentista en la Península Ibérica." In *Text und Kontext. Romanische Literaturen und Allgemeine*, edited by Klaus W. Hempfer, Gerhard Regn, and Sunita Scheffel, 141–146. Stuttgart: Franz Steiner Verlag, 2005.

Friedman, John B. "Cultural Conflict in Medieval World Maps." In *Implicit Understandings: Observing Reporting and Reflecting on the Encounters between Europeans and Other Peoples in the Early Modern Era*, edited by Stuart B. Schwartz, 64–95. New York: Cambridge University Press, 1994.

Fromont, Cécile. *The Art of Conversion: Christian Visual Culture in the Kingdom of Kongo*. Chapel Hill, NC: University of North Carolina Press, 2014.

Furtado, Júnia Ferreira. *Chica da Silva: A Brazilian Slave of the Eighteenth Century*. New York: Cambridge University Press, 2009.

Garcia, José Manuel. *O livro de Francisco Rodrigues: o primeiro atlas do mundo moderno*. Porto: Editora da Universidade do Porto, 2008.

Garcia-Ballester, Luís, Jon Arrizabalaga, Montserrat Cabré, Lluís Cifuentes, and Fernando Salmón, eds. *Galen and Galenism: Theory and Medical Practice from Antiquity to the European Renaissance*. London: Ashgate, 2002.

Ghantkar, Gajanana Shantaram Sinai. *History of Goa through Gōykanadi Script*. Panaji: Prabhakar Bhide and Rajhauns Vitaran, 1993.

Glacken, Clarence J. *Traces on the Rhodian Shore: Nature and Culture in Western Thought from Ancient Times to the End of the Eighteenth Century.* Berkeley, CA: University of California Press, 1967.

Glassie, John. *A Man of Misconceptions: The Life of an Eccentric in an Age of Change.* New York: Riverhead Books, 2012.

Godinho, Vitorino Magalhães. "A ideia de descobrimento e os descobrimentos e expansão." *Anais do Club Militar Naval* 120 (October–December 1990): 627–642.

Gómez, Pablo F. *The Experiential Caribbean: Creating Knowledge and Healing in the Early Modern Atlantic.* Chapel Hill, NC: University of North Carolina Press, 2017.

González, Ondina E., and Bianca Premo, eds. *Raising an Empire: Children in Early Modern Iberia and Colonial Latin America.* Albuquerque, NM: University of New Mexico Press, 2007.

Good, Byron J. "How Medicine Constructs Its Objects." In *Medicine, Rationality, and Experience: An Anthropological Perspective,* 65–87. New York: Cambridge University Press, 1994.

Goodman, David C. *Power and Penury: Government, Technology and Science in Philip II's Spain.* Cambridge: Cambridge University Press, 1988.

Goodyear, James D. "Agents of Empire: Portuguese Doctors in Colonial Brazil and the Idea of Tropical Disease." PhD diss., Johns Hopkins University, 1985.

Grafton, Anthony. *Defenders of the Text: The Traditions of Scholarship in an Age of Science, 1450–1800.* Cambridge, MA: Harvard University Press, 1991.

Grafton, Anthony, with April Shelford and Nancy Siraisi. *New Worlds, Ancient Texts: The Power of Tradition and the Shock of Discovery.* Cambridge, MA: Harvard University Press, 1995.

Grant, Edward. "The Partial Transformation of Medieval Cosmology by Jesuits in the Sixteenth and Seventeenth Centuries." In *Jesuit Science and the Republic of Letters,* edited by Mordechai Feingold, 127–155. Cambridge, MA: MIT Press, 2003.

Green, Monica H. *Making Women's Medicine Masculine: The Rise of Male Authority in Pre-Modern Gynaecology.* New York: Oxford University Press, 2008.

Green, Toby. *The Rise of the Trans-Atlantic Slave Trade in Western Africa, 1300–1589.* New York: Cambridge University Press, 2011.

Greenblatt, Stephen. "Invisible Bullets: Renaissance Authority and its Subversions, *Henry IV* and *Henry V.*" *Glyph* 8 (1981): 40–61.

Marvelous Possessions: The Wonder of the New World. Chicago: Chicago University Press, 1991.

Grove, Richard. *Green Imperialism: Colonial Expansion, Tropical Island Edens, and the Origins of Environmentalism, 1600–1860.* Cambridge: Cambridge University Press, 1995.

"Indigenous Knowledge and the Significance of South-West India for Portuguese and Dutch Constructions of Tropical Nature." *Modern Asian Studies* 30 (1996): 121–143.

Grover, Mark L. "The Book and the Conquest: Jesuit Libraries in Colonial Brazil." *Libraries and Culture* 28 (1993): 266–283.

Gruzinski, Serge. *The Mestizo Mind: The Intellectual Dynamics of Colonization and Globalization.* Translated by Deke Dusinberre. New York: Routledge, 2002.

Gschwend, Annemarie Jordan. "Catarina de Áustria: Colecção e *Kunstkammer* de uma Princesa Renascentista." *Oceanos* 16 (1993): 62–70.

"A Procura Portuguesa por Animais Exóticos/The Portuguese Demand for Exotic Animals." In *Cortejo Triunfal com Girafas: animais exóticos ao service do poder/Triumphal Procession with Giraffes: exotic animals at the service of power*, 33–77. Lisbon: N.p., n.d.

"As Maravilhas do Oriente: Colecções de Curiosidades Renascentista em Portugal/The Marvels of the East: Renaissance Curiosity Collections in Portugal." In *A Herança de Rauluchantim/The Heritage of Rauluchantim*, edited by N. V. Silva, 82–127. Lisbon: Museo de São Roque, 1996.

Gschwend, Annemarie Jordan, and K. J. P. Lowe, eds. *The Global City: On the Streets of Renaissance Lisbon.* London: Paul Holberton, 2015.

Guerra, Francisco. "Aleixo de Abreu (1568–1630), Author of the earliest book on Tropical Medicine describing Amoebiasis, Malaria, Typhoid Fever, Scurvy, Yellow Fever, Dracontiasis, Trichuriasis and Tungiasis in 1623." *The Journal of Tropical Medicine ad Hygiene* 71 (1968): 55–69.

Gunther, Robert T., ed. *The Greek Herbal of Dioscorides.* Translated by John B. Goodyear. New York: Hafner Publishing Company, 1968 [1934]).

Gupta, Ashin Das. "Indian Merchants and Trade in the Indian Ocean." *The World of the Indian Ocean Merchant, 1500–1800.* New Delhi: Oxford University Press, 2001.

Gurgel, Cristina. *Doenças e curas: o Brasil nos primeiros séculos.* São Paulo: Contexto, 2010.

Hair, P. E. H. "The Early Sources on Guinea." *History in Africa* 21 (1994): 87–126.

The Founding of the Castelo de São Jorge da Mina: An Analysis of the Sources. Madison, WI: African Studies Program and the University of Wisconsin Press, 1994.

Halikowski-Smith, Stefan. "Perceptions of Nature in Early Modern Portuguese India." *Itinerario* 31 (2007): 17–49.

"Demystifying a Change in Taste: Spices, Space, and Social Hierarchy in Europe, 1380–1750." *The International History Review* 29 (2007): 237–257.

Hamlin, Christopher. *More than Hot: A Short History of Fever.* Baltimore, MD: Johns Hopkins University Press, 2014.

Hanson, Carl A. *Economy and Society in Baroque Portugal, 1668–1703.* Minneapolis, MN: University of Minnesota Press, 1981.

Harkness, Deborah. *The Jewel House: Elizabethan London in the Scientific Revolution.* New Haven, CT: Yale University Press, 2007.

"Managing an Experimental Household: the Dees of Mortlake and the Practice of Natural Philosophy." *Isis* 88 (1997): 247–262.

Harris, Steven J. "Confession-Building, Long Distance Networks, and the Organization of Jesuit Science." *Early Science and Medicine* 1 (1996): 287–318.

"Long-Distance Corporations, Big Sciences, and the Geography of Knowledge." *Configurations* 6 (1998): 269–304.

"Jesuit Scientific Activity in the Overseas Missions, 1540–1773." *Isis* 96 (2005): 71–79.

"Transposing the Merton Thesis: Apostolic Spirituality and the Establishment of the Jesuit Scientific Tradition." *Science in Context* 3 (1989): 29–67.

Harrison, Mark. *Climates and Constitutions: Health, Race, Environment and British Imperialism in India, 1600–1850.* New York: Oxford University Press, 1999.

"A Global Perspective: Reframing the History of Health, Medicine, and Disease." *Bulletin of the History of Medicine* 89 (2015): 639–689.

Contagion: How Commerce Has Spread Disease. New Haven, CT: Yale University Press, 2012.

Medicine in an Age of Commerce and Empire: Britain and its Tropical Colonies, 1660–1830. New York: Oxford University Press, 2010.

Hays, J. N. *The Burdens of Disease: Epidemics and Human Response in Western History.* New Brunswick, NJ: Rutgers University Press, 1998.

Headrick, Daniel R. *Power over Peoples: Technology, Environments, and Western Imperialism, 1400 to the Present.* Princeton, NJ: Princeton University Press, 2012.

The Tools of Empire: Technology and European Imperialism in the Nineteenth Century. New York: Oxford, 1981.

Hemming, John. *Naturalists in Paradise: Wallace, Bates, and Spruce in the Amazon.* London: Thames and Hudson, 2015.

Red Gold: The Conquest of the Brazilian Indians. Cambridge, MA: Harvard University Press, 1978.

Henderson, John. *The Renaissance Hospital: Healing the Body and Healing the Soul.* New Haven, CT: Yale University Press, 2006.

Herrero Massari, José Manuel. *Libros de viajes de los siglos XVI-XVII en España y Portugal: lecturas y lectores.* Madrid: Fundación Universitaria Española, 1999.

Herson, Bella. *Cristãos-novos e seus desvendentes na medicina brasileira, 1500–1850.* São Paulo: Edusp, 1996.

Hinderaker, Eric and Rebecca Horn. "Territorial Crossings: Histories and Historiographies of the Early Americas." *William and Mary Quarterly* 67 (2010): 395–432.

Hodgen, Margaret T. *Early Anthropology in the Sixteenth and Seventeenth Centuries.* Philadelphia, PA: University of Pennsylvania Press, 1964.

Hodgson, Marshall. *Rethinking World History: Essays on Europe, Islam, and World History,* edited and with an introduction by Edmund Burke III. New York: Cambridge University Press, 1993.

Holanda, Sérgio Buarue de. *Visão do paraíso: Os motivos edenicos no descobrimento e colonização do Brasil.* 2nd edn. São Paulo: Companhia Editora Nacinoal, 1969.

Hsia, Florence C. *Sojourners in a Strange Land: Jesuits and their Scientific Missions in Late Imperial China.* Chicago: University of Chicago Press, 2009.

Ikram, S. M. *Muslim Civilization in India.* New York: Columbia University Press, 1964.

Jaggi, O. P. *Dawn of Indian Science.* Delhi: Atma Ram and Sons, 1969.

Jardine, N[ick], J. A. Secord, and E. C. Spary, eds. *Cultures of Natural History*. New York: Cambridge University Press, 1996.

Jasanoff, Maya. *Edge of Empire: Lives, Culture, and Conquest in the East*. New York: Vintage, 2005.

Jennings, Eric T. *Curing the Colonizers: Hydrotherapy, Climatology, and French Colonial Spas*. Durham, NC: Duke University Press, 2006.

Johns, Adrian. *The Nature of the Book: Print and Knowledge in the Making*. Chicago: University of Chicago Press, 1998.

Johnson, H. B. "The settlement of Brazil, 1500–1580." In Leslie Bethell, ed. *Colonial Brazil*. New York: Cambridge University Press, 1987.

Jordan, Annemarie. "Diplomata e dealer de arte." *L+arte* 20 (2006): 58–60.

Kehlmann, Daniel. *Measuring the World: A Novel*. Translated by Carol Brown Janeway. New York: Vintage Books, 2006.

Kennedy, Dane. *The Magic Mountains: Hill Stations and the British Raj*. Berkeley, CA: University of California Press, 1996.

Kiple, Kenneth F. *The Caribbean Slave: A Biological History*. New York: Cambridge University Press, 1984.

Kisling, Vernon N. Jr. "The Origin and Development of American Zoological Parks to 1899." In *New Worlds, New Animals: From Menagerie to Zoological Park in the Nineteenth Century*, edited by R. J. Hoage and William A. Deiss, 109–125. Baltimore, MD: Johns Hopkins University Press, 1996.

Kupperman, Karen Ordahl. *The Jamestown Project*. Cambridge, MA: Belknap Press, 2007.

"The Puzzle of the American Climate in the Early Colonial Period." *American Historical Review* 87 (1982): 1262–1289.

Kusukawa, Sachiko. "Illustrating Nature." In *Books and the Sciences in History*, edited by Marina Frasca-Spada and Nick Jardine, 90–113. New York: Cambridge University Press, 2000.

"Leonhart Fuchs on the Importance of Pictures." *Journal of the History of Ideas* 58 (1997): 403–427.

Lach, Donald F. *Asia in the Making of Europe*. 3 vols. Chicago: University of Chicago Press, 1965–1993.

Lambert, David. *Mastering the Niger: James MacQueen's African Geography and the Struggle over Atlantic Slavery*. Chicago: University of Chicago Press, 2013.

Lameira, António. *Do Informalismo ao Formalismo na Ciência Setecentista em Portugal. Do Conde da Ericeira à Academia Real das Ciências de Lisboa*. MA thesis, Faculdade de Ciências e Tecnologia da Universidade Nova de Lisboa, 2000.

Langfur, Hal. *The Forbidden Lands: Colonial Identity, Frontier Violence, and the Persistence of Brazil's Eastern Indians, 1750–1830*. Stanford, CA: Stanford University Press, 2006.

Latour, Bruno. "On the Partial Existence of Existing *and* Nonexisting Objects." In *Biographies of Scientific Objects*, edited by Lorraine Daston, 247–269. Chicago: University of Chicago Press, 2000.

Pandora's Hope: Essays on the Reality of Science Studies. Cambridge, MA: Harvard University Press, 1999.

Science in Action: How to Follow Scientists and Engineers through Society. Cambridge, MA: Harvard University Press, 1987.

Lattis, James M. *Between Copernicus and Galileo: Christoph Clavius and the Collapse of Ptolemaic Cosmology.* Chicago: University of Chicago Press, 1994.

Law, John. "On the methods of long distance control: vessels, navigation, and the Portuguese route to India." In *Power, Action, and Belief: A New Sociology of Knowledge,* edited by John Law, 234–263. New York: Routledge, 1986.

Lawrence, Christopher, and Michael Brown. "Quintessentially Modern Heroes: Surgeons, Explorers, and Empire, c. 1840–1914." *Journal of Social History* 50 (2016): 148–178.

Lawrence, Jeremy. "The Middle Indies: Damião de Góis on Prester John and the Ethiopians." *Renaissance Studies* 6 3/4 (1992): 306–324.

Leask, Nigel. *Curiosity and the Aesthetics of Travel Writing, 1770–1840.* New York: Oxford University Press, 2002.

Leitão, Henrique. *A ciência na Aula da Esfera do Colégio de Santo Antão, 1590–1759.* Lisbon: Comissariado Geral das Comemorações do V Centenário do Nascimento de S. Francisco Xavier, 2007.

"Jesuit Mathematical Practice in Portugal, 1540–1759." In *The New Science and Jesuit Science: Seventeenth Century Perspectives,* edited by Mordechai Feingold, 229–247. Dordrecht: Kluwer Academic Publishers, 2003.

Pedro Nunes, 1502–1578: novas terras, novos mares e o que mays he: novo ceo e novas estrellas. Lisbon: Biblioteca Nacional de Portugal 2002.

Leite, Serafim. *Artes e ofícios dos Jesuítas no Brasil (1549–1760).* Rio de Janeiro: Livros de Portugal, 1953.

História da Companhia de Jesus no Brasil. 10 vols. Rio de Janeiro: Lisbon, 1938–1950.

Lemos, Maximiano. *O "Auto dos físicos" de Gil Vicente: Comentario medico.* Porto: N.p., 1921.

Archivos de Historia da Medicina Portuguesa. 2 vols. Lisbon, 1887–1888.

História da medicina em Portugal: doutrinas e instituições. 2 vols. Lisbon: N.p., 1899.

Lev, Efraim, and Zohar Amar. *Practical* Materia Medica *of the Medieval Eastern Mediterranean According to the Cairo Genizah.* Boston: Brill, 2008.

Lévi-Strauss, Claude. *Tristes Tropiques.* Translated by John and Doreen Weightman. New York: Penguin, 1992 [1955].

Levinson, Jay A., ed. *Circa 1492: Art in the Age of Exploration.* New Haven, CT: Yale University Press, 1991.

Lewis, Martin W. and Kären E. Wigen. *The Myth of Continents: A Critique of Metageography.* Berkeley, CA: University of California Press, 1997.

Linschoten, Jan Huygen van. *The Voyage of John Huyghen Van Linschoten to the East Indies.* 2 vols. Translated and edited by Arthur Coke Burnell and P. A. Tiele. London: Hakluyt Society, 1885.

Livingstone, David N. "Tropical Climate and Moral Hygiene: The Anatomy of a Victorian Debate." *The British Journal for the History of Science* 32 (1999): 93–110.

Lloyd, G.E.R. *Early Greek Science: Thales to Aristotle.* New York: Norton, 1974.

Lloyd, G.E.R., ed. *Hippocratic Writings*. New York: Penguin 1983.

Lonie, Iain M. "Fever Pathology in the Sixteenth Century: Tradition and Innovation." *Medical History* 1 (1981): 19–44.

Lopes Andrade, António Manuel, Carlos de Miguel Mora, and João Manuel Nunes Torrão, eds., *Humanismo e Ciência: Antiguidade e Renascimento*. Coimbra: The University of Aveiro and the University of Coimbra Press, 2015.

Loureiro, Rui Manuel. "Information Networks in the *Estado da Índia*, A Case Study: Was Garcia de Orta the Organizer of the *Codex Casanatense* 1889?" *Anais de História de Além-Mar* 13 (2012): 41–72.

Maclean, Ian. *Learning and the Market Place: Essays in the History of the Early Modern Book*. Boston: Brill, 2009.

MacLeod, Roy. "On Visiting the Moving Metropolis: Reflections on the Architecture of Imperial Science." *Historical Records of Australian Science* 5 (1982): 1–16.

Marcgocsy, Daniel. *Commercial Visions: Science, Trade, and Visual Culture in the Dutch Golden Age*. Chicago: University of Chicago Press, 2014.

Marchant, Alexander. *From Barter to Slavery: The Economic Relations of Portuguese and Indians in the Settlement of Brazil, 1500–1580*. Gloucester, MA: P. Smith, 1966.

Markham, Clements R., ed. and trans. *Colloquies on the Simples and Drugs of India by Garcia da Orta*. London: Henry Sotheran and Company, 1913.

Marques, Alfred Pinheiro. *Origem e Desenvolvimento da Cartografia Portuguesa na época dos Descobrimentos*. Lisbon: Imprensa Nacional-Casa da Moeda, 1987.

Martínez, María Elena. *Genealogical Fictions: Limpieza de Sangre, Religion, and Gender in Colonial Mexico*. Stanford, CA: Stanford University Press, 2008.

Martins, José F. Ferreira. ed., *Historia da Misericordia de Goa (1520–1620)*. 2 vols. Nova Goa: Imprensa Nacional, 1910.

Martins, Mário. "Experiência religiosa e analogia sensorial." *Brotéria: cultura e informação* 78 (1964): 552–561.

Mathew, K. M. *History of the Portuguese Navigation in India*. Delhi: Mittal Publications, 1988.

Matta, Roberto da. *A casa e a rua: Espaço, cidadania, mulher, e morte no Brasil*. São Paulo: Brasiliense, 1985.

McCleery, Iona. "Both 'Illness and Temptation of the Enemy': Melancholy, the Medieval Patient and the Writing of King Duarte of Portugal." *Journal of Medieval Iberian Studies* 1 (2009): 163–178.

"Medical 'Emplotment' and Plotting Medicine: Health and Disease in Late Medieval Portuguese Chronicles." *Social History of Medicine* 24 (2011): 125–141.

"'Christ More Powerful than Galen'? The Relationship between Medicine and Miracles." In *Contextualizing Miracles in the Christian West, 1100–1500*, edited by M. M. Mesley and L. E. Wilson, 127–154. Oxford: Medium Aevum, 2014.

"Medical Licensing in Late Medieval Portugal." In *Medicine and the Law in the Middle Ages*, edited by W. J. Turner and S. M. Butler, 196–219. Leiden: Brill, 2014.

"From the Edge of Europe to Global Empire: Portuguese Medicine Abroad (Thirteenth to Sixteenth Centuries)." In *Travels and Mobilities in the Middle Ages: From the Atlantic to the Black Sea*, edited by Marianne O'Doherty and Felicitas Schmieder, 55–90. Turnhout: Brepols, 2015.

McClellan, James E., and François Regourd. "The Colonial Machine: French Science and Colonization in the Ancien Régime." *Osiris* 15 (2000): 31–50.

McNeil, J. R. *Mosquito Empires: Ecology and War in the Greater Caribbean, 1620–1914*. New York: Cambridge University Press, 2010.

McVaugh, Michael R. *Medicine before the Plague: Practitioners and their Patients in the Crown of Aragon, 1285–1345*. New York: Cambridge University Press, 1993.

Meadow, Mark A. "Merchants and Marvels: Hans Jacob Fugger and the Origins of the Wunderkammer." In *Merchants and Marvels: Commerce, Science, and Art in Early Modern Europe, edited* by Pamela H. Smith and Paula Findlen, 182–200. New York: Routledge, 2002.

Meilink-Roelofsz, M. A. P. *Asian trade and European influence in the Indonesian archipelago between about 1500 and about 1630*. The Hague: Martinus Nijhoff, 1962.

Mejía, Carmen. "*El libro del Infante don Pedro de Portugal*: estudio crítico y problemas de transmisión." *Revista de Filología Románica* 15 (1998): 215–232.

Melo, Arnaldo Sousa. "Women and Work in the Household Economy: The Social and Linguistic Evidence from Porto, c. 1340–1450." In *The Medieval Household in Christian Europe, c. 850–1550: Managing Power, Wealth, and the Body*, edited by Cordelia Beattie, 249–269. Turnhout: Brepols, 2003.

Mendes, Maria Valentina C. A. Sul. "O livro quinhentista espanhol em bibliotecas portuguesas." In *O livro antigo em Portugal e Espanha, séculos XVI-XVIII*, a special issue of *Leituras. Revista da Biblioteca Nacional* 9/10 (2002): 223–236.

Merchant, Carolyn. *The Death of Nature: Women, Ecology, and the Scientific Revolution*. New York: Harper Collins, 1980.

Metcalf, Alida. C. *Go-Betweens and the Colonization of Brazil, 1500–1600*. Austin, TX: University of Texas Press, 2005.

"Millenarian Slaves? The Santidade de Jaguaripe and Slave Resistance in the Americas." *American Historical Review* 104 (1999): 1531–1559.

Mignolo, Walter. *The Darker Side of the Renaissance: Literacy, Territoriality, and Colonization*. Ann Arbor: University of Michigan Press, 1995.

Miller, Joseph C. *Poder Político e Parentesco: Os antigos Estados Mbundu em Angola*. Luanda, Angola: Arquivo Histórico Nacional and the Ministério da Cultura, 1995 [1976].

Way of Death: Merchant Capitalism and the Angolan Slave Trade, 1730–1830. Madison, WI: University of Wisconsin Press, 1988.

Mitchell, Piers. "Retrospecitve Diagnosis and the Use of Historical Texts for Investigating Disease in the Past." *Journal of International Palaeopathology* 1 (2011): 81–88.

Mokyr, Joel. "Induced Medical Innovation and Medical History: An Evolutionary Approach." *Journal of Evolutionary Economics* 8 (1998): 119–137.

Monteiro, John M. "The Crisis and Transformation of Invaded Societies: Coastal Brazil in the Sixteenth Century." In *The Cambridge History of the Native Peoples of the Americas*, 3 vols, edited by Frank Salomon and Stuart B. Schwartz, vol. 3, part 1, 973–1023. New York: Cambridge University Press, 1996.

"The Heathen Castes of Sixteenth-Century Portuguese America: Unity, Diversity, and the Invention of the Brazilian Indians." *Hispanic American Historical Review* 80 (2000): 697–719.

Morrison, Kathleen D. *Daroji Valley: Landscape History, Place, and the Making of a Dryland Reservoir*. New Delhi: Manohar, 2009.

Moura, Vasco Graça. *Sobre Camões, Gândavo e Outras Personagens*. Lisbon: Campo das Letras, 2000.

Mundy, Barbara E. *The Mapping of New Spain: Indigenous Cartography and the Maps of the Relaciones Geográficas*. Chicago: University of Chicago Press, 1996.

Murphy, Trevor. *Pliny the Elder's Natural History: The Empire in the Encyclopedia*. New York: Oxford University Press, 2004.

Myrup, Erik Lars. "To Rule from Afar: The Overseas Council and the Making of the Brazilian West, 1642–1807." PhD Thesis, Yale University, 2006.

Navarro Brotóns, Victor, and William Eamon. eds. *Más allá de la Leyenda Negra: España y la Revolución Científica*. Valencia: Instituto de Historia de la Ciencia y Documentación López Piñero of the University of Valencia and CSIC, 2007.

Nayeem, M. A. *The Heritage of the Adil Shahis of Bijapur*. Hyderabad: Hyderabad Publishers, 2008.

Neill, Deborah J. *Networks in Tropical Medicine: Internationalism, Colonialism, and the Rise of a Medical Specialty, 1890–1930*. Stanford, CA: Stanford University Press, 2012.

Nelson, Roxanne. "The Last Worm: A dreaded tropical disease is on the verge of eradication." *Scientific American* 307 (2012): 24.

Newitt, Malyn. *A History of Portuguese Overseas Expansion, 1400–1668*. New York: Routledge, 2005.

Newman, William R. *Promethean Ambitions: Alchemy and the Quest to Perfect Nature*. Chicago: University of Chicago Press, 2004.

Newman, William R. and Anthony Grafton, eds. *Secrets of Nature: Astrology and Alchemy in Early Modern Europe*. Cambridge, MA: MIT Press, 2001.

Nicholson, Malcolm. "Alexander von Humboldt and the Geography of Vegetation." In *Romanticism and the Sciences*, edited by Andrew Cunningham and Nicholas Jardine, 169–186. New York: Cambridge University Press, 1990.

Nieto Olarte, Mauricio. *Las máquinas del imperio y el reino de Dios: reflexiones sobre la ciencia, tecnología y religión en el mundo Atlántico del siglo XVI*. Bogotá: Universidad de los Andes, 2013.

Remedios para el imperio: historia natural y la apropiación del Nuevo Mundo. Bogota: Universidad de los Andes, 2006.

Nogueira, Fernando A. R. "Garcia de Orta, Physician and Scientific Researcher." In *The Great Maritime Discoveries and World Health*, edited by Mário Gomes Marques and John Cule, 227–236. Lisbon: Escola Nacional de Saúde Pública, 1991.

Norton, Marcy. *Sacred Gifts, Profane Pleasures: A History of Tobacco and Chocolate in the Atlantic World*. Ithaca, NY: Cornell University Press, 2008.

"The Chicken or the *Iegue*: Human-Animal Relationships and the Columbian Exchange." *American Historical Review* 120 (2015): 28–60.

Novoa, James Nelson. "Unicorns and Bezoars in a Portuguese house in Rome. António da Fonseca's Portuguese Inventories." *Ágora. Estudos Clássicos em Debate* 14 (2012): 91–111.

Nowell, Charles E. "The Historical Prester John." *Speculum* 28 (1953): 435–445.

Nutton, Vivian. "Books Erudition and Medicine, 1450–1700." In *Percursos na História* do Livro Médico (1450–1800), edited by Palmira Fontes da Costa and Adelino Cardoso, 33–44. Lisbon: Edições Colibri, 2011.

"The Reception of Fracastoro's Theory of Contagion: The Seed That Fell among Thorns?" *Osiris* 2nd series, 6 (1990): 196–234.

"The Seeds of Disease: An Explanation of Contagion and Infection from the Greeks to the Renaissance." *Medical History* 27 (1983): 1–34.

Ogilvie, Brian. "Image and Text in Natural History, 1500–1700." In *The Power of Images in Early Modern Science*, edited by Wolfgang Lefèvre et al., 141–166. Boston: Birkhäuser Verlag, 2003.

The Science of Describing: Natural History in Renaissance Europe Chicago: The University of Chicago Press, 2006.

O'Gorman, Edmundo. *La invención de América*. Mexico City: Fondo de Cultura Económica, 1986.

Okihiro, Gary Y. "Unsettling the Imperial Sciences." *Environment and Planning D: Society and Space* 28 (2010): 745–758.

O'Malley, John W. *The First Jesuits*. Cambridge, MA: Harvard University Press, 1993.

Osborne, Michael A. *The Emergence of Tropical Medicine in France*. Chicago: University of Chicago Press, 2014.

"Zoos in the Family: The Geoffroy Saint-Hilaire Clan and the Three Zoos of Paris." In *New Worlds, New Animals: From Menagerie to Zoological Park in the Nineteenth Century*, edited by R. J. Hoage and William A. Deiss, 33–42. Baltimore, MD: Johns Hopkins University Press, 1996.

Nature, the Exotic, and the Science of French Colonialism. Bloomington, IN: Indiana University Press, 1994.

Osseo-Asare, Abena Dove. *Bitter Roots: The Search for Healing Plants in Africa*. Chicago: University of Chicago Press, 2014.

Outram, Dorinda. *Georges Cuvier: Vocation, Science, and Authority in Post-Revolutionary France*. Manchester: Manchester University Press, 1984.

Packard, Randall M. *The Making of a Tropical Disease: A Short History of Malaria*. Baltimore, MD: Johns Hopkins University Press, 2007.

Padrón, Ricardo. *The Spacious Word: Cartography, Literature, and Empire in Early Modern Spain*. Chicago: University of Chicago Press, 2004.

Pagden, Anthony. *European Encounters with the New World: From Renaissance to Romanticism*. New Haven, CT: Yale University Press, 1993.

The fall of natural man: The American Indian and the origins of comparative ethnology. New York: Cambridge University Press, 1982.

Paiva, José Pedro. *Bruxaria e superstição num país sem 'caça às bruxas: Portugal, 1600–1774*. Lisbon: Editorial Notícias, 1997.

Palladino, Palo and Michael Worboys. "Science and Imperialism." *Isis* 84 (1993): 91–102.

Pandit, Heta. *Hidden Hands: Master Builders of Goa.* Goa: Heritage Network, 2003.

Park, Kathryn. *Doctors and Medicine in Early Renaissance Florence.* Princeton, NJ: Princeton University Press, 1985.

Secrets of Women: Gender, Generation, and the Origins of Human Dissection. Brooklyn, NY: Zone Books, 2006.

Park, Katharine, and Lorraine Daston, eds. *The Cambridge History of Science. Volume 3: Early Modern Science.* New York: Cambridge University Press, 2003.

Parrish, Susan Scott. *American Curiosity: Cultures of Natural History in the Colonial British Atlantic World.* Chapel Hill, NC: University of North Carolina Press, 2006.

Parry, J. H. *The Discovery of the Sea.* Berkeley, CA: University of California Press, 1981.

Pearson, Michael. "Locating Garcia de Orta in the Port City of Goa and the Indian Ocean World." In *Medicine, Trade and Empire: Garcia de Orta's Colloquies on the Simples and Drugs of India (1563) in Context*, edited by Palmira Fontes da Costa, 33–48. Burlington, VT: Ashgate, 2015.

Coastal Western India: Studies from the Portuguese Records. New Delhi: Concept Publishing Company, 1981.

"First Contacts between Indian and European Medical Systems: Goa in the Sixteenth Century." In *Warm Climates and Western Medicine: The Emergence of Tropical Medicine, 1500–1900*, edited by David Arnold, 20–41. Atlanta, GA: Rodopi, 1996.

"The Thin End of the Wedge: Medical Relativities as a Paradigm of Early Modern Indian-European Relations." *Modern Asian Studies* 29 (1995): 141–170.

Merchants and Rulers in Gujarat: The Response to the Portuguese in the Sixteenth Century. Berkeley, CA: University of California Press, 1976.

The Portuguese in India. New York: Cambridge University Press, 1987.

Pedreira, Jorge M. "Costs and Financial Trends, 1415–1822." In *Portuguese Oceanic Expansion, 1500–1800*, edited by Francisco Bethencourt and Diogo Ramado Curto, 49–87. New York: Cambridge University Press, 2007.

Penrose, Boies. *Goa—Rainha do Oriente.* Lisbon: Comemorações do V centenário da Morte do Infante D. Henrique, and the Comissão Ultramarina, 1960.

Phillips, Seymour. "The Outer World of the European Middle Ages." In *Implicit Understandings: Observing Reporting and Reflecting on the Encounters between Europeans and Other Peoples in the Early Modern Era*, edited by Stuart B. Schwartz, 23–63. New York: Cambridge University Press, 1994.

Pickstone, John V. "Working Knowledges Before and After circa 1800: Practices and Disciplines in the History of Science, Technology, and Medicine." *Isis* 98 (2007): 489–516.

Pimentel, Juan. *El Rinoceronte y el Megaterio. Un ensayo de morfología histórica.* Madrid: Abada Editores. 2010.

"The Iberian Vision: Science and Empire in the Framework of a Universal Monarchy, 1500–1800." *Osiris*, 2nd series, 15 (2000): 17–30.

Pina, Luiz de. *História da Medicina Imperial Portuguesa (Angola)*. Lisbon: Agência Geral das Colónias, 1943.

Piper, Anson C. "Jorge Ferreira de Vasconcellos: Defender of the Portuguese Vernacular." *Hispania* 37 (1954): 400–405.

Polónia, Amélia. "Global Interactions: Representations of the East and the Far East in Portugal in the Sixteenth Century." In *Networks in the First Global Age, 1400–1800*, edited by Rila Mukherjee, 263–301. New Delhi: Primus Books, 2011.

Portuondo, María M. *Secret Science: Spanish Cosmography and the New World*. Chicago: University of Chicago Press, 2009.

Pratt, Mary Louise. *Imperial Eyes: Travel Writing and Transculturation*. 2nd edn. New York: Routledge, 2008.

Prestage, Edgar. *As relações diplomáticas de Portugal com a França, Inglaterra e Holanda, de 1640 a 1668*. Coimbra: Imprensa da Universidade, 1928.

Prieto, Andrés I. *Missionary Scientists: Jesuit Science in Spanish South America, 1570–1810*. Nashville, TN: Vanderbilt University Press, 2011.

Principe, Lawrence M. *The Secrets of Alchemy* Chicago: University of Chicago Press, 2013.

Priolkar, A[nant]. K[akba]. *The Goa Inquisition. Being a Quatercentenary Commemoration Study of the Inquisition in India*. Bombay: V.G. Moghe at the Bombay University Press, 1961.

Proctor, Robert N. and Londa Schiebinger. *Agnotology: The Making and Unmaking of Ignorance*. Stanford, CA: Stanford University Press, 2008.

Raffles, Hugh. *In Amazonia: A Natural History*. Princeton, NJ: Princeton University Press, 2002.

Ragab, Ahmed. "'In a Clear Arab Tongue': Arabic and the Making of a Science-Language Regime." *Isis* 108 (2017): 612–620.

Raj, Kapil. "The Historical Anatomy of a Contact Zone: Calcutta in the Eighteenth Century." *The Indian Economic and Social History Review* 48 (2011): 55–82.

Relocating Modern Science: Circulation and the Construction of Knowledge in South Asia and Europe, 1650–1900. New York: Palgrave Macmillan, 2007.

Rankin, Alisha. *Panaceia's Daughters: Noblewomen as Healers in Early Modern Germany*. Chicago: University of Chicago Press, 2013.

Rau, Virginia. *Política Economica e Mercantilismo na Correspondência de Duarte Ribeiro de Macedo (1668–1676)*. Lisbon: n.p., 1968.

Reff, Daniel T. *Disease, Depopulation, and Culture Change in Northwestern New Spain, 1518–1764*. Salt Lake City, UT: University of Utah Press, 1991.

Reichenbach, Herman. "A Tale of Two Zoos: The Hamburg Zoological Garden and Carl Hagenbeck's Tierpark." In *New Worlds, New Animals: From Menagerie to Zoological Park in the Nineteenth Century*, edited by R. J. Hoage and William A. Deiss, 51–62. Baltimore, MD: Johns Hopkins University Press, 1996.

Reid, Anthony. "From Betel-Chewing to Tobacco Smoking in Indonesia." *The Journal of Asian Studies* 44 (1985): 529–532.

Richardson, Lind Deer. "The Generation of Diseases: Occult Causes and Diseases of the Total Substance." In *The medical renaissance of the sixteenth century*, edited by A. Wear, R. K. French, and I. M. Lonie, 175–194. New York: Cambridge University Press, 1985.

Riddle, John M. *Dioscorides on Pharmacy and Medicine*. Austin, TX: University of Texas Press, 1985.

Ritvo, Harriet. *The Animal Estate: The English and Other Creatures in the Victorian Age*. Cambridge, MA: Harvard University Press 1987.

Roberts, Lissa. "Situating Science in Global History: Local Exchanges and Networks of Circulation." *Itinerario* 33 (2009): 9–30.

Robinson, Rowena. "Some Neglected Aspects of the Conversion of Goa: A Socio-Historical Perspective." In *Sociology of Religion in India*, edited by Rowena Robison, 177–198. New Delhi: Sage, 2004.

Rodrigues, Lisbeth de Oliveira, and Isabel dos Guimarães Sá. "Sugar and Spices in Portuguese Renaissance Medicine." *Journal of Medieval Iberian Studies* 7 (2015): 176–196.

Rodrigues, Lopes. *Anchieta e a Medicina*. Bello Horizonte: Edições Apollo, 1934.

Romo, Eduardo Javier Alonso. "Português e Castelhano no Brasil Quinhentista: À Volta dos Jesuítas." *Revista de Indias* 65 (2005): 491–510.

Rothfels, Nigel. *Savages and Beasts: The Birth of the Modern Zoo*. Baltimore, MD: Johns Hopkins University Press, 2002.

Roxburgh, William. "Aquilaria." *The Transactions of the Linnean Society of London* 21 (1855): 206.

Rubiés, Joan-Pau. *Travel and Ethnology in the Renaissance: South India through European Eyes, 1250–1625*. New York: Cambridge University Press, 2000.

"Instructions for Travellers: Teaching the Eye to See." *History and Anthropology* 9 (1996): 139–190.

Rupke, Nicolaas A. "Humboldtian Medicine." *Medical History* 40 (1996): 293–310.

Russell, Peter. *Prince Henry 'the Navigator': A Life*. New Haven, CT: Yale University Press, 2001.

Russell-Wood, A. J. R. *The Portuguese Empire, 1415–1808: A World on the Move*. Baltimore, MD: Johns Hopkins University Press, 1992.

Russo, Alessandra. "Cortés's Objects and the Idea of New Spain: Inventories as Spatial Narratives." *Journal of the History of Collections* 23 (2011): 229–252.

Sá, Isabel dos Guimarães. *Quando o rico se faz pobre: Misericórdias, caridade e poder no Império Português, 1500–1800*. Lisbon: Comissão Nacional para as Comemoracões dos Descobrimentos Portugueses, 1997.

Sachs, Aaron. *The Humboldt Current: Nineteenth-Century Exploration and the Roots of American Environmentalism*. New York: Penguin, 2006.

Safier, Neil. *Measuring the New World: Enlightenment Science in South America* Chicago: University of Chicago Press, 2008.

"The Tenacious Travels of the Torrid Zone and the Global Dimensions of Geographical Knowledge in the Eighteenth Century." *Journal of Early Modern History* 18 (2014): 141–172.

Said, Edward. *Orientalism.* New York: Pantheon, 1978.

Sack, Robert D. *Human Territoriality: Its Theory and History.* New York: Cambridge University Press, 1986.

Sallares, Robert. *Malaria and Rome: A History of Malaria in Ancient Italy.* New York: Oxford University Press, 2002.

Sandman, Alison. "Mirroring the World: Sea Charts, Navigation, and Territorial Claims in Sixteenth-Century Spain." In *Merchants and Marvels: Commerce, Science, and Art in Early Modern Europe*, edited by Pamela H. Smith and Paula Findlen, 83–108. New York: Routledge, 2002.

Santos, Boaventura de Sousa. "Between Prospero and Caliban: Colonialism, Post-Colonialism, and Inter-identity." *Luso-Brazilian Review* 39 (2002): 9–43.

Saunders, A. C. de C. M. *A Social History of Black Slaves and Freedmen in Portugal, 1441–1555.* New York: Cambridge University Press, 1982.

Scafi, Alessandro. *Mapping Paradise: A History of Heaven on Earth.* Chicago: University of Chicago Press, 2006.

Schiebinger, Londa. *The Mind Has No Sex? Women in the Origins of Modern Science.* Cambridge, MA: Harvard University Press, 1989.

Nature's Body: Gender in the Making of Modern Science. 2nd ed. New Brunswick, NJ: Rutgers University Press, 2004.

Plants and Empire: Colonial Bioprospecting in the Atlantic World. Cambridge, MA: Harvard University Press, 2004.

Schiebinger, Londa, and Claudia Swan, eds. *Colonial Botany: Science Commerce, and Politics in the Early Modern World.* Philadelphia, PA: The University of Pennsylvania Press, 2005.

Schmidt, Benjamin. *Innocence Abroad: The Dutch Imagination and the New World, 1570–1670.* New York: Cambridge University Press, 2001.

"'Imperfect Chaos': Tropical Medicine and Exotic Natural History c. 1700." In *Medicine and Religion in Enlightenment Europe*, edited by Ole Peter Grell and Andrew Cunningham, 145–173. Burlington, VT: Ashgate, 2007.

Inventing Exoticism: Geography, Globalism, and Europe's Early Modern World. Philadelphia: University of Pennsylvania Press, 2015.

Schwartz, Stuart B. *All Can be Saved: Religious Tolerance and Salvation in the Iberian Atlantic World.* New Haven, CT: Yale University Press, 2008.

"A Commonwealth within Itself: The Early Brazilian Sugar Industry, 1550–1670." In *Tropical Babylons: Sugar and the Making of the Atlantic World, 1450–1680*, edited by Stuart B. Schwartz, 1158–1200. Chapel Hill, NC: University of North Carolina Press, 2004.

"The Formation of a Colonial Identity in Brazil." In *Colonial Identity in the Atlantic World, 1500–1800*, edited by Nicholas Canny and Anthony Pagden, 15–50. Princeton, NJ: Princeton University Press, 1987.

"Indian Labor and New World Plantations: European Demands and Indian Responses in Northeastern Brazil." *American Historical Review* 83 (1978): 43–79.

"The King's Processions: Municipal and Royal Authority and the Hierarchies of Power in Colonial Salvador." In *Portuguese Colonial Cities in the Early Modern World*, edited by Liam Matthew Brockey, 177–203. Burlington, VT: Ashgate, 2008.

Sovereignty and Society in Colonial Brazil: The High Court of Bahia and Its Judges, 1609–1751. Berkeley, CA: University of California Press, 1973.

"The Voyage of the Vassals: Royal Power, Noble Obligations, and Merchant Capital before the Portuguese Restoration of Independence." *American Historical Review* 96 (1991): 735–762.

Sugar Plantations in the Formation of Brazilian Society: Bahia, 1550–1835. New York: Cambridge University Press, 1985.

ed. *A Governor and His Image in Baroque Brazil: The Funereal Eulogy of Afonso Furtado de Castro do Rio de Mondonça by Juan Lopes Sierra*. Translated by Ruth Jones. Minneapolis, MN: University of Minnesota Press, 1979.

ed. *Implicit Understandings: Observing Reporting and Reflecting on the Encounters between Europeans and Other Peoples in the Early Modern Era*. New York: Cambridge University Press, 1994.

ed. *Tropical Babylons: Sugar and the Making of the Atlantic World, 1450–1680*. Chapel Hill, NC: University of North Carolina Press, 2004.

Secord, James A. "Knowledge in Transit." *Isis* 95 (2004): 654–672.

Seed, Patricia. "Navigating the Mid-Atlantic; or, What Gil Eanes Achieved." In *The Atlantic in Global History, 1500–2000*, eds., Jorge Cañizares Esguerra and Erik R. Seeman, 77–89. Upper Saddle River, NJ: Prentice Hall, 2007.

Ceremonies of Possession in Europe's Conquest of the New World, 1492–1640. New York: Cambridge University Press, 1995.

Shapin, Steven. "The House of Experiment in Seventeenth Century England." *Isis* 79 (1988): 373–404.

Shapin, Steven and Simon Schaffer. *Leviathan and the Air Pump: Hobbes, Boyle, and the Experimental Life*. Princeton, NJ: Princeton University Press, 1989.

Shapiro, Barbara J. *A Culture of Fact: England, 1550–1720*. Ithaca, NY: Cornell University Press, 2000.

Silva, Vítor de Albuquerque Freire da. "*O Hospital Real de Goa (1510–1610): Contribuição para o estudo da sua história e regimentos*." 2 vols. MA thesis, University of Lisbon, 1997.

Siraisi, Nancy G. "Medicine, 1450–1620, and the History of Science." *Isis* 103 (2012): 491–514.

Slater, John, Maríaluz López-Terrada, and José Pardo-Tomás, eds. *Medical Cultures of the Early Modern Spanish Empire*. New York: Routledge, 2014.

Smith, Andrew F. *Sugar: A Global History*. London: Reaktion, 2015.

Smith, Catherine Delano. "Cartographic Signs on European Maps and Their Explanation before 1700." *Imago Mundi* 37 (1985): 9–29.

Smith, Pamela H. *The Body of the Artisan: Art and Experience in the Scientific Revolution*. Chicago: University of Chicago Press, 2004.

The Business of Alchemy: Science and Culture in the Holy Roman Empire. Princeton, NJ: Princeton University Press, 1994.

Smith, Pamela H. and Paula Findlen. *Merchants and Marvels: Commerce, Science, and Art in Early Modern Europe*. New York: Routledge, 2002.

Sobral, Luís de Moura. "The Expansion and the Arts: Transfers, Contaminations, Innovations." In *Portuguese Oceanic Expansion, 1400–1800*, edited by Francisco Bethencourt and Diogo Ramada Curto, 390–428. New York, 2007.

Sousa, Bernardo Vasconcelos e. "Medieval Portuguese Royal Chronicles: Topics in a Discourse of Identity and Power." *e-Journal of Portuguese History* 5 (2007): 1–7.

Souza, Teotonio R. de. "The Council of Trent (1545–1563): Its Reception in Portuguese India." In *Transcontinental Links in the History of Non-Western Christianity*, edited by Klaus Koschorke, 189–202. Wiesbaden: Harrassowitz Verlag, 2002.

Souza, Laura de Mello E. *The Devil and the Land of the Holy Cross: Witchcraft, Slavery, and Popular Religion in Colonial Brazil*. Translated by Diane Grosklaus Whitty. Austin, TX: University of Texas Press, 2003 [1986].

Inferno Atlântico: Demonologia e colonização, séculos XVI-XVIII. São Paulo: Companhia das Letras, 1993.

Speck, Reinhard S. "Cholera." In *The Cambridge World History of Human Disease*, edited by Keneth Kiple, 642–649. New York: Cambridge University Press, 1993.

Spence, Jonathan D. *The Memory Palace of Matteo Ricci*. New York: Penguin, 1984.

Stepan, Nancy Leys. *Picturing Tropical Nature*. Ithaca, NY: Cornell University Press, 2001.

Stevens-Arroyo, Anthony. "The Inter-Atlantic Paradigm: The Failure of Spanish Medieval Colonization of the Canary and Caribbean Islands." *Comparative Studies in Society and History* 35 (1993): 515–543.

Studnicki-Gizbert, Daviken. *A Nation Upon the Ocean Sea*. New York: Oxford University Press, 2007.

Subrahmanyam, Sanjay. *Explorations in Connected History: From the Tagus to the Ganges*. New Delhi: Oxford University Press, 2005.

Explorations in Connected History: Mughals and Franks. New Delhi: Oxford University Press, 2005.

"Holding the World in Balance: The Connected Histories of the Iberian Overseas Empires, 1500–1640." *American Historical Review* 112 (2007): 1359–1385.

Improvising Empire: Portuguese Trade and Settlement in the Bay of Bengal, 1500–1700. Delhi: Oxford University Press, 1990.

"On World Historians in the Sixteenth Century." *Representations* 91 (2005): 26–57.

The Political Economy of Commerce: Southern India, 1500–1650. New York: Cambridge University Press, 1990.

The Portuguese Empire in Asia. New York: Norton, 1993.

Subrahmanyam, Sanjay, ed. *Sinners and Saints: The Successors of Vasco da Gama*. Delhi: Oxford University Press, 1998.

Sweet, James H. *Domingos Álvares: African Healing and the Intellectual History of the Atlantic World*. Chapel Hill, NC: University of North Carolina Press, 2011.

"Mutual Misunderstandings: Gesture, Gender and Healing in the African Portuguese World." *Past and Present* (2009): Supplement 4, 128–143.

Recreating Africa: Culture, Kinship, and Religion in the African-Portuguese World, 1441–1770. Chapel Hill, NC: University of North Carolina Press, 2003.

Tavares, Célia Cristina da Silva. *"A Cristandade Insular: Jesuítas e Inquisidores em Goa (1540–1682)."* PhD diss., Universidade Federal Fluminense, 2002.

Temkin, Oswei. *Galenism: Rise and Decline of a Medical Philosophy*. Ithaca, NY: Cornell University Press, 1973.

Thomas, Nicholas. *Entangled Objects: Exchange, Material Culture, and Colonialism in the Pacific*. Cambridge, MA: Harvard University Press, 1991.

Thornton, John K. *Africa and Africans in the Making of the Atlantic World, 1450–1800*. New York: Cambridge University Press, 1998.

"The Development of an African Catholic Church in the Kingdom of Kongo, 1491–1750." *Journal of African History* 25 (1984): 147–167.

"Les États de l'Angola et la formation de Palmares (Brésil)." *Annales* 63 (2008): 769–797.

"The Portuguese in Africa." In *Portuguese Oceanic Expansion, 1400–1800*, edited by Francisco Bethencourt and Diogo Ramado Curto, 138–160. New York: Cambridge University Press, 2007.

Tilley, Helen. *Africa as a Living Laboratory: Empire, Development, and the Problem of Scientific Knowledge, 1870–1950*. Chicago: University of Chicago Press, 2011.

Tobin, Beth Fowkes. *Colonizing Nature: The Tropics in British Arts and Letters, 1760–1820*. Philadelphia, PA: University of Pennsylvania Press, 2005.

Todorov, Tzvetan. *The Conquest of America: The Question of the Other*. Translated by Richard Howard. New York: Harper & Row, 1984 [1982].

Townsend, Camilla. "Burying the White Gods: New Perspectives on the Conquest of Mexico." *American Historical Review* 108 (2003): 659–687.

Toulmin, Stephen. *Cosmopolis: The Hidden Agenda of Modernity*. Chicago: University of Chicago Press, 1992.

Tudela, A. Pérez de and Annemarie Jordan Gschwend. "Luxury Goods for Royal Collectors: Exotica, princely gifts, and rare animals exchanged between the Iberian courts and Central Europe in the Renaissance (1560–1612)." In *Exotica. Portugals Entdeckungen im Spiegel fürstlicher Kunst- und Wunderkammern der Renaissance. Die Beiträge des am 19, und 20. Mai 2000 vom Kunsthistorischen Museum Wien veranstalteten Symposiums, Jahrbuch des Kunsthistorischen Museums Wien 3*, edited by H. Trnek and S. Haag, 1–127. Mainz: P. von Zabern, 2001.

"Renaissance Menageries. Exotic Animals and Pets at the Habsburg Courts in Iberia and Central Europe." In *Early Modern Zoology: The Construction of Animals in Science, Literature and the Visual Arts*, edited by Karl A. E. Enenkel and Paul J. Smith, 419–445. Boston: Brill, 2007.

Tuer, Dot. "Old Bones and Beautiful Words: The Spiritual Contestation between Shaman and Jesuit in the Guaraní Missions." In Alan Greer and Jodi Bilinkoff, eds. *Colonial Saints: Discovering the Holy in the Americas, 1500–1800*. New York: Routledge, 2002.

Turnbull, David. "Travelling knowledge: narratives, assemblage, encounters." In *Instruments, Travel, and Science: Itineraries of precision from the seventeenth to the twentieth century*, edited by Marie-Noëlle Bourguet, Christian Licoppe, and H. Otto Sibum, 273–294. New York: Routledge, 2002.

Vainfas, Ronaldo. *A heresia dos Indios: Catolicismo e rebeldia no Brasil colonial*. São Paulo: Companhia das Letras, 1995.

Trópico dos pecados: moral, sexualidade, e Inquisição no Brasil. Rio de Janeiro: Editora Campus, 1997.

Van Veen, Ernst. *Decay or Defeat?: An Inquiry into the Portuguese Decline in Asia, 1580–1645*. Leiden: Research School of Asian, African, and Amerindian Studies of the University of Leiden: 2000.

Veloso, Caetano. *Tropical Truth: A Story of Music and Revolution in Brazil*. Cambridge, Mass.: Da Capo Press, 2002 [1997].

Ventura, Maria da Graça Mateus, ed. *Viagens e viajantes no Atlântico quinhentista*. Lisbon: Edições Colibri, 1996.

Vilches, Elvira. *New World Gold: Cultural Anxiety and Monetary Disorder in Early Modern Spain*. Chicago: University of Chicago Press, 2010.

Vos, Paula de. "The Science of Spices: Empiricism and Economic Botany in the Early Spanish Empire." *Journal of World History* 17 (2006): 399–427.

Wadsworh, James E. *Agents of Orthodoxy: Honor, Status, and the Inquisition in Colonial Pernambuco, Brazil*. New York: Rowman and Littlefield, 2006.

Walker, Timothy D. "The Medicines Trade in the Portuguese Atlantic World: Acquisition and Dissemination of Healing Knowledge from Brazil (c. 1580–1800)." *Social History of Medicine* (2013): 403–431.

Doctors, Folk Medicine, and the Inquisition: The Repression of Magical Healing in Portugal During the Enlightenment. Leiden: Brill, 2005.

"Acquisition and Circulation of Medical Knowledge within the Early Modern Portuguese Colonial Empire." In *Science in the Spanish and Portuguese Empires*, edited by Daniela Bleichmar, Paula de Vos, Kristin Huffine, and Kevin Sheehan, 247–270. Stanford, CA: Stanford University Press, 2008.

"Stocking Colonial Pharmacies: Commerce in South Asian Indigenous Medicines from their Native Sources in the Portuguese Estado da Índia." In *Networks in the First Global Age, 1400–1800*, edited by Rila Mukherjee, 113–136. New Delhi: Primus Books, 2011.

"The Role and Practices of the Female Folk Healer in the Early Modern Portuguese Atlantic World." In *Women of the Iberian Atlantic*, edited by Sarah E. Owens and Jane E. Mangan, 148–173. Baton Rouge, LA: Louisiana State University Press, 2012.

Wald, Priscilla *Contagious: Cultures, Carriers, and the Outbreak Narrative*. Durham, NC: Duke University Press, 2008.

Walter, Jaime. "Garcia de Orta. Relance da sua vida." *Separata* of *Garcia de Orta. Revista da Junta de Investigações do Ultramar* 11 (1963): 619–622.

"Dimas Bosque, físico-mor da Índia e as Sereias." *Studia* 12 (1963): 261–271.

"O Infante D. Henrique e a medicina." *Studia* 13/14 (1964): 31–39.

Wear, Andrew. "Explorations in Renaissance Writings on the Practice of Medicine." In *The Medical Renaissance of the Sixteenth Century*, edited by A. Wear, R. K. French, and I. M. Lonie, 118–145. New York: Cambridge University Press, 1985.

"Place, Health, and Disease: The *Airs, Waters, Places* Tradition in Early Modern England and North America." *Journal of Medieval and Early Modern Studies* 38 (2008): 443–465.

Knowledge and Practice in English Medicine, 1550–1680. New York: Cambridge University Press, 2000.

Webb, James L. A. *Humanity's Burden: A Global History of Malaria.* New York: Cambridge University Press, 2009.

Weber, David J. *Bárbaros: Spaniards and Their Savages in the Age of Enlightenment.* New Haven, CT: Yale University Press, 2005.

Wey Gómez, Nicolás. *The Tropics of Empire: Why Columbus Sailed South to the Indies.* Cambridge, MA: MIT Press 2008.

Winsor, Mary P. *Reading the Shape of Nature: Comparative Zoology at the Agassiz Museum.* Chicago: University of Chicago Press, 1991.

Wintroub, Michael. "The Translations of a Humanist Ship Captain: Jean Parmentier's 1529 Voyage to Sumatra." *Renaissance Quarterly* 68 (2015): 98–132.

Wood, Denis. "How Maps Work." *Cartographica* 29 (1992): 66–74.

Worboys, Michael. "Germs, Malaria, and the Invention of Mansonian Tropical Medicine: From 'Diseases in the Tropics' to 'Tropical Diseases.'" In *Warm Climates and Western Medicine: The Emergence of Tropical Medicine, 1500–1900*, edited by David Arnold, 181–207. Atlanta, GA: Rodopi, 1996.

"The Emergence of Tropical Medicine: a Study in the Establishment of a Scientific Specialty." In *Perspectives on the Emergence of Scientific Disciplines*, edited by Gerard Lemaine, Roy Macleod, Michael Mulkay, and Peter Weingart, 75–98. The Hague: Mouton, 1976.

Wragge-Morley, Alexander. "The Work of Verbal Picturing for John Ray and Some of His Contemporaries." *Intellectual History Review* 20 (2010): 165–179.

Wujastyk, Dagmar. *Well-Mannered Medicine: Medical Ethics and Etiquette in Classical Ayurveda.* New York: Oxford University Press, 2012.

"Traditional Indian Systems of Healing and Medicine: Ayurveda." In *Encyclopedia of Religion*, 2nd edn., edited by Lindsay Jones, 3852–3858. New York: Macmillan, 2005.

Wulf, Andrea. *The Invention of Nature: Alexander von Humboldt's New World.* New York: Alfred A. Knopf, 2015.

Xavier, Ângela Barreto and Ines Županov. *Catholic Orientalism: Portuguese Empire, Indian Knowledge (16th to 18th Centuries).* New Delhi: Oxford University Press, 2014.

Yule, Henry, and Arthur Coke Burnell. *Hobson-Jobson: A Glossary of Anglo-Indian Words and Phrases.* London: J. Murray, 1886.

Županov, Ines G. *Disputed Missions: Jesuit Experiments and Brahmanical Knowledge in Seventeenth-Century India*. New Delhi: Oxford University Press, 1999.

"Drugs, Health, Bodies and Souls in the Tropics: Medical Experiments in Sixteenth-Century Portuguese India." *Indian Economic and Social History Review* 39 (2002): 1–43.

Missionary Tropics: The Catholic Frontier in India (16th-17th Centuries). Ann Arbor, MI: University of Michigan Press, 2005.

"Garcia de Orta's *Colóquios*: Context and Afterlife of a Dialogue." In *Medicine, Trade and Empire: Garcia de Orta's* Colloquies on the Simples and Drugs of India *(1563) in Context*, edited by Palmira Fontes da Costa, 49–65. Burlington, VT: Ashgate, 2012.

Index

Clusius translation, 106–107
his empiricism, 119, 120
idea of experiment, 131

Pagden, Anthony, 89
Pahang (Myanmar), 91
pain relievers, 96
pajés (Tupí shamans), 200–201, 203, 243
Palembang (Sumatra), 69
Panjim (in Goa), 273
paradise
discussion of its location, 54–55
Paraíba (Brazil), 233, 242
parakeets, 11
paralysis, 288
Paris, 18, 169, 254, 265
parrots, 4, 11, 201, 210
passion fruit, 237
pearls, 69, 121
Pedro II (King of Portugal), 255
Pegu (Myanmar), 11, 69, 96, 159
pepper, 62, 81, 84, 86, 92, 114, 120, 237,
259, 261
trade, 66–67, 83, 258
varieties, 99–100, 102, 120
white, 100
Pereira, Duarte Pacheco, 27, 29, 31, 36, 42,
44–45, 49–50, 231, 263
Esmeraldo de situ orbis, 31, 49
Pereira, Rui (SJ), 196–197
Pernambuco (Brazilian captaincy), 16, 85,
182, 220–221, 233, 245–246, 252,
259, 288–289
perspectivism, 201
Peru, 121, 276
pestilence, 31
pharmacopoeia, 231, 241, 310
Philadelphia, 4
Philip I (King of Portugal), 217
Philip III (King of Portugal), 215
philosopher's stone, 305–306
physicians, 10, 12–16, 19, 23, 33, 46, 60,
86–87, 95, 111–112, 129, 135,
139–140, 143, 156, 188, 195–196,
199, 211–212, 214–215, 217, 221,
240, 252, 256, 271, 273, 279–280,
284, 298, 307
físico-mor of Goa, 146
Greek, 113
Hindu, 135–138, 143
Indian, 62

Islamic, 113
non-Christian, 142, 146, 160
and politics, 271
and print culture, 269, 271
proper conduct of, 231
writing, 277
pilots, 38, 51, 70, 89, 101, 137, 165, 203,
264, 305
Pina, Rui de, 32
Pinto, Francisco (SJ), 240
Pinto, Thomas, 133
Piratininga (Brazil), 185, 202
Pires, Francisco (SJ), 182–183, 186, 197, 200
Pires, Tomé, 86–90, 92, 94–95, 102, 110,
116, 137–138, 140, 152, 157, 252
Suma Oriental, 87, 89, 264
Pirez, Sancho (Portuguese renegade), 159
Piso, Willem. *See* Marcgraff, Georg
Historia naturalis Brasiliae, 252
plague, 211, 235
plantains, 11
plantation agriculture, 217, 221
Pliny, 37, 99, 211
Natural History, 37
poison, 96, 148, 159, 300
porcelain, 210
Portuguese
vernacular language (use of), 274
Portuguese fleets, 70
Portuguese print culture, 14
Portuguese Restoration (1640), 258, 265
Potosí, 216
mines, 261
pox, 24, 174, 206, 211, 226, 228, 235, 253,
279, 289–292, 294, 307
causes, 291
epidemics, 293
great pox (*morbo gallico*), 211, 279–280, 307
identification, 290
Prester John, 37, 39–42, 45, 53, 307
Principe island, 27
print culture, 275
in Goa, 63
Ptolemy, 35, 37, 45, 54–55, 234, 240
Geography, 36
purgatives, 96
pythons, 4

quarantine, 221
quinine, 5
Quintanilha, João de, 241